Screening for Diseases

Screening for Diseases

Prevention in Primary Care

VINCENZA SNOW, MD, FACP
AMERICAN COLLEGE OF PHYSICIANS
EDITOR

AMERICAN COLLEGE OF PHYSICIANS
PHILADELPHIA

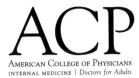

Clinical Consultant: David R. Goldmann, MD
Manager, Books Program: Diane McCabe
Production Supervisor: Allan S. Kleinberg
Design and Layout: Lorraine Lostracco, Wendy Smith

Printed in the United States of America
Printing/binding by Versa Press

Library of Congress Cataloging-in-Publication Data
Screening for diseases: prevention in primary care / Vincenza Snow, editor.
    p. ; cm.
    Includes bibliographical references.
    ISBN: 1-930513-56-9
    1. Medical screening. 1. Snow, Vincenza, 1961-
[DNLM: 1. Diagnostic Services. 2. Primary Health Care—methods.
3. Preventive Health Services. 4. Primary Prevention—methods.
5. Treatment Outcome. WA 243 S433 2004]
RA427.5.S365 2004
616.07'5—dc22   2004041115

N.B. All screening/prevention evidence reviews except Hypertension and
      Depression are the work of the United States Preventive Services Task
      Force and have previously been published in *Annals of Internal
      Medicine.* The introductory chapter by David M. Eddy has previously
      appeared in the ACP publication *Common Screening Tests.*

04 05 06 07 08 / 9 8 7 6 5 4 3 2 1

Contents

Preface

In 1991, the American College of Physicians published *Common Screening Tests.* Quickly becoming one of the best-selling publications in the history of the College, it provided clinicians with rigorous and thorough data analysis and recommendations based on only the highest-quality evidence.

Common Screening Tests comprised eleven guidelines approved by ACP through its Clinical Efficacy Assessment Project (CEAP). The latter began in 1981 as a three-year grant. Its goals were three-fold: to assemble and review the clinical literature on a specified topic; to identify the best scientific papers; and to analyze, reformulate, and present such information so that practitioners can readily determine the usefulness of diagnostic tests, procedures, or treatments.

The initial charge to CEAP was the evaluation of medical technology. Thus early ACP guidelines emphasized screening and diagnostic tests. Because of CEAP's success, particularly of its screening guidelines, the program was given permanent status. CEAP is administered by the Clinical Efficacy Assessment Subcommittee (CEAS), a subcommittee of the Education Committee. Through the work of CEAS/CEAP, the College has become recognized as a premier producer of evidence-based guidelines.

The CEAS continues to issue evidence-based guidelines; however, the last screening guideline (thyroid disease) was published in 1998. The cessation was a result of the work of the United States Preventive Services Task Force (USPSTF), which is in its third iteration. In November 1998, the Agency for Healthcare Research and Quality (then the Agency for Health Care Policy and Research) convened the current USPSTF to update existing Task Force assessments and recommendations and to address new topics. Release of USPSTF recommendations and supporting evidence began in the spring of 2001. Because the USPSTF follows a stringent and thorough methodology in its evidence reviews, the CEAS concluded that there was no need to duplicate its efforts and that CEAS resources would be better directed towards developing guidelines covering other areas of Internal Medicine interest.

The present volume, which may be considered an updated edition of the 1991 work, has been retitled. *Screening for Diseases: Prevention in Primary Care* recognizes the change in screening strategies, which no longer are all "tests", and the fact that chemoprophylaxis can be used for the prevention of disease. The reader will find herein seven USPSTF evidence reviews (all previously published in *Annals of Internal Medicine*) and two new chapters (Depression and Hypertension) commissioned especially for this book.

Key Points summarize the basic "take-home" messages. A two-page table at the back of the book provides an easily accessible guide to over 20 preventive services. As a bonus, David Eddy's superb introduction to *Common Screening Tests,* long unavailable, precedes the chapters.

Vincenza Snow, MD, FACP

How to Think About Screening

David M. Eddy, MD, PhD

Making recommendations about screening is one of the most difficult problems in clinical medicine. Screening, by definition, involves testing persons, usually in large numbers, who have no symptoms of the condition being searched for. Most persons who are screened will receive no benefit because they do not have the target condition. But many persons will suffer risks, and all will face some inconvenience, anxiety, personal cost, and sometimes discomfort. In short, the stakes are high. This fact places a special burden on any individual or group that wants to recommend a screening test. They must determine that screening can in fact deliver benefits and that the potential benefits outweigh the harms and justify the costs.

The main issues in the evaluation of screening tests and the design of screening policies are discussed in this chapter. The issues are described from the point of view of the individual or organization that is designing the screening policy. The purpose of this chapter is to help practitioners who actually do screening to evaluate the rationale for the recommendations offered to them.

Definitions

Screening

Screening is the application of a test to detect a potential disease or condition in a person who has no known signs or symptoms of that disease or condition. There are two main purposes for screening. One is to detect a disease early in its natural history when treatment might be more effective, less expensive, or both. The other purpose is to detect risk factors that put a person at a higher than average risk for developing a disease, with the goal of modifying the risk factor or factors to prevent the disease. Screening for high cholesterol levels to prevent a myocardial infarction is one example. (Hereinafter, the term "condition" will be used in a general sense to describe any disease, risk factor, or other condition that is the target of screening.)

Asymptomatic

For the purpose of defining screening, a person is asymptomatic if, at the time screening is done, he or she has no known signs or symptoms of the target condition. The person might have signs or symptoms of which he or she is unaware, in which case screening might result in discovery of those hidden signs or symptoms. For example, a woman might be unaware of a tiny breast mass that could be found during a breast physical examination. The persons being screened might also have other signs or symptoms suggestive of other conditions. The crucial point is that, at the time of screening, neither the patient nor the practitioner is aware of any signs or symptoms of the target condition.

Patient

In a physician's practice many if not most of the persons being screened will have other medical problems. The term "patient" therefore will be used in a general sense to describe the persons being screened.

Practitioner

Many types of health care professionals, for example, physicians, nurses, and specially trained assistants, can do screening. For simplicity, the term "practitioner" will be used to include anyone who does the screening test.

Screening Tests

A condition can be detected by a variety of methods, including patient history, blood tests, physical examinations, invasive procedures, and imaging tests. The term "test" will be used in a general sense to include any screening method.

Policymaker

An individual, a group of individuals, or an organization can develop a recommendation for screening. Frequently, as was the case for this book, the process will require all three: Individual authors will draft papers for review by one or more committees and final approval by an organization. In this chapter, the term "policymakers" will be used to describe the collection of persons that produced a screening recommendation. "Policymaking" will refer to the process.

Steps

Once a condition has been selected for analysis, designing a screening recommendation for that condition has two main steps. The first is to estimate the health and economic outcomes of the proposed screening strategy—the benefits, harms, and costs. The second step is to compare those outcomes to determine whether the benefits outweigh the harms and whether the health outcomes (benefits and harms combined) are worth the costs.

It is important to keep the two steps separate. The first step is a question of science and is anchored to evidence. Different parties should be able to agree on the evidence and on the estimated outcomes of screening. In contrast, the second step is not a question of science but a question of personal values. It is anchored not to evidence but to the preferences and desires of the persons receiving the screening tests. Different persons have different preferences, and it might well be that no single screening recommendation is best for everyone. When designing a screening policy, policymakers must take into account not only the evidence of benefits and harms but the range of patients' preferences about the outcomes.

Both of these main steps can be divided into several smaller steps. To estimate the outcomes, policymakers must formulate the screening problem; identify the health outcomes that are important to the persons who will be screened (hereinafter called "patients"); search for evidence for the effect of screening on each health outcome; interpret the pieces of evidence; and synthesize or combine the evidence to estimate the effect of the test on health and economic outcomes. When making value judgments, policymakers must determine who should compare the benefits, harms, and costs; actually make the comparisons; and design the policy.

Important issues arise in the performance of these steps. These issues, which will be discussed in turn, include the formulation of a screening strategy; the types of outcomes affected by screening tests; the types of evidence commonly used to evaluate screening tests; biases that typically affect evidence for screening tests; techniques used to synthesize the evidence; the comparison of benefits, harms, and costs; and techniques for incorporating uncertainty about outcomes and variability of preferences in the design of a policy.

Formulating a Screening Strategy

Before the appropriateness of a screening program can be analyzed, the program must be defined. Variables to be considered include which persons will be targeted for screening (for example, groupings based on gender, age, risk factors, geographic regions, or socioeconomic status); which tests will be used; the order and frequency of testing; and the setting in which screening will be offered (for example, who will do the screening, where, and under what circumstances). Defining variables of the program in advance is important because the benefits, harms, and costs of screening depend acutely on these factors. For example, the outcome of screening high-risk women 50 to 65 years of age with an annual, breast physical examination and mammography in practitioners' offices is very different from the value of screening average-risk women 40 to 50 years of age with biennial "low-cost" mammography. Indeed, the category of "screening with mammography" is so general that it cannot be evaluated without further specification.

When identifying screening strategies, it is important not to be limited by tradition or convention. For example, many screening tests have been offered annually based on no better logic than the fact that the earth circles the sun every year. The frequency of screening depends on the natural history of the condition—how long it takes to develop from first detectability to signs or symptoms—not on astronomy, and it might be that frequencies other than once a year are more appropriate. Similarly, just because two or more tests are available to screen for a condition does not mean they all have to be used. Decisions about combinations of tests depend on the properties and dependencies of the tests, not on their availability.

Frequently, it will be appropriate to identify several different screening strategies so that they can be compared. Decisions about a particular screening strategy should be based on the strategy's benefits, harms, and costs compared with those of adjacent strategies (what economists call "marginal" benefits, harms, and costs). The benefits, harms, and costs of a screening strategy should not be evaluated in comparison with no screening (what economists call "average" benefits, harms, and costs). For example, screening for hypertension every 5 years should be compared with 4-year screening and 6-year screening, not with no screening. To ensure that the proper strategies are being compared, several adjacent strategies must be identified and analyzed.

Types of Outcomes

Health Outcomes

The purpose of screening, indeed, the purpose of all medical interventions, is to improve health outcomes. Health outcomes are outcomes that patients experience and care about. These outcomes can affect length and quality of life and may cause pain, anxiety, death, or functional disability and affect appearance or peace of mind.

Screening typically affects several types of health outcomes, such as the immediate side effects of screening: the inconvenience, anxiety, and possible discomfort associated with the test. These outcomes are experienced by everyone who gets the screening test, although different patients might react to them differently. Another type of health outcome affected by screening is any potential risks of the tests (for example, perforation of the colon by a sigmoidoscope or the potential radiation effects of mammography).

Other outcomes affected by the performance of the test are outcomes associated with the test results. When a screening test is done on a patient, four results are possible: The test might correctly indicate the presence of the target condition (a true-positive result); it might incorrectly indicate that the condition is absent when in fact it is present (a false-negative result); it might correctly indicate the absence of the condition (a true-negative result); or it might falsely indicate that the condition is present when in fact it is absent (a false-positive result). Each of these results affects health outcomes. A true-positive result controls the potential benefits of screening-the possible reduction in morbidity and mortality. However, the other three test results can also affect health outcomes. A false-negative result can lead to a false sense of security. A false-positive result can cause great anxiety, can label a patient, and can require that additional testing be done, with its attendant side effects, risks, and costs. A true-negative result can provide reassurance, which for many people is the main reason to be screened. It is important to recognize that the first result—the benefit from detecting an existing condition—is experienced by only a few of the people who are screened, those who happen to have the condition. In contrast, the harms of screening are experienced by many more people.

Intermediate Outcomes or Measures

In addition to health outcomes, screening tests have intermediate outcomes or measures that policymakers might use to help evaluate screening. Intermediate outcomes and, measures cannot be directly experienced by patients and are important to patients only to the extent that they provide information about the probabilities or magnitudes of health outcomes. Examples of intermediate outcomes and measures frequently used to help evaluate screening tests include the probability that the screening test will detect a condition if it is present (the sensitivity or true-positive rate of the test); the proportion of screened people who are found to have the condition (the "yield" of screening in a population); the predictive values of the test (the probability that patients who test positive actually have the condition, and the probability that people who test negative do not actually have the condition); and the shift in the state of the condition at the time of detection (for example, an increase in the proportion of patients who have cancer detected in the early stages).

When information about intermediate outcomes is used as the basis for decisions about screening, some assumptions must be made about how the intermediate outcomes and measures affect the health outcomes. For example, finding a condition in 5% of a population does not by itself determine whether screening is good or bad. To decide that, assumptions must be made about whether the discovery of the condition changes management, whether the change in management changes health outcomes, and whether the magnitude of the expected change in health outcomes is worth the side effects, risks, and costs.

Types of Evidence

It is rare that all the outcomes of screening can be learned from a single source. More commonly, a policymaker must examine many sources and types of evidence to document the benefits of screening and to estimate the magnitude of benefits, harms, and costs.

The harmful outcomes of a screening test—side effects, risks, and false-positive results—are usually learned by simply observing what happens when a large population is tested. Patients can be asked about anxiety and discomfort; the frequency of short-term risks such as perforations can be noted; and the frequency of false-positive test results can be counted. For some screening tests, the potential risks are more difficult to estimate, particularly when they occur with low frequency or over long periods of time, or both. An example of this type of outcome is the potential radiation hazard of mammography. For this type of risk, indirect evidence and mathematical models are usually required.

Given that virtually all screening tests have potential for harm, it is essential to determine that the test can also yield benefit. Documenting the benefits of screening can be extremely difficult, far more difficult than for a treatment. The effect of screening on health outcomes is inherently indirect, requiring a sequence of actions and outcomes. The primary effect of screening is to provide information about the probability a patient has the targeted condition. A positive test result increases the probability that the patient has the condition; a nega

Figure 1.

Apply the screening test	→	Detect the possible presence of the condition	→	Confirm the presence of the condition	→	Change the timing of treatment	→	Change the health outcomes

tive result decreases the probability. In order for the screening test to have any effect on health outcomes, a positive test result must lead to a diagnostic workup to confirm the presence of the condition; which in turn must cause a change in the choice or timing of treatment; which in turn must cause a change in health outcomes. Thus, many links must be in place to connect screening to an improvement in health outcomes (Figure 1).

If any of these links is broken, the value of screening to a patient can be nullified. For example, the screening center might neglect to follow up a positive result; a patient might decline to return for a diagnostic workup; the practitioner might not choose the correct treatment; or the treatment might not change health outcomes. To document that screening will in fact improve health outcomes, there must be evidence for all of these links. That evidence can be either direct or indirect.

Direct Evidence

The most desirable type of evidence directly connects the application of the screening test with the occurrence of health outcomes. (That is, direct evidence spans from one end of Figure 1 to the other.) The prototype for direct evidence is the randomized controlled trial. Because exposure to the screening tests is determined by the investigator and because both the screened and control groups are essentially similar in all other respects, any differences in health outcomes between the two groups can be attributed to screening. Unfortunately, this type of evidence is rare; usually because huge numbers of people must be screened to generate a sufficient number of outcomes for statistical analysis, and because many of the outcomes are chronic and require long follow-up times. Examples of conditions for which randomized controlled trials have been done are screening for cancers of the breast, colon, and lung. Each of these trials followed tens of thousands of patients over decades.

Occasionally, nonrandomized controlled trials are used to provide evidence for screening. These trials usually involve comparisons of convenience. For example, screening might be offered to persons who live in one town, with persons who live in an adjacent town serving as controls. The value of this design depends on the similarities between the two groups and the extent to which any differences in outcomes can be attributed to screening as opposed to other uncontrollable factors (for example, differences in the population or differences in the available treatments). Statistical techniques can sometimes be used to adjust for such differences. The Edinburgh trial of breast cancer screening is an example.

Another type of direct evidence used to evaluate screening tests is the case-control study. In this design, the investigators identify patients, or "cases," who have had the outcome of interest (for example, who have died of breast cancer). The investigators also identify a group of persons (the "controls") who have not had the outcome (for example, who have not died of breast cancer), but who are similar in other respects such as age and socioeconomic status. The investigators then retrospectively review the histories of both the cases and controls to determine what proportion of persons in each group had received the screening test. From these proportions, an odds ratio can be calculated to compare the odds of the outcome (for example, the odds of dying of breast cancer) in screened as opposed to unscreened people. This design has several advantages: It does not require randomization; it can take advantage of natural experiments; and it can be conducted more quickly and less expensively than randomized controlled trials. A major disadvantage is the high potential for patient-selection biases and errors in retrospectively determining screening histories. Case-control studies have been used to evaluate screening for cervical cancer, breast cancer, and osteoporosis.

The uncontrolled study is a fourth type of direct evidence. A typical design is to offer screening to a population, follow the patients who are screened, and observe the outcomes. Uncontrolled studies of screening are common because they are the easiest and least expensive type of design. This design is useful for determining outcomes that can occur only with screening, such as side effects, risks, false-positive results, and the immediate financial costs of screening and workups. Uncontrolled studies are also useful for estimating these outcomes because the occurrence of these outcomes in the absence of screening is known with certainty—they never occur. Thus, for these outcomes no control group is needed. However, the uncontrolled study is far less useful for determining the potential benefits of screening, such as the potential reduction in morbidity or mortality of the disease; without a control group there is no way to know for certain what would have happened without screening. To use this type of evidence to estimate the benefits of screening, some comparison must be found. For such comparisons, policymakers usually turn to historical observations, national statistics, or other uncontrolled studies that did not involve screening. In addition to being vulnerable to patient-selection biases, uncontrolled studies are also subject to a variety of biases that affect screening programs in particular.

Indirect Evidence

When there is no evidence that directly relates the performance of a screening test to health outcomes, a policymaker has two choices. One choice is to insist on direct evidence and decline to recommend any screening test for which there is no direct evidence of benefit. This approach is safe because it decreases the chance of recommending an ineffective test, and it has a clean, if somewhat rigid, line of defense. However, if this approach were applied uniformly to all medical interventions, very few would be recommended because very few have been documented by well-designed controlled trials. Thus, this approach is not particularly helpful to practitioners who must make decisions with or without direct evidence.

The other option for policymakers is to use indirect evidence. Evidence is called indirect if it addresses individual links in the chain that connects the act of screening to the changes in health outcomes (Figure 1). To use indirect evidence, several bodies of evidence (for each link or component of a model) must be integrated.

Interpretation of indirect evidence always requires the use of a model. Two types of models, subjective and formal, are commonly used to interpret evidence about screening tests. In a subjective or mental model (also known as clinical judgment or clinical intuition), policymakers attempt to mentally absorb information about each factor described in Figure 1 and subjectively determine the effect of the screening test on health outcomes. For screening tests, this process involves integrating information about factors such as the incidence and prevalence of the condition; risk factors that affect the incidence and prevalence of the condition; risk factors that affect the incidence and prevalence for particular patients; the natural history of the condition; the sensitivity and specificity of the screening test; compliance to screening; the stages in which a disease is likely to be detected with and without screening; the effectiveness of treatment as a function of the stage of a condition; compliance to treatment; and the differences in outcomes caused by different screening strategies (for example, the order and frequency of tests). Needless to say, digesting all of this information is exceedingly difficult. This process is vulnerable to the inherent limitations of the human mind and to a variety of professional and personal biases.

A formal model attempts to formalize the subjective process by explicitly identifying and describing all the factors that would ideally be included in a subjective model and by using quantitative tools to process that information. Many types of formal models have proven useful for analyzing screening problems. Perhaps the most common models are probability trees and decision trees, examples of which are found in the analyses of screening for coronary heart disease and osteoporosis. These models are most helpful for analyzing one-shot screening, in which the patient either has the condition or does not have it and the test is done only once. Probability and decision trees are less useful for analyzing sequential or intermittent screening of chronic conditions, where the patient can develop the condition at any time; the condition can change over time (for example, a cancer can grow); the probability that a screening test will detect the condition (its sensitivity) is not constant but rather is a function of the state of the condition's development at the time of screening (for example, the size of a cancer or the level of blood pressure); and screening is done more than once (for example, every other year). To the extent that a policymaker wants to take these dynamic features into account, these problems require dynamic models such as Markov processes or models specifically built to analyze screening problems.

Formal models are helpful because they provide a structure that integrates the important factors and enable policymakers to focus on one factor at a time. These models provide quantitative tools for integrating all the factors according to accepted axioms of mathematics and probability theory. Formal models make explicit the important assumptions and reasoning and provide a tool for exploring the implications of uncertainty about any parameter (sensitivity analysis).

When subjective models are used, there is great risk of oversimplification, errors in reasoning, and personal and professional bias. An example of oversimplification is to use a highly condensed model: "The test can detect the condition; therefore screening should be recommended"; or, "This is a serious disease; we have little else to offer. Therefore . . ." Examples of errors in reasoning are confusing sensitivity, specificity, and predictive values; confusing the incidence of a disease with the prevalence of occult disease; and misestimating the effect of prevalence on predictive value. Examples of professional and personal biases are well known. Because of these problems, screening recommendations based on clinical and expert judgment are highly suspect. Additionally, recommendations based on clinical judgment and mental models are difficult to document, verify, and defend.

Interpreting the Evidence

Unfortunately, all types of evidence suffer from biases. These biases can work in either direction—sometimes causing ineffective screening tests to appear effective, sometimes causing effective tests to appear ineffective. Biases can affect both the internal validity of a study (its accuracy for estimating the effect of a screening test in the setting of the study) and the external validity of a study (its accuracy for estimating the effect of the screening test in other settings).

Biases Affecting Controlled Studies

The main biases affecting the internal validity of randomized controlled trials are dilution and contamination: Some of the patients offered screening might not receive the test (dilution), and some of the patients not offered screening might receive the test anyway (contamination). To the extent dilution and contamination occur, the observed results of the trial will tend to underestimate the true effect of screening. Several biases affect the external validity of randomized controlled trials. The trials might be done in experimental settings that do not accurately reflect what happens in community practice. Investigators might take measures to improve compliance, causing the compliance observed in trials to overstate that which can be expected in realistic settings. Investigators might take extraordinary pains to interpret the screening tests, causing the sensitivity of the test observed in a trial to exceed the sensitivity of the test in realistic settings. The screening technology might change during or after completion of a trial. The trials might deal with narrowly defined populations such as particular high-risk groups. Finally, the trials might use a particular screening protocol (for example, annual mammography and breast physical examination) that is different from the protocol of interest to the policymaker (for example, physical examination alone or mammography done every 2 years). All of these biases can work in either direction, understating or overstating the true effect of the screening test depending on the circumstances.

Nonrandomized controlled trials tend to be more realistic than randomized controlled trials. Investigators tend to be less aggressive in promoting compliance, tend to include broader groups of people, and tend to be less intrusive in terms of affecting how the screening is done. However, the lack of randomization causes a greater chance of patient-selection bias. This bias can work in either direction.

The main bias affecting case-control studies is patient-selection bias. Another problem is that there can be errors in the retrospective review of patients' histories, that is, in determining who was screened and whether a patient actually had the outcome of interest. Sorting out the net effects of these potential biases can be difficult, which is why policymakers tend to assign less "weight" to case-control studies than to prospective designs.

Biases Affecting Uncontrolled Studies

Uncontrolled studies obviously face a serious threat from patient-selection biases. In addition, uncontrolled studies are affected by several other biases that are peculiar to screening, particularly lead-time bias, length bias, and over-diagnosis. The interval between the moment a condition is detected and the moment that condition would have been detected (after signs or symptoms) is known as the "lead time." (By the definition of screening, any condition detected by a screening test is found before it would ordinarily have become apparent through signs or symptoms.) This lead time will automatically increase the time between the moment of detection and the occurrence of some outcome, such as death. This increase occurs whether or not the outcome has actually been postponed. Thus, the observation of a longer survival time from diagnosis might be due only to advancing the time of diagnosis, not to postponing the time of death. Because of this, a comparison of survival rates in screened or unscreened populations can be misleading.

Another problem affecting the interpretation of uncontrolled studies that follow patients with conditions detected by screening is the so-called "length bias." Conditions detected by a test in a periodic screening program tend to have longer preclinical intervals than average. The preclinical interval is the interval between the time a screening test could detect a condition and the time a patient would seek care for signs or symptoms in the absence of screening. The duration of this interval is related to the growth rate and other biological characteristics of the condition, the effectiveness of the screening test, and the patient's awareness of signs or symptoms. Several of these factors can influence how long a patient survives from the time of diagnosis. For example, conditions with longer preclinical intervals might have slower growth rates, be less aggressive, and have inherently better prognoses. Thus, observations of longer survival times in uncontrolled studies might be due to the selection of patients with longer preclinical intervals rather than to any real improvement in survival. This bias can be overcome by tracking all patients offered screening, not just those whose conditions were detected through screening.

A third problem that can confuse the interpretation of data from uncontrolled studies is overdiagnosis. The purpose of screening is to find conditions in their earliest stages. Unfortunately, there is often no sharp boundary between normal findings and the earliest stages of a condition, and it is possible to overdiagnose an atypical but essentially normal finding as a very early case of the condition. As well as increasing the number of "conditions" detected, overdiagnosis can inflate the number of conditions thought to be detected in the earliest stages. Because these cases would never have become clinically significant, this can inflate survival statistics.

Adjusting for Biases

When any of these biases is believed to exist, policymakers must determine the potential effect of each bias on the results of the study. If the policymakers intend to estimate the actual magnitudes of benefits and harms, they must go on to make quantitative estimates of how the biases affect the studies' results. At present, the most common approach for dealing with biases is the "all or nothing" approach; the policymaker determines either that the biases are so great that the study should be discarded or that the biases are sufficiently small that they can be ignored and the study can be taken at face value. Obviously, both choices are oversimplifications. A second approach is to attempt to adjust subjectively for the biases. This approach is not only difficult technically, but introduces the possibility of professional or personal biases. A third approach is to use formal statistical techniques to adjust for biases, but these techniques are still relatively new and not widely available. Currently, the most common approach is to estimate a range of uncertainty for important variables. The range of uncertainty should incorporate both the design of the trial (for example, sample size) and the presence of biases. Then sensitivity analyses are done to explore the impact of uncertainty about specific variables on the outcomes of interest.

Synthesizing Evidence

After the experimental evidence has been identified and pieces of evidence have been interpreted, the evidence must be synthesized. For any variable—whether it is a health outcome that can be estimated directly from the evidence or a variable to be used in a model of indirect evidence—there are frequently multiple pieces of evidence that show slightly different, sometimes conflicting results. The policymaker must reconcile these differences to develop a "best" estimate of the health outcome or variable based on the combined results. The most common approach is to calculate a weighted average of the results of separate pieces of evidence or to combine the evidence subjectively. In the latter, the policymaker surveys all of the evidence and attempts to "sense" the best estimate and an appropriate range of uncertainty. As with techniques for adjusting for biases, formal statistical techniques for synthesizing evidence from multiple sources are becoming available (called "meta-analysis").

After the evidence has been interpreted and synthesized, the resulting estimates can then be used directly to estimate the benefits, harms, and costs of the screening program (if the evidence is direct) or to execute a model that in turn estimates the health and economic outcomes (if the evidence is indirect). The ranges of uncertainty are used to do sensitivity analyses.

Comparing Benefits, Harms, and Costs

Three main issues arise when comparing benefits, harms, and costs: obtaining estimates of benefits, harms, and costs; making the comparisons; and avoiding pitfalls.

The Importance of Estimating Outcomes

Ideally, a decision to recommend a screening test will be based on an explicit comparison of the test's benefits, harms, and costs. Making such a comparison obviously requires estimates of the magnitudes of the benefits, harms, and costs. Without such estimates of health outcomes, there is no solid basis for the comparison. In particular, when an analysis of a screening test describes only intermediate outcomes, such as the sensitivity, yield, or predictive values of the screening test, a truly informed comparison of benefits and harms is not possible. In such cases, judgments about the desirability of screening based on intermediate outcomes require making many assumptions, usually unstated, about what the detection of a disease (an intermediate outcome) implies about the morbidity and mortality of the disease (the health outcomes). To the extent that the actual magnitudes of health and economic outcomes are not explicitly estimated, there is greater uncertainty about the appropriateness of a screening recommendation.

Who Should Make the Comparisons?

Comparison of the benefits, harms, and costs of screening should ideally be done by the people who will actually receive the benefits and harms and pay the costs (that is, the patients themselves). Information about their preferences could be learned through such methods as polls, interviews, focus groups, or even experiments. At present, these methods are virtually never used. For screening recommendations (or recommendations about any health intervention, for that matter), representatives of patients are not systematically surveyed for their preferences. Rather, policymakers commonly use their own personal judgments to weigh the benefits and harms of screening. The implicit assumption is either that the policy-maker's personal preferences match the preferences of patients, or that the policy-makers are separating their personal values from the values of patients, are trying to represent patients (act as their agents), and accurately know how patients feel about the benefits, harms, and costs. Both of these assumptions are questionable, and some day the standard practice will be to consult representatives of patients for their preferences before developing recommendations for a screening test. Learning the spectrum of preferences by surveying representatives of patients differs from the individualized decision-making described below. In the spirit of market research, these surveys would provide essential information about how patients, in general, value the benefits, harms, and costs of a screening test.

Psychological Biases

Comparing the benefits and harms of any intervention can be affected by many psychological traps. This comparison involves not only processing complex information, but explicitly addressing issues that have powerful emotional connotations. In addition, few people readily want the responsibility of making a decision that will affect the lives of hundreds of thousands of people. As a consequence policymakers have a powerful psychological drive to find some simplifying principle that will make the decision obvious and minimize the need for personal exposure. Unfortunately, most of the simplifying principles are misleading. Some examples of common traps are the following: picking a single outcome and using it as the sole basis for a decision, and ignoring the other outcomes such as harms ("Screening reduces mortality, therefore it should be recommended"); using statistical significance as a proxy for the desirability of an outcome ("The benefits of screening were statistically significant, therefore it should be recommended," or conversely, "There is no randomized controlled trial proving the test is effective, therefore it cannot be recommended"); ignoring costs; using spurious tricks to tip the balance ("I cannot decide if this screening test is desirable for average-risk people; but if it is a tossup for average-risk people, it must be desirable for high-risk people"); ignoring the actual magnitude of an outcome ("If there is any benefit, screening must be worthwhile," or "If only one life is saved, the effort will have been worthwhile"); retreating to generalities ("Cancer is bad, therefore any intervention that combats cancer must be worthwhile"); or following the herd ("Other groups have recommended for [or against] screening; they must know what they are doing," or "Most practitioners are [or are not] using this test; therefore it must be appropriate [or inappropriate]"). The last pitfall—following the herd—is especially dangerous. It assumes that others have systematically evaluated the evidence; estimated the benefits, harms, and costs; and assessed patients' preferences. This assumption is rarely the case.

Making a Recommendation

After the policymaker has evaluated the evidence and has gone as far as possible to estimate the health and economic outcomes of screening, the policymaker is in a position to make a recommendation. The general direction of the recommendation will follow from the estimates of benefits, harms, and costs: Screening strategies for which the benefits outweigh the harms and are worth the costs can be recommended; screening strategies for which the harms and costs outweigh the benefits will not be recommended. However, several additional factors must be considered when designing the actual recommendation.

Degrees of Flexibility

Two factors are particularly important. First, depending on the quality of the evidence and the ability of the policymaker to estimate actual health outcomes instead of just intermediate outcomes, the policymaker will have different degrees of conviction about the consequences of screening. If the evidence is poor, or if the analysis stopped at estimating intermediate outcomes instead of health outcomes, the policymaker might be uncertain about the actual outcomes of screening and might be uneasy about making a firm recommendation. Conversely, if the evidence is superb and the analysis has been carried through to estimates of health and economic outcomes, the policymaker might be confident about the accuracy of the analysis. The second factor concerns the degree of unanimity of patient preferences for the health and economic outcomes (assuming that the outcomes have been estimated) as perceived by the policymaker. For some screening strategies, the benefits might so far outweigh the harms and costs that virtually everyone will find the screening strategy desirable (or vice versa). On the other hand, the benefits, harms, and costs might be close enough that some people will find screening desirable, and others will not.

Both of these factors must be incorporated in the final recommendation. Policymakers must describe the degree of conviction with which the screening recommendation is made or the intended degree of flexibility for the recommendation. There are several ways to do this. The most common is to simply insert the appropriate words directly into the recommendation. For example, a recommendation might begin "We strongly recommend that . . ." or "Due to the lack of direct evidence, it is difficult to make any firm recommendation . . ." A second approach is to use some grading system, such as that used by the Canadian Task Force on Preventive Medicine and United States Preventive Services Task Forces (1). For example, a recommendation issued with great conviction and rigidity might be labeled an "A" recommendation, whereas recommendations intended to be more ambiguous and flexible might be labeled "C." A third approach is to issue the recommendation as a "standard," "guideline," or "option," depending on the degree of uncertainty about outcomes and the perceived degree of unanimity of patients' preferences (2).

Standards, Guidelines, and Options

Standards are intended to be rigid. They must be followed, with exceptions being rare and difficult to justify. Deviation from a standard could well imply malpractice. Guidelines are intended to be more flexible; they should be followed in most cases. Guidelines, however, can and should be tailored to fit individual needs, depending on the patient, setting, and other factors. Deviations will be fairly common and can be justified by individual circumstances. Options are intended to be neutral. They recommend neither for nor against the use of an intervention but merely note that different interventions are available and that practitioners are free to choose any course. Several different types of options are possible depending on whether outcomes and patients' preferences are known and on the degree of unanimity of preferences.

Most of the screening tests evaluated in this book are options, or at most, guidelines. When a recommendation is issued as either a guideline or option, it is important to describe the rationale: the evidence, areas of uncertainty, best-estimates of outcomes, and value judgments. This description enables practitioners to interpret the facts for themselves and tailor a recommendation to fit particular circumstances.

Taxonomy

The terminology used to describe screening is among the most confusing in medicine. Terms include "detection," "diagnosis," "screening," "early detection," "mass screening," "routine screening," and "case-finding." Currently, different authors use these terms in different ways, with no universally accepted set of definitions. This section gives one set of definitions.

The most general term is "detection," which is the application of a test to a person for the purpose of finding a potential disease, or finding a condition that increases the probability the person has or will develop a disease. The two main types of detection, "diagnosis" and "screening," are distinguished by whether the person has known signs or symptoms of the target condition. Diagnosis occurs when the person to whom the test is being applied has known signs or symptoms of the target condition. On the other hand, if at the time of testing the person does not have any known signs or symptoms suggestive of the condition, then the application of the test is termed "screening." Thus, the definition of screening is the application of a test to detect a potential disease or condition in a person who has no known signs or symptoms of that condition at the time the test is done. In this definition, it does not matter where screening is done (for example, in a practitioner's office or a shopping center), whether the patient has signs or symptoms suggestive of other conditions, whether the patient has risk factors, or who initiates the request (the patient or the practitioner). "Early detection" refers to the detection of a disease or condition before the appearance of obvious signs or symptoms and therefore is synonymous with "screening."

Several qualifying adjectives are frequently used to describe screening such as "routine," "general," "selective," "individual," and "mass." These qualifiers can be explained by identifying several dimensions that distinguish them.

One dimension is whether the screening is to be done in a setting in which the decision to screen can take into account an individual patient's concerns and preferences (for example, in practitioners' offices) or in a setting in which individualized decision-making is not anticipated (for example, in shopping centers). Screening done in the second type of setting is called "mass screening," where large numbers of people are screened under fairly impersonal circumstances and costs can be minimized. This type of screening provides little opportunity for individualized decision-making. Because the criteria for determining who should be screened must be simple and easily elicited, the type of screening being done must not require a face-to-face discussion of complex issues relating to the quality of the evidence, the magnitudes of benefits and harms, or personal preferences. "Individualized screening" occurs in a setting where the decision to screen takes into account the concerns of individual patients.

Another dimension that distinguishes types of screening is the presence of risk factors. Some screening recommendations are intended only for patients who have specific risk factors, such as a family history of the disease. This type of screening is called "selective." In contrast, some screening is intended to be applied to all persons who fit very general criteria (for example, gender or age). When the recommendation to screen does not depend on the presence of risk factors, the term "general screening" will be used. Some authors consider age to be a risk factor, whereas other authors do not. In this book, age will be considered a general criterion for identifying candidates for screening and will not be considered a risk factor. Otherwise, all screening would be "selective."

Another frequently used term is "routine screening." Although the term has never been well defined, it generally denotes automatic, repetitive, unthinking behavior. Because of this connotation, many organizations, including the Blue Cross and Blue Shield Association and the American College of Physicians, have recommended against routine screening.

The term "case-finding" is perhaps the most confusing of all. It has been used to distinguish between screening that takes place in a practitioner's office and screening in other settings, screening of high-risk patients and screening of average-risk patients, or screening done at a patient's request and screening initiated by the practitioner. Because it has no uniform definition and because its important concepts can be described by other qualifying terms, the term "casefinding" should be avoided where possible.

The distinction between these terms can be important. The overall goal is to ensure that for every patient who is screened, the benefits outweigh the harms to that patient and the health outcomes are worth the costs. That is, the goal is to ensure that every patient who is screened comes out ahead. This goal should be sought whether screening is to be done one-on-one in practitioners' offices or through mass screening in shopping centers. The fact that all screening has this common goal suggests that the criteria for screening should be the same for all settings and circumstances.

However, depending upon the screening test, the nature of the evidence of benefits and harms, the magnitudes of the benefits and harms, and the uniformity of patient preferences, screening recommendations might be different for different settings. There are two main factors that determine these differences: how and where screening is to be done, and the nature of the benefits, harms, and costs. How and where screening is done can affect both the quality and the cost of screening. These factors in turn affect the benefits, harms, and costs, which might affect the recommendation to screen. For example, in a mass screening program, economies of scale that decrease costs are usually achieved, but the quality of screening done on a mass basis might be lower than the quality of screening offered on an individualized basis.

The nature of the benefits, harms, and costs can affect the need for individualized decision-making. If the evidence of benefits is strong and if the benefits far outweigh the harms and costs, then it is safe to assume that everyone would want to be screened. In such cases individualized decision-making is unnecessary, and screening might well be done on a "mass" basis. On the other hand, if the evidence of benefit is not clearcut, or if the benefits do not unequivocally outweigh the harms and costs, then different patients might have different views about the value of screening. The need for individualized decision-making would increase. For this type of screening, blanket national recommendations or mass screening is usually not appropriate. Rather the appropriate strategy is "Talk to your doctor."

References

1. Guide to Clinical Preventive Services: Report of the U.S. Preventive Services Task Force. Baltimore: Williams & Wilkins; 1989.
2. Eddy DM. Designing a practice policy: standards, guidelines and options. JAMA. 1990; 263:3077,3081,3084.

Type 2 diabetes mellitus

❏ It has not been demonstrated that beginning diabetes control early (in the preclinical stage) as a result of screening provides an incremental benefit compared with initiating treatment after clinical diagnosis.

❏ Intensive control of glycemia in patients with clinically detected (not screening detected) diabetes can reduce the progression of microvascular disease; however, it takes about 15 years to see benefits.

❏ In patients with clinically detected diabetes, intensive control of blood pressure and lipids produces significant benefits in cardiovascular morbidity and mortality. This benefit is seen in a shorter time frame (about 5 years).

❏ Screening for diabetes in patients with hypertension and/or hypercholesterolemia is reasonable.

Screening Adults for Type 2 Diabetes: A Review of the Evidence for the U.S. Preventive Services Task Force

Russell Harris, MD, MPH; Katrina Donahue, MD, MPH; Saif S. Rathore, MPH; Paul Frame, MD; Steven H. Woolf, MD, MPH; and Kathleen N. Lohr, PhD

Background: Type 2 diabetes mellitus is associated with a heavy burden of suffering. Screening for diabetes is controversial.

Purpose: To examine the evidence that screening and earlier treatment are effective in reducing morbidity and mortality associated with diabetes.

Data Sources: MEDLINE, the Cochrane Library, reviews, and experts, all of which addressed key questions about screening.

Study Selection: Studies that provided information about the existence and length of an asymptomatic phase of diabetes; studies that addressed the accuracy and reliability of screening tests; and randomized, controlled trials with health outcomes for various treatment strategies were selected.

Data Extraction: Two reviewers abstracted relevant information using standardized abstraction forms and graded articles according to U.S. Preventive Services Task Force criteria.

Data Synthesis: No randomized, controlled trial of screening for diabetes has been performed. Type 2 diabetes mellitus includes an asymptomatic preclinical phase; the length of this phase is unknown. Screening tests can detect diabetes in its preclinical phase. Over the 10 to 15 years after clinical diagnosis, tight glycemic control probably reduces the risk for blindness and end-stage renal disease, and aggressive control of hypertension, lipid therapy, and aspirin use reduce cardiovascular events. The magnitude of the benefit is larger for cardiovascular risk reduction than for tight glycemic control. The additional benefit of starting these treatments in the preclinical phase, after detection by screening, is uncertain but is probably also greater for cardiovascular risk reduction.

Conclusions: The interventions that are most clearly beneficial during the preclinical phase are those that affect the risk for cardiovascular disease. The magnitude of additional benefit of initiating tight glycemic control during the preclinical phase is uncertain but probably small.

The prevalence of type 2 diabetes mellitus (diabetes) in the United States is growing (1, 2); the burden of suffering caused by its complications is heavy (3) and may also be growing. These complications include increased risk for cardiovascular disease (CVD) (4), end-stage renal disease (ESRD) (5, 6), blindness (7), and amputation of the lower extremities (8, 9). The magnitude of the risk for these complications varies among persons with a new clinical diagnosis of diabetes. After 10 years, more than 20% of such persons will have had a major cardiovascular event (for example, myocardial infarction [MI], stroke, heart failure, or sudden death), fewer than 5% will have developed blindness, and fewer than 2% will have developed ESRD or had lower-extremity amputation (10).

Three general approaches to reducing the complications of diabetes are 1) preventing the occurrence of diabetes in the first place, 2) improving care for persons who have already received a diagnosis, and 3) screening asymptomatic persons for diabetes (11). By *asymptomatic*, we mean persons without both the direct symptoms of hyperglycemia (for example, polyuria) and the symptoms of associated conditions (for example, infections or angina pectoris). We distinguish between detection of diabetes due to the presence of these symptoms and detection of diabetes by screening, either systematic screening or the haphazard screening that occurs with frequent use of multichannel chemistry profiles. Our review focuses on the evidence for the effectiveness of systematic screening for diabetes as opposed to no screening.

Interest in screening has been prompted by research showing that approximately one third of persons who meet criteria for diabetes have not received a diabetes diagnosis (12). In 1996, the U.S. Preventive Services Task Force (USPSTF) found insufficient evidence to recommend for or against screening for diabetes (13). Since that USPSTF review, new evidence concerning the effectiveness of various treatments to prevent complications has fueled continued controversy about the effectiveness of screening (14–22). To assist the USPSTF in updating its recommendation, we performed a systematic review of the evidence concerning screening adults for diabetes.

METHODS

To guide our literature search, we used USPSTF methods to develop an analytic framework with linkages that represent five key questions in a logical chain between screening and health outcomes (23). We developed eligibility criteria for admissible evidence for each key question, focusing on screening strategies that are feasible in a primary care environment and on high-quality evidence about health outcomes (as contrasted with intermediate outcomes) of treatment for newly diagnosed diabetes.

We examined the critical literature from the 1996 USPSTF review and searched MEDLINE and the Cochrane Library for reviews and relevant studies published in English between 1 January 1994 and 30 July 2002. We also examined key articles published before 1994 and arti-

Table 1. **Randomized, Controlled Trials of Tight Glycemic Control***

Study, Year (Reference)	Quality	Length of Study, y	Groups (Patients)	Glycemic Control	Renal Failure
UGDP, 1971 (48), 1978 (49)	Fair	8.75	Placebo (*n* = 204) Insulin variable (*n* = 198)	22.8% increase vs. 13.5% decrease†	NR
UKPDS 33, 1998 (10)	Good	10	Conventional therapy (*n* = 1138) Intensive therapy (*n* = 2729)	7.9% vs. 7.0%‡	<1% vs. <1% (*P* > 0.2)
UKPDS 34, 1998 (47)	Good	10.7	Conventional therapy, primarily diet (*n* = 411) Intensive therapy with metformin (*n* = 342)	8.0% vs. 7.4%‡	<1% vs. <1% (*P* > 0.2)
Kumamoto, 1995 (55), 2000 (51)	Fair	8	Conventional therapy (*n* = 50) Intensive therapy (*n* = 52)	9.4% vs. 7.1%‡	NR
VA CSDM, 1997 (52), 1996 (54), 1995 (56), 1999 (50), 2000 (57)	Fair	2.25	Standard therapy (*n* = 78) Intensive therapy (*n* = 75)	9.2% vs. 7.1%‡	NR
Steno 2, 1999 (53)	Fair	3.8	Standard therapy (*n* = 80) Intensive therapy (*n* = 80)	9.0% vs. 7.6%‡	0% vs. 0%

* CVD = cardiovascular disease; ECG = electrocardiographic; MI = myocardial infarction; NR = not reported; NS = nonsignificant; Steno = Steno type 2 randomized study; UGDP = University Group Diabetes Program; UKPDS = U.K. Prospective Diabetes Study; VA CSDM = VA Cooperative Study on Glycemic Control and Complications in Type 2 Diabetes.
† Change in fasting blood glucose from baseline.
‡ Median hemoglobin A_{1C} level.

cles found by examining the reference lists of pertinent reviews or suggested by experts.

The first author and at least one coauthor or trained assistant reviewed abstracts and articles to find those that met eligibility criteria (**Appendix Table 1**, available at www.annals.org). For included studies, two reviewers abstracted relevant information using standardized abstraction forms and graded the quality of the study according to USPSTF criteria (23). Important articles on which a recommendation could rest were examined and discussed by all authors. We distributed a draft systematic evidence review for external peer review, soliciting comments from experts, relevant professional organizations, and federal agencies, and made revisions based on feedback. A more complete account of the methods used in this review can be found in the Appendix (available at www.annals.org). The complete systematic evidence review is available on the Agency for Healthcare Research and Quality Web site (www.ahrq.gov) (24).

This evidence report was funded through a contract to the Research Triangle Institute–University of North Carolina Evidence-based Practice Center from the Agency for Healthcare Research and Quality. Staff of the funding agency and members of the USPSTF contributed to the study design, reviewed draft and final manuscripts, and made editing suggestions.

RESULTS

For the USPSTF to conclude that screening reduces diabetic complications, the evidence must demonstrate that feasible screening tests can detect diabetes during a preclinical phase and that the knowledge of the diagnosis of diabetes in this phase will lead to earlier treatment that will reduce complications more than would treatment be-

gun after clinical detection. Furthermore, the magnitude of this "additional benefit" (that is, the reduction in complications from initiation of treatment in the preclinical phase minus the reduction in complications from starting treatment after clinical diagnosis) must be great enough to outweigh the harms and effort of screening.

Does Diabetes Have an Asymptomatic Preclinical Phase, and How Long Is It?

The natural history of diabetes includes an asymptomatic preclinical phase. Many people who meet criteria for diabetes have not received a diabetes diagnosis. In the third National Health and Nutrition Examination Study (NHANES III), conducted between 1988 and 1994, the prevalence of diagnosed diabetes among persons 20 years of age and older was 5.1%; the prevalence of previously undiagnosed diabetes was 2.7% (12). Rates of diagnosed diabetes for non-Hispanic black and Mexican-American persons were 1.6 and 1.9 times the rate for non-Hispanic white persons, and the rates of undiagnosed diabetes were similarly higher.

The length of this asymptomatic period is less clear. No study has compared a screened with a comparable unscreened sample to determine the difference in the time at which diabetes is diagnosed. One group used an indirect approach to calculate this interval. After making assumptions about the rate of development of diabetic retinopathy early in diabetes, Harris and colleagues (25, 26) estimated that the preclinical period lasted between 10 and 12 years. According to this calculation, screening a previously unscreened population would detect diabetes an average of 5 to 6 years before clinical diagnosis. Even if this estimate is accurate, however, it represents a mean value. Some people will have a longer and some a shorter asymptomatic period.

Table 1—**Continued**

Severe Visual Impairment	Myocardial Infarction	Stroke	Amputation	All-Cause Mortality
11.2% vs. 11.4% for acuity ≤ 20/200 in either eye (NS)	20% vs. 17.6% for significant ECG abnormality (NS)	NR	1.5% vs. 1.6% (NS)	26.3% vs. 24.0% (NS)
11% vs. 11% for vision too poor to drive (NS)	16.3% vs. 14.2% ($P = 0.052$)	4.8% vs. 5.4% ($P > 0.2$)	1.6% vs. 1.0% ($P = 0.099$)	18.7% vs. 17.9% ($P > 0.2$)
3.2% vs. 3.5% for blindness in one eye ($P > 0.2$)	17.8% vs. 11.4% ($P = 0.001$)	5.6% vs. 3.5% ($P = 0.13$)	2.2% vs. 1.8% ($P > 0.2$)	21.7% vs. 14.6% ($P = 0.011$)
NR	1.3 events/100 person-years vs. 0.6 events/100 person-years for major CVD event (NS)			NR
9.0% vs. 6.7% for unilateral or bilateral visual impairment (NS)	5.1% vs. 6.7% (NS)	2.6% vs. 6.7% (NS)	0% vs. 1.3% (NS)	5.1% vs. 6.7% (NS)
9.0% vs. 1.3% for blindness in one eye ($P = 0.03$)	5.1% vs. 5.2% for nonfatal MI (NS)	10.2% vs. 1.3% for nonfatal stroke (NS)	5.1% vs. 5.2% (NS)	2.6% vs. 5.2% (NS)

The true mean length of this period and the distribution of its length are unknown.

How Accurate Are the Screening Tests?

Determining the accuracy of screening tests for diabetes is complicated by uncertainty about the most appropriate reference standard. Two standards of diagnosis are in general use: one based on the 2-hour postload plasma glucose test and the other based on the fasting plasma glucose (FPG) test (27–29). The standard cut-point for the 2-hour postload plasma glucose test is 11.1 mmol/L (200 mg/dL); the FPG cut-point is 7.0 mmol/L (126 mg/dL). Both tests require a second confirmation. Hemoglobin A_{1c}, using various cut-points, is a third test that has been proposed as a standard reference for diagnosing diabetes (30–32).

It is not clear which of these tests and cut-points most closely predict diabetic complications (33). The cut-point for the 2-hour postload plasma glucose test was based on a threshold that predicted retinopathy prevalence in several studies (27, 28). The FPG cut-point was chosen to correspond to that for the 2-hour postload plasma glucose test (27, 28). All three tests (2-hour postload plasma glucose, FPG, and hemoglobin A_{1c}) are associated with future cardiovascular events in a linear fashion both above and below the present diabetes cut-points, with no obvious threshold (34–39). However, experts have set the point at which hyperglycemia is termed diabetes without considering CVD prediction.

When a 2-hour postload glucose level of at least 11.1 mmol/L (≥200 mg/dL) is used as the reference standard, the specificity of an FPG level with a cut-point of 7.0 mmol/L (126 mg/dL) is greater than 95%; the sensitivity is about 50% and may be lower for persons older than 65 years of age (40). Among a general, previously nondiabetic sample of persons 40 to 74 years of age, a person with an FPG level of 7.8 mmol/L or greater (≥140 mg/dL) has a 91% probability of having a 2-hour postload plasma glucose level at least 11.1 mmol/L (≥200 mg/dL). For an FPG level between 7.0 mmol/L (126 mg/dL) and 7.8 mmol/L (140 mg/dL), the probability is 47% (41). Hemoglobin A_{1c} level is more closely related to FPG than to 2-hour postload plasma glucose level (42), but it is not sensitive to low levels of hyperglycemia (30). Reliability is higher for FPG than for hemoglobin A_{1c} or 2-hour postload plasma glucose level (43–45). Although the reliability of the hemoglobin A_{1c} assay has been a concern, it is now not as grave a problem (43).

In clinical practice, requiring a screening test to be fasting (as with the FPG) or postload (as with the 2-hour plasma glucose test) presents logistical problems. In a recent study in primary care settings, random capillary blood glucose with a cut-point of 6.7 mmol/L (120 mg/dL) had a sensitivity of 75% and a specificity of 88% for detecting persons who have positive results on FPG assay or on 2-hour postload plasma glucose assay (46).

Does Earlier Knowledge of Diabetes after Screening Lead to Better Treatment and Improved Health Outcomes?

We examine here the extent to which earlier application of available treatments for diabetes would improve health outcomes.

Tight Glycemic Control

Five randomized, controlled trials (RCTs) have compared health outcomes in groups that differ with respect to glycemic control (10, 47–57) (**Table 1**). Four of these studies (48–56), although generally well conducted, were small and lacked power to detect clinically important differences between groups. The longest and largest study was

Table 2. **Studies of Intensity of Treatment with Antihypertensive Medications***

Study, Year (Reference)	Quality	Population	Length of Study	Patient Age	Groups (Patients)	Blood Pressure Control
			y			*mm Hg*
UKPDS 38, 1998 (60)	Fair	Patients with diabetes and hypertension	8.4	56–57	Less tight blood pressure control (*n* = 390) Tight blood pressure control (*n* = 758)	154/87 vs. 144/82
HOT, 1998 (59)	Fair	Diabetes subgroup	3.8	61.5	Target DBP ≤ 90 mm Hg (*n* = 501) Target DBP ≤ 85 mm Hg (*n* = 501) Target DBP ≥ 80 mm Hg (*n* = 499)	143.7/85.2 vs. 141.4/83.2 vs. 139.7/81.1
ABCD, 2000 (61)	Fair	Patients with hypertension and diabetes	5	57	Moderate blood pressure control (*n* = 233) Intensive blood pressure control (*n* = 237)	138/86 vs. 132/78
ABCD, 2002 (62)	Fair	Normotensive patients with diabetes	5.35	58–59	Moderate blood pressure control (*n* = 243) Intensive blood pressure control (*n* = 237)	137/81 vs. 128/75

* ABCD = Appropriate Blood Pressure Control in Diabetes; CVD = cardiovascular disease; DBP = diastolic blood pressure; ESRD = end-stage renal disease; HOT = Hypertension Optimal Treatment; NR = not reported; UKPDS = U.K. Prospective Diabetes Study.

the United Kingdom Prospective Diabetes Study (UKPDS), an RCT of 3867 people with newly diagnosed diabetes over 10 years (10). Because the UKPDS intervention was not blinded, outcomes that involve clinician judgment (such as whether to use retinal photocoagulation) could have been biased (58).

The primary UKPDS analysis found a nonsignificant trend (relative risk, 0.84 [95% CI, 0.71 to 1.0]) toward a reduction in MI for tight versus less tight glycemic control groups but no difference in any other cardiovascular outcome (10). The absolute difference in MI events was 2.1% over 10 years, entirely in nonfatal events. Three other studies found no statistically significant difference in cardiovascular outcomes from tight glycemic control (48, 49, 51, 52, 56). The most positive study, a UKPDS analysis, had puzzling results (47). It found that metformin reduced MI and all-cause mortality compared with conventional glycemic control (**Table 1**). Further analyses, however, showed that these benefits were out of proportion to the achieved glycemic control and disappeared when all patients taking metformin (including those who had metformin added to another treatment) were considered (47).

In three of the studies, tight glycemic control reduced the progression of albuminuria and retinopathy (10, 51, 57). Although this important finding in intermediate outcomes may herald future clinical benefits, few people in any group in these trials developed the clinical outcomes of ESRD or blindness (**Table 1**). One study of a multifactorial intervention that included more than tight glycemic control (53) found a statistically significant reduction in

severe visual impairment in the intervention group; in the other studies, groups did not differ in the development of severe visual impairment or ESRD.

Only two of these trials included persons with diabetes who had received recent diagnoses (10, 49); in neither study was diabetes detected primarily by screening. Thus, these studies provide information about the effect of tight glycemic control among persons whose diabetes has been detected clinically. Compared with tight glycemic control after clinical detection, the added benefit of earlier tight glycemic control after detection by screening (at a time when glycemic levels are often only slightly elevated) is unknown but probably small over at least 15 years after diagnosis.

Antihypertensive Treatment

Earlier knowledge of diabetes status could affect treatment for hypertension during the preclinical period by changing the intensity of treatment or the choice of antihypertensive drug. The optimal target blood pressure is lower for hypertensive patients with diabetes than for those without. The Hypertension Optimal Treatment (HOT) trial found that diabetic persons randomly assigned to a target diastolic blood pressure of 80 mm Hg had a reduction in CVD and all-cause mortality compared with diabetic persons in the group with a target of 90 mm Hg, but there were no differences among nondiabetic persons randomly assigned to the same blood pressure target groups (**Table 2**) (59). Three other randomized, controlled trials (one in normotensive diabetic persons) support the conclu-

Table 2—Continued

Myocardial Infarction	Stroke	Death from CVD Events	Non-CVD Outcomes
23.5 vs. 18.6 per 1000 person-years ($P = 0.13$)	11.6 vs. 6.5 per 1000 person-years ($P = 0.013$)	20.3 vs. 13.7 per 1000 person-years for diabetes-related death ($P = 0.019$)	2.3 vs. 1.4 per 1000 person-years for ESRD ($P > 0.2$) 19.4% vs. 10.2% for marked deterioration in vision ($P = 0.004$)
7.5 vs. 4.3 vs. 3.7 per 1000 person-years ($P = 0.11$)	9.1 vs. 7.0 vs. 6.4 per 1000 person-years ($P > 0.2$)	11.1 vs. 11.2 vs. 3.7 per 1000 person-years for CVD death ($P = 0.016$)	NR
No difference	No difference	10.7% vs. 5.5% for all-cause mortality ($P = 0.037$)	No difference in vision, ESRD, neuropathy
6.2% vs. 8.0% ($P > 0.2$)	5.4% vs. 1.7% ($P = 0.03$)	8.2% vs. 7.6% for all-cause mortality ($P > 0.2$)	No difference in creatinine clearance; vision not reported

sion that more intensive blood pressure control reduces stroke, diabetes-related death, and all-cause mortality in persons with diabetes (**Table 2**) (60–62).

These four RCTs were acceptable in quality. Although blinding caregivers and participants was difficult, end point assessment was blinded in all four trials. Four percent of participants or fewer were lost to follow-up for mortality end points. The trials used various antihypertensive drugs.

Ten RCTs and three meta-analyses have compared clinical outcomes among diabetic persons treated with various antihypertensive agents (62–76) (**Tables 3** and **4**). Two issues addressed by these studies are whether calcium antagonists provide less benefit to diabetic persons than to nondiabetic persons (and thus should be avoided) and whether agents that interrupt the renin–angiotensin system (for example, angiotensin-converting enzyme [ACE] inhibitors or angiotensin-receptor blocking [ARB] agents) provide greater benefit to diabetic than to nondiabetic persons (and thus should be prescribed).

The evidence concerning the effects of calcium antagonists among diabetic persons is mixed. Hypertensive persons taking calcium antagonists compared with those taking other drugs may have a somewhat increased risk for MI and congestive heart failure and a decreased risk for stroke; drug groups do not differ in all-cause mortality (**Tables 3** and **4**). Although these trends may be slightly more pronounced for diabetic persons, the effects of calcium antagonists are not qualitatively different between persons with and without diabetes (73).

Some evidence suggests that, compared with most other antihypertensive drugs, ACE inhibitors or ARBs provide better protection against CVD events (more so for MI than for stroke) and renal disease, an effect that may be partly independent of blood pressure reduction. Five of six RCTs that have compared ACE inhibitors or ARBs with other agents in diabetic persons with hypertension have found a reduction in some CVD outcomes in the ACE inhibitor or ARB group, even after adjusting for differences in blood pressure (**Table 3**) (62–64, 66–68, 74–76). The Losartan Intervention for Endpoint reduction study, for example, found that, for diabetic patients with hypertension, the ARB losartan reduced all-cause mortality compared with the β-blocker atenolol, a result that was less certain for hypertensive patients without diabetes (75). Angiotensin-converting enzyme inhibitors or ARBs also reduce the development of diabetic nephropathy (77–82) and its progression to ESRD (71, 83, 84) more than most other antihypertensive agents.

One large study of hypertensive diabetic persons showed no benefit of an ACE inhibitor compared with a β-blocker for either CVD or renal outcomes (63); another study of normotensive diabetic persons found no difference in outcomes between treatment with an ACE inhibitor compared with a calcium antagonist (**Table 3**) (62). The discrepancy between these results and those of other studies has not been satisfactorily explained. The benefits of ACE inhibitors and ARBs over other antihypertensive drugs are also unclear for nondiabetic persons (68, 72, 74–76), especially those at lower CVD risk. A large meta-analysis of studies of predominantly nondiabetic persons

Table 3. **Studies Comparing One Antihypertensive Drug with Another***

Study, Year (Reference)	Quality	Population	Length of Study	Patient Age	Groups (Patients)	Blood Pressure Control	Myocardial Infarction
			y			*mm Hg*	
UKPDS-39, 1998 (63)	Fair	Patients with diabetes	8.4	56	Captopril (*n* = 400) Atenolol (*n* = 358)	144/83 vs. 143/81	20.2 vs. 16.9 per 1000 person-years (*P* > 0.2)
CAPPP, 1999 (76), 2001 (68)	Fair	Diabetes subgroup	6.1	55–56	Captopril (*n* = 309) Conventional (*n* = 263)	155.5/89 vs. 153.5/88	3.9% vs. 10.3% (*P* = 0.002)
STOP-2, 2000 (66)	Fair	Diabetes subgroup	5.3	75–76	ACE inhibitors (*n* = 235) CA (*n* = 231) Conventional with diuretics and/or β-blockers (*n* = 253)	161.3/80.3 vs. 161.8/79.1 vs. 161.3/81.2	15.3 vs. 29.6 vs. 22.2 per 1000 person-years (*P* = 0.025)
ABCD, 1998 (64)	Fair	Patients with diabetes	5	57	Nisoldipine (*n* = 235) Enalapril (*n* = 235)	135/82 vs. 135/82	10.6% vs. 2.1% (*P* = 0.001)
FACET, 1998 (67)	Fair	Patients with diabetes	2.5	62–63	Fosinopril (*n* = 189) Amlodipine (*n* = 191)	157/88 vs. 153/86	1.8 vs. 2.4 per 100 person-years (*P* > 0.1)
NORDIL, 2000 (70)	Fair	Diabetes subgroup	4.5	60–61	Diltiazem (*n* = 351) Diuretics and/or β-blockers (*n* = 376)	152.2/87.6 vs. 149.1/87.4	11.2 vs. 11.1 per 1000 person-years (*P* > 0.2)
INSIGHT, 2000 (69)	Fair	Diabetes subgroup	4	65	Nifedipine (GITS) (*n* = 649) Co-amilozide (diuretic) (*n* = 653)	138/82 vs. 138/82	NR
Lewis et al., 2001 (71)	Good	Patients with diabetes	2.6	58–59	Irbesartan (*n* = 579) Amlodipine (*n* = 567) Placebo (*n* = 569)	140/77 vs. 141/77 vs. 144/80	NR
ABCD, 2002 (62)	Fair	Patients with diabetes	5.3	58–59	Nisoldipine (*n* = 234) Enalapril (*n* = 246)	132.1/78.0 vs. 132.4/78.0	7.7% vs. 6.5% (*P* > 0.2)
LIFE, 2002 (74, 75)	Good	Diabetes subgroup	4.7	67	Losartan (*n* = 586) Atenolol (*n* = 609)	146/79 vs. 148/79	7% vs. 8% (*P* > 0.2)

* ABCD = Appropriate Blood Pressure Control in Diabetes; ACE = angiotensin-converting enzyme; CA = calcium antagonist; CAPPP = Captopril Prevention Project; CV = cardiovascular; CVD = cardiovascular disease; ESRD = end-stage renal disease; FACET = Fosinopril versus Amlodipine Cardiovascular Events Randomized Trial; GITS = gastrointestinal-transport system; INSIGHT = Intervention as a Goal in Hypertension Treatment; LIFE = Losartan Intervention for Endpoint reduction in hypertension study; NORDIL = Nordic Diltiazem Study; NR = not reported; NS = nonsignificant; STOP-2 = Swedish Trial in Old Patients with Hypertension-2; UKPDS = U.K. Prospective Diabetes Study.
† Myocardial infarction, stroke, cardiovascular death, amputation, congestive heart failure.
‡ Doubling of creatinine concentration, ESRD, any death.

found that ACE inhibitors provided no CVD benefit over other types of drugs (mostly diuretics and β-blockers) in the treatment of hypertension (**Table 4**) (72) (see Addendum).

We should be cautious in drawing conclusions from these studies for several reasons. First, many trial participants required more than a single drug to attain their target blood pressures, making head-to-head comparisons of particular drugs difficult. Second, the meta-analyses grouped specific drugs within a class together. Drugs within a class, however, may have different effects. Third, the patients studied in these trials differed in many respects, including age, presence of comorbid conditions, degree of hypertension, duration of diabetes, and presence of other cardiovascular risk factors. Nonetheless, the meta-analyses compared results across trials. Drug effects that vary by patient group make it more difficult to identify the effects of a single drug or drug class. Finally, although these trials are generally acceptable in quality, they vary in such important issues as blinding procedures and withdrawal rates (**Table 3**).

Thus, the current evidence favors the conclusion that diabetic patients benefit from more intensive blood pres-

Table 3—Continued

Stroke	CVD Events and Mortality	Non-CVD Outcomes	Adherence and Withdrawal	Blinding and Comments
6.8 vs. 6.1 per 1000 person-years ($P > 0.2$)	15.2 vs. 12.0 per 1000 person-years for diabetes-related death ($P > 0.2$)	No difference in vision, ESRD	22% vs. 35% for discontinuation of the study drug	Open-label; blinded outcome assessment
7.4% vs. 7.2% ($P > 0.2$)	6.5% vs. 12.9% for all-cause mortality ($P = 0.034$)	NR	One patient lost to follow-up; adherence to medications not reported	Open-label; blinded outcome assessment
31.6 vs. 26.9 vs. 34.7 per 1000 person-years ($P > 0.2$)	49.0 vs. 43.9 vs. 55.5 per 1000 person-years for all-cause mortality ($P = 0.20$)	NR	61.3% vs. 66.2% vs. 62.3% for taking study drug at study end; 0% withdrew	Open-label; blinded outcome assessment
4.7% vs. 3.0% (NS)	4.3% vs. 2.1% for CVD death (NS)	No difference in vision, ESRD	39.1% vs. 34.9% for discontinuation of the study drug	Double-blind; MI was a secondary end point; blinded outcome assessment
0.7 vs. 1.9 per 100 person-years ($P > 0.1$)	2.6 vs. 5.0 per 100 person-years for major CVD event ($P = 0.03$)	NR	19.0% vs. 27.2% for discontinuation of the study drug; 1% withdrew	Open-label; blinded outcome assessment
13.3 vs. 12.3 per 1000 person-years ($P > 0.2$)	29.8 vs. 27.7 per 1000 person-years for CVD events ($P > 0.2$)	NR	77% vs. 93% for taking study drug at study end; <1% withdrew	Open-label; blinded outcome assessment
NR	8.3% vs. 8.4% for CVD events (NS)	NR	33.1% vs. 39.9% for discontinuation of the study drug; 2.4% withdrew	Double-blind; blinded outcome assessment; randomization imbalance in diabetic subgroup
NR	23.8% vs. 22.6% vs. 25.3% for CV outcome† (NS)	32.6% vs. 41.1% ($P = 0.006$) vs. 39.0% for renal outcome ($P = 0.02$ for all)‡	<1% withdrew	Double-blind; blinded outcome assessment; randomized by central office
4.7% vs. 2.4% ($P = 0.18$)	8.1% vs. 7.7% for all-cause mortality ($P > 0.2$)	No differences in renal and visual outcomes	Participants were taking study drug approximately 70% of the time	Double-blind; placebo-controlled; blinded outcome assessment
9% vs. 11% ($P = 0.20$)	11% vs. 17% for all-cause mortality ($P = 0.002$)	NR	73% vs. 68% for taking study drug at study end	Double-blind; blinded outcome assessment

sure control than do nondiabetic persons. It remains uncertain whether diabetic patients should be treated with different antihypertensive medications than those given to nondiabetic persons. Although the studies reviewed included diabetic persons whose disease presumably had been detected clinically, CVD risk is still increased twofold or more among people with undiagnosed diabetes (34–39, 85). Direct evidence shows that among diabetic persons with this degree of risk, an aggressive approach is beneficial within a 5-year time frame, the estimated mean time before clinical diagnosis.

Treatment of Dyslipidemia and the Use of Aspirin

Although persons with diabetes do not have higher total cholesterol or low-density lipoprotein (LDL) cholesterol levels than similar nondiabetic persons, they have higher levels of triglycerides and lower levels of high-density lipoprotein (HDL) cholesterol (86). They may also have a tendency toward thrombosis (87, 88). Knowledge of diabetes during the preclinical period could influence treatment for coronary heart disease (CHD) risk by changing the use of aspirin or the intensity or type of treatment for dyslipidemia.

Table 4. **Meta-Analyses of Comparisons of Antihypertensive Drugs***

Study, Year (Reference)	Quality	Population	Inclusion Criteria	Studies, *n*
Blood Pressure Trialists, 2000 (72)	Good	Patients with and without diabetes	Random assignment of patients between antihypertensive regimens; minimum of 1000 patient-years in each group; prespecified outcomes	8
Pahor et al., 2000 (73)	Good	Patients with and without diabetes	Studied patients with hypertension; compared CA with another drug; assessed CVD events; included 100 persons or more	9
Pahor et al., 2000 (65)	Good	Patients with diabetes only	RCT of ACE inhibitor vs. other drug for hypertensive patients with diabetics; 2-y follow-up; CVD outcomes	4 (ABCD, CAPPP, FACET, UKPDS) (heterogeneity)

* ABCD = Appropriate Blood Pressure Control in Diabetes; ACE = angiotensin-converting enzyme; CA = calcium antagonist; CAPPP = Captopril Prevention Project; CHD = coronary heart disease; CHF = congestive heart failure; CVD = cardiovascular disease; FACET = Fosinopril versus Amlodipine Cardiovascular Events Randomized Trial; MI = myocardial infarction; OR = odds ratio; RCT = randomized, controlled trial; RR = relative risk; UKPDS = U.K. Prospective Diabetes Study.
† Values <1.0 favor CAs.
‡ Values <1.0 favor ACE inhibitors.

Randomized, controlled trials of both primary and secondary prevention have shown that 3-hydroxy-3-methylglutaryl coenzyme A reductase inhibitors (statins) and fibric acid derivatives (fibrates) lower the risk for CHD events; relative risk reduction is similar (about 25% to 30%) in both diabetic persons and nondiabetic persons (89–101). Aspirin also effectively reduces CHD events in both diabetic persons and nondiabetic persons with a similar relative risk reduction (about 30%) (102–106).

To determine the value of knowing about diabetes status for lipid treatment, a study would ideally randomly assign both diabetic persons and nondiabetic persons without established vascular disease to groups that differed in target LDL cholesterol levels or class of drug. It could then be determined whether diabetic persons should be treated differently from other groups. No such trial has been completed.

Two other studies provide mixed evidence about this issue. A secondary analysis of two secondary prevention studies found that diabetic persons but not nondiabetic persons with LDL cholesterol levels below 3.2 mmol/L (<125 mg/dL) benefited from statin treatment (107). A recent large study of statin treatment that included diabetic persons without established vascular disease as well as nondiabetic persons with vascular disease found a similar relative risk reduction in CHD mortality for all groups, including those with initial levels of LDL cholesterol below 3.0 mmol/L (<116 mg/dL) (99). Thus, it is not clear whether clinicians should treat high levels of LDL cholesterol more aggressively in diabetic persons than in nondiabetic persons. Absolute benefit may be determined by overall CHD risk rather than diabetes status itself.

Furthermore, it is not certain whether the most effective target for diabetic persons is LDL cholesterol levels (which might lead to initial statin treatment) or HDL cholesterol levels (which might lead to initial fibrate treatment) and whether different strategies should be used in diabetic and nondiabetic persons. Expert groups recommend that lipid and aspirin treatment be based on CHD risk, for which diabetes status is an important determining factor (108). Thus, persons without previously diagnosed diabetes who would cross a threshold for initiation of aggressive treatment of lipids or use of aspirin in the presence of diabetes could potentially benefit from screening and earlier treatment.

The magnitude of added benefit from earlier detection of diabetes for treatment of lipids or the use of aspirin is uncertain. If one considers that undetected diabetes increases CHD risk by a factor of two or more and that aspirin and lipid treatment are clearly effective in reducing CHD events over 5 years, then the magnitude of this added benefit is potentially substantial.

Counseling for Diet, Physical Activity, and Smoking Cessation

For both diabetic persons and nondiabetic persons, dietary change, increased physical activity, and smoking cessation are important behavioral steps to reduce adverse health events. No study has found that counseling is more effective in changing long-term behavior for diabetic persons than for nondiabetic persons or that effective behav-

Table 4—**Continued**

	Comparators		Comments
Calcium Antagonists	ACE Inhibitors	Calcium Antagonists	
RR vs. diuretics or β-blockers† CHD: 1.12 (1.00–1.26) Stroke: 0.87 (0.77–0.98) CHF: 1.12 (0.95–1.33) CVD events: 1.02 (0.95–1.10) Mortality: 1.01 (0.92–1.11)	No difference for any outcome vs. diuretics of β-blockers	RR vs. ACE inhibitors† CHD: 1.23 (1.03–1.47) Stroke: 0.98 (0.83–1.18) CHF: 1.22 (1.00–1.49) CVD events: 1.09 (0.99–1.20) Mortality: 0.97 (0.85–1.10)	Heterogeneity in trials comparing CAs and ACE inhibitors
OR vs. all other drugs, all participants† MI: 1.26 (1.11–1.43) Stroke: 0.90 (0.80–1.02) CHF: 1.25 (1.07–1.46) CVD events: 1.10 (1.02–1.18) Mortality: 1.03 (0.94–1.13)	OR vs. CAs, all participants† MI: 1.43 (1.15–1.76) Stroke: 1.01 (0.84–1.23) CHF: 1.24 (1.00–1.55) CVD events: 1.18 (1.04–1.33) Mortality: 0.97 (0.83–1.13)	OR vs. all other drugs, diabetic patients† MI: 1.53 (1.01–2.31) Stroke: 1.37 (0.86–2.20) CHF: 1.76 (0.97–3.21) CVD events: 1.44 (1.09–1.91) Mortality: 1.24 (0.84–1.83)	Diabetic patients were qualitatively the same as all participants, but with higher ORs
NA	RR vs. diuretics or β-blockers or CAs‡ MI: 0.37 (0.24–0.57) Stroke: 0.76 (0.48–1.22) CVD events: 0.49 (0.36–0.67) Mortality: 0.57 (0.38–0.87)	NA	Heterogeneity when UKPDS added; results are for other 3 trials without UKPDS

ioral change programs for diabetic persons should be designed differently from programs for nondiabetic persons.

Foot Care Programs

Although foot care programs may decrease the risk for amputation among persons with long-standing diabetes (109–111), no study has shown that initiation of such programs during the preclinical period provides additional benefit. Because the risk for amputation in the 10 years after clinical diagnosis is low (112), the additional benefit from starting such programs in the preclinical phase is uncertain but likely to be small.

Do Diagnosis and Treatment of Impaired Fasting Glucose or Impaired Glucose Tolerance Improve Health Outcomes?

Impaired fasting glucose and *impaired glucose tolerance* are terms for conditions among persons who do not meet criteria for diabetes but whose fasting glucose level or 2-hour postload plasma glucose level is in the top few percentiles of the nondiabetic population (12). These people have an increased risk for diabetes in the future but do not usually develop diabetic visual, neurologic, or renal complications while in this intermediate state. People with impaired fasting glucose or impaired glucose tolerance, however, have more CVD risk factors and higher CVD risk than nondiabetic persons (34–39, 85, 113–115). People with impaired fasting glucose or impaired glucose tolerance do not have symptoms of hyperglycemia; their state can be detected only by screening. In screening studies, more than twice as many persons have impaired fasting glucose or

impaired glucose tolerance as have undiagnosed diabetes (12, 41).

If interventions at the stage of impaired fasting glucose or impaired glucose tolerance can reduce diabetic complications, this would be a potential benefit of screening. Five RCTs have reported results from lifestyle or drug interventions in people with impaired fasting glucose or impaired glucose tolerance, using progression to diabetes as the relevant outcome (116–120). Three of these trials (the largest ones with the most intensive interventions) found that intensive lifestyle interventions reduced the development of diabetes by 42% to 58% over 3 to 6 years (117, 119, 120). In the largest, U.S.-based study, for example, the intensive behavioral and social program included a case manager with frequent meetings, group and individual support, diet and physical activity training, and enrollment at an exercise facility (121).

Although these trials convincingly demonstrate that intensive behavioral and social interventions can reduce the progression from impaired fasting glucose or impaired glucose tolerance to diabetes, determining the magnitude of additional health benefit from screening and intervening at this stage rather than waiting to intervene at clinical diagnosis is complex. The trials do not permit a clear estimate of the added impact on diabetic complications. Because the risk for severe visual impairment, ESRD, or amputation is low until 15 years or more after diabetes diagnosis, any benefit of treatment of impaired fasting glucose or impaired glucose tolerance to prevent these complications would be small for at least this period. The effect of life-

Table 5. **Number Needed To Screen for Diabetes To Prevent One Adverse Event***

Prevalence of Undiagnosed Diabetes	Additional Time of Intensive Treatment Due to Screening	Tight Glycemic Control To Prevent One Case of Blindness in One Eye (Screening 1000 People with Given Prevalence)†		Tight Blood Pressure Control To Prevent One CVD Event (Screening 1000 Hypertensive Persons with Given Prevalence)‡	
		Increase in Persons with Tight Glycemic Control Due to Screening	Case of Blindness Averted (NNS)	Increase in Persons with Tight Blood Pressure Control Due to Screening	CVD Events Averted (NNS)
%	y	%	n (n)	%	n (n)
6	5	25	0.07 (15 400)	25	0.56 (1800)
		50	0.13 (7700)	50	1.13 (900)
		90	0.23 (4300)	90	2.03 (500)
3	2.5	25	0.02 (61 400)	25	0.14 (7200)
		50	0.04 (30 700)	50	0.28 (3600)
		90	0.07 (17 000)	90	0.51 (2000)

* CVD = cardiovascular disease; NNS = number needed to screen.
† Assumptions: 1.5% 5-year risk for blindness in one eye with no glycemic control; relative risk reduction for blindness with tight glycemic control is the same as relative risk reduction for photocoagulation (10).
‡ Assumptions: 7.5% 5-year risk for CVD event with usual blood pressure control (60); 50% relative risk reduction in CVD events with tight blood pressure control (59). Usual blood pressure control is equivalent to a diastolic goal of 90 mm Hg; tight blood pressure control is equivalent to a diastolic goal of 80 mm Hg. Hypertension is blood pressure ≥140/90 mm Hg.

style interventions on CVD events, independent of other risk factor modification, is also uncertain. Finally, the cost-effectiveness of offering lifestyle interventions only to persons who have positive results on a glucose screening test compared with offering these programs more generally to persons with such risk factors for diabetes as obesity or sedentary lifestyle is uncertain.

What Are the Harms of Screening and Treatment, and How Frequently Do They Occur?

Screening for diabetes could potentially cause harm in several ways. One way is by labeling people as diabetic. One study in a Veterans Affairs Medical Center screened a convenience sample of 1253 outpatients for diabetes and also administered a global measure of quality of life (122). The study found no differences in quality of life at baseline or 1 year later between patients newly detected by screening to have diabetes and those not found to have diabetes. Whether more sensitive measures in healthier samples would have similar findings is unclear. No study has examined the psychological effects of diabetes detection by screening compared with clinical detection. Because few studies have examined the harmful effects of screening, the possibility of labeling effects remains a potential harm. False-positive diagnoses may also cause unnecessary treatment and difficulty obtaining life or health insurance. Between 30% and 50% of people who receive a diagnosis of impaired glucose tolerance will revert to normoglycemia (123–128). Two studies found that between 12.5% and 42% of men who were found to have diabetes on screening reverted to normoglycemia after 2.5 to 8 years (129, 130).

Another potential harm of screening is subjecting patients to a potentially harmful or unnecessary treatment for a longer time. On the whole, treatments for diabetes are relatively safe. Tight glycemic control, especially at a time when glycemic levels are low (that is, the time between

screening and clinical detection), can induce hypoglycemia. In the UKPDS, 2.3% of persons taking insulin had a major hypoglycemic episode each year, as did 0.4% to 0.6% of persons taking oral hypoglycemic agents (10). The most common side effect of ACE inhibitors, a reversible cough, occurs in 5% to 20% of patients and is dose related (131). Angiotensin-converting enzyme inhibitors have fewer side effects than most antihypertensive agents and are associated with high rates of adherence. Statins also have low rates of serious adverse effects (132, 133).

Although the effect of tight glycemic control on quality of life has been a concern, three RCTs have indicated that better glycemic control actually improves quality of life (134–136). These studies were conducted in persons with a clinical diagnosis of diabetes, whose glycemic levels were presumably higher than those of persons who would be detected by screening.

DISCUSSION

No RCT of screening for diabetes has been performed. The natural history of diabetes includes an asymptomatic preclinical phase, and currently available screening tests can detect the disease during this period. The mean length and distribution of lengths of this preclinical period are unknown. A longer preclinical period provides a better opportunity for early treatment to reduce complications.

Early detection by screening could allow clinicians to offer a variety of interventions during the preclinical period, including tight glycemic control; more intensive use and targeted choice of antihypertensive agents; more aggressive use of lipid treatment and aspirin; institution of foot care programs; and counseling for dietary change, physical activity, and smoking cessation. Direct evidence shows that many of these interventions improve health outcomes when initiated after clinical diagnosis. The magnitude of added benefit to initiating them earlier, during the preclinical period, however, must be extrapolated from indirect evidence.

The effect of earlier initiation of these interventions depends on the magnitude of the absolute risk reduction of the complications that they target. The impact of earlier initiation of interventions, such as tight glycemic control, that target blindness, ESRD, or lower-extremity amputation—complications that occur in a substantial number of diabetic persons only 15 years or more after diagnosis—is uncertain but probably small for some years. By contrast, the impact of earlier initiation of interventions, such as intensive blood pressure control, that target CVD events—complications that occur sooner and at a higher rate than blindness—is likely to be larger within the first 10 years after diagnosis.

Table 5 considers the number needed to screen (NNS) to prevent one case of blindness in one eye or one CVD event over 5 years, given various assumptions. Given favorable assumptions, including that tight glycemic control yields a 29% reduction in the risk for blindness in one eye among diabetic persons identified by screening (the relative risk reduction in retinal photocoagulation in the UKPDS trial) (10) and that screening increases the percentage of persons with tight control by 90%, then the NNS to prevent one case of blindness by tight glycemic control for 5 years is about 4300. Less optimistic assumptions result in higher NNS estimates.

If one screened only people with hypertension for diabetes, estimates of the NNS to prevent one CVD event with 5 years of intensive hypertension treatment events are lower. Realistic assumptions of the risk for CVD and the relative risk reduction from intensive hypertension control lead to an NNS estimate of 900, even with an increase of only 50% in the percentage of new diabetic persons with tight blood pressure control. With less favorable assumptions, the NNS calculations for preventing one CVD event are still lower than those for preventing blindness in one eye. The initial assumptions for the CVD calculations are based more on direct evidence and less on extrapolation than those in the blindness example.

Special Populations

A systematic review in 1994 found that nearly all minority groups in the United States have a higher prevalence of diabetes than white persons (137). Many of these groups also have a higher incidence and prevalence of such diabetic complications as ESRD and higher overall mortality rates (138). The RCTs of interventions cited in this review include predominantly white patients. Thus, the relative risk reduction for diabetic complications in minority groups must be extrapolated from data on white samples.

Assuming that the effectiveness of the interventions is similar in various ethnic groups, the most important issue from the standpoint of benefit from screening is whether the rates of development of diabetic complications in minority groups are different from those of persons in the intervention trials. If, for example, ESRD in minority groups occurs earlier and in a larger proportion of diabetic persons than in the study samples, and if intervening earlier with tight glycemic control or more intensive blood pressure control substantially reduces the development of these complications, then screening might well be more beneficial in these groups. However, the evidence on these issues is insufficient to draw a conclusion.

Future Research

The most important gap in our understanding of screening for diabetes is our knowledge of the added benefit of starting various interventions earlier, during the preclinical period, compared with at clinical detection. Ideally, an RCT of screening, especially in populations that are not otherwise at high CVD risk, should be considered. Mounting such a study, although expensive and difficult, could teach us much about preventing diabetic complications and could assist us in developing the most effective and efficient strategy to reduce the burden of diabetes. Because some of these complications occur many years after clinical diagnosis, this study should include long-term follow-up.

In the absence of a trial of screening, natural experiments should be examined. Areas that adopt an aggressive screening approach (for example, among Native American groups) could be compared with areas that offer little screening. Registries of diabetic complications, including CVD events, should be established for monitoring. Because not all persons with abnormal results on glycemic tests are at equal risk for diabetic complications, studies that help define and identify high- and low-risk groups are needed to better target such interventions as screening.

Until we have better evidence about its benefits, harms, and costs, the role of screening as a strategy to reduce the burden of suffering of diabetes will remain uncertain. Current evidence suggests that the benefits of screening are more likely to come from modification of CVD risk factors rather than from tight glycemic control.

Addendum: The recently reported ALLHAT trial provides further evidence that ACE inhibitors have no special benefit, and calcium-channel blockers have no special adverse effects, in diabetic compared with nondiabetic patients. (Major outcomes in high-risk hypertensive patients randomized to angiotensin-converting enzyme inhibitor or calcium channel blocker vs diuretic: The Antihypertensive and Lipid-Lowering Treatment to Prevent Heart Attack Trial (ALLHAT). JAMA. 2002;288:2981-97. [PMID: 12479763]).

From University of North Carolina at Chapel Hill, Chapel Hill, and Research Triangle Institute, Research Triangle Park, North Carolina; Yale University Medical School, New Haven, Connecticut; Tri-County Family Medicine, Cohocton, New York; and Virginia Commonwealth University, Fairfax, Virginia.

Disclaimer: The authors of this article are responsible for its contents, including any clinical or treatment recommendations. No statement in this article should be construed as an official position of the U.S. Agency for Healthcare Research and Quality or the U.S. Department of Health and Human Services.

Grant Support: This study was conducted by the Research Triangle Institute–University of North Carolina Evidence-based Practice Center under contract to the Agency for Healthcare Research and Quality, Rockville, Maryland (contract no. 290-97-0011, task order 3).

Requests for Single Reprints: Reprints are available from the Agency for Healthcare Research and Quality Web site (www.ahrq.gov/clinic/uspstffix.htm) or the Agency for Healthcare Research and Quality Publications Clearinghouse.

Current author addresses are available at www.annals.org.

References

1. **Boyle JP, Honeycutt AA, Narayan KM, Hoerger TJ, Geiss LS, Chen H, et al.** Projection of diabetes burden through 2050: impact of changing demography and disease prevalence in the U.S. Diabetes Care. 2001;24:1936-40. [PMID: 11679460]

2. **Geiss LS.** Diabetes Surveillance, 1999. Centers for Disease Control and Prevention. Washington, DC: U.S. Department of Health and Human Services; 1999.

3. Economic consequences of diabetes mellitus in the U.S. in 1997. American Diabetes Association. Diabetes Care. 1998;21:296-309. [PMID: 9539999]

4. **National Diabetes Data Group, ed.** Diabetes in America. 2nd ed. Bethesda, MD: National Institutes of Health, National Institute of Diabetes and Digestive and Kidney Diseases; 1995:429-56. NIH publication no. 95-1468.

5. **National Diabetes Data Group, ed.** Diabetes in America. 2nd ed. Bethesda, MD: National Institutes of Health, National Institute of Diabetes and Digestive and Kidney Diseases; 1995:349-400. NIH publication no. 95-1468.

6. **Perneger TV, Brancati FL, Whelton PK, Klag MJ.** End-stage renal disease attributable to diabetes mellitus. Ann Intern Med. 1994;121:912-8. [PMID: 7978716]

7. **Klein R, Klein BEK.** Vision disorders in diabetes. In: National Diabetes Data Group, ed. Diabetes in America. 2nd ed. Bethesda, MD: National Institutes of Health. National Institute of Diabetes and Digestive and Kidney Diseases; 1995:293-338. NIH publication no. 95-1468.

8. **National Diabetes Data Group, ed.** Diabetes in America. 2nd ed. Bethesda, MD: National Institutes of Health, National Institute of Diabetes and Digestive and Kidney Diseases; 1995:339-48. NIH publication no. 95-1468.

9. **National Diabetes Data Group, ed.** Diabetes in America. 2nd ed. Bethesda, MD: National Institutes of Health, National Institute of Diabetes and Digestive and Kidney Diseases; 1995:401-28. NIH publication no. 95-1468.

10. Intensive blood-glucose control with sulphonylureas or insulin compared with conventional treatment and risk of complications in patients with type 2 diabetes (UKPDS 33). UK Prospective Diabetes Study (UKPDS) Group. Lancet. 1998;352:837-53. [PMID: 9742976]

11. **Clark CM, Fradkin JE, Hiss RG, Lorenz RA, Vinicor F, Warren-Boulton E.** Promoting early diagnosis and treatment of type 2 diabetes: the National Diabetes Education Program. JAMA. 2000;284:363-5. [PMID: 10891969]

12. **Harris MI, Flegal KM, Cowie CC, Eberhardt MS, Goldstein DE, Little RR, et al.** Prevalence of diabetes, impaired fasting glucose, and impaired glucose tolerance in U.S. adults. The Third National Health and Nutrition Examination Survey, 1988-1994. Diabetes Care. 1998;21:518-24. [PMID: 9571335]

13. **U.S. Preventive Services Task Force.** Guide to Clinical Preventive Services. 2nd ed. Washington, DC: Office of Disease Prevention and Health Promotion; 1996.

14. **Wareham NJ, Griffin SJ.** Should we screen for type 2 diabetes? Evaluation against National Screening Committee criteria. BMJ. 2001;322:986-8. [PMID: 11312236]

15. **Engelgau MM, Aubert RE, Thompson TJ, Herman WH.** Screening for NIDDM in nonpregnant adults. A review of principles, screening tests, and recommendations. Diabetes Care. 1995;18:1606-18. [PMID: 8722060]

16. **Harris MI, Modan M.** Screening for NIDDM. Why is there no national program. Diabetes Care. 1994;17:440-4. [PMID: 8062613]

17. **Marshall KG.** The folly of population screening for type 2 diabetes [Editorial]. CMAJ. 1999;160:1592-3. [PMID: 10374003]

18. **Goyder E, Irwig L.** Screening for diabetes: what are we really doing? BMJ. 1998;317:1644-6. [PMID: 9848909]

19. **Davidson MB.** The case for screening for type 2 diabetes in selected populations. BMJ USA. 2001;1:297-8.

20. ACE Consensus Conference on Guidelines for Glycemic Control. American Association of Clinical Endocrinologists. Endocr Pract. 2002;8(Suppl 1):5-11.

21. **American Diabetes Association.** Screening for diabetes. Diabetes Care. 2001; 24:S21-4.

22. **Engelgau MM, Narayan KM, Herman WH.** Screening for type 2 diabetes. Diabetes Care. 2000;23:1563-80. [PMID: 11023153]

23. **Harris RP, Helfand M, Woolf SH, Lohr KN, Mulrow CD, Teutsch SM, et al.** Current methods of the US Preventive Services Task Force: a review of the process. Am J Prev Med. 2001;20:21-35. [PMID: 11306229]

24. **Harris R, Donahue K, Rathore S, Frame P, Woolf SH, Lohr KN.** Screening Adults for Type 2 Diabetes Mellitus. Systematic Evidence Review No. 19. Rockville, MD: Agency for Healthcare Research and Quality; 2002. Available at www.ahrq.gov/clinic/serfiles.htm.

25. **Harris MI, Klein R, Welborn TA, Knuiman MW.** Onset of NIDDM occurs at least 4-7 yr before clinical diagnosis. Diabetes Care. 1992;15:815-9. [PMID: 1516497]

26. **Jarrett RJ.** Duration of non-insulin-dependent diabetes and development of retinopathy: analysis of possible risk factors. Diabet Med. 1986;3:261-3. [PMID: 2951182]

27. Report of the Expert Committee on the Diagnosis and Classification of Diabetes Mellitus. Diabetes Care. 1997;20:1183-97. [PMID: 9203460]

28. **Alberti KG, Zimmet PZ.** Definition, diagnosis and classification of diabetes mellitus and its complications. Part 1: diagnosis and classification of diabetes mellitus provisional report of a WHO consultation. Diabet Med. 1998;15:539-53. [PMID: 9686693]

29. **American Diabetes Association.** Report of the expert committee on the diagnosis and classification of diabetes mellitus. Diabetes Care. 2001;24:S5-20.

30. **Davidson MB, Schriger DL, Peters AL, Lorber B.** Relationship between fasting plasma glucose and glycosylated hemoglobin: potential for false-positive diagnoses of type 2 diabetes using new diagnostic criteria. JAMA. 1999;281:1203-10. [PMID: 10199430]

31. **Rohlfing CL, Little RR, Wiedmeyer HM, England JD, Madsen R, Harris MI, et al.** Use of GHb (HbA1c) in screening for undiagnosed diabetes in the U.S. population. Diabetes Care. 2000;23:187-91. [PMID: 10868829]

32. **Peters AL, Davidson MB, Schriger DL, Hasselblad V.** A clinical approach for the diagnosis of diabetes mellitus: an analysis using glycosylated hemoglobin levels. Meta-analysis Research Group on the Diagnosis of Diabetes Using Glycated Hemoglobin Levels. JAMA. 1996;276:1246-52. [PMID: 8849753]

33. **Barr RG, Nathan DM, Meigs JB, Singer DE.** Tests of glycemia for the diagnosis of type 2 diabetes mellitus. Ann Intern Med. 2002;137:263-72. [PMID: 12186517]

34. **Meigs JB, Nathan DM, Wilson PW, Cupples LA, Singer DE.** Metabolic risk factors worsen continuously across the spectrum of nondiabetic glucose tolerance. The Framingham Offspring Study. Ann Intern Med. 1998;128:524-33. [PMID: 9518396]

35. **Coutinho M, Gerstein HC, Wang Y, Yusuf S.** The relationship between glucose and incident cardiovascular events. A metaregression analysis of published data from 20 studies of 95,783 individuals followed for 12.4 years. Diabetes Care. 1999;22:233-40. [PMID: 10333939]

36. **Bjørnholt JV, Erikssen G, Aaser E, Sandvik L, Nitter-Hauge S, Jervell J, et al.** Fasting blood glucose: an underestimated risk factor for cardiovascular death. Results from a 22-year follow-up of healthy nondiabetic men. Diabetes Care. 1999;22:45-9. [PMID: 10333902]

37. **Balkau B, Bertrais S, Ducimetiere P, Eschwege E.** Is there a glycemic threshold for mortality risk? Diabetes Care. 1999;22:696-9. [PMID: 10332668]

38. **Saydah SH, Loria CM, Eberhardt MS, Brancati FL.** Subclinical states of

glucose intolerance and risk of death in the U.S. Diabetes Care. 2001;24:447-53. [PMID: 11289466]

39. Khaw KT, Wareham N, Luben R, Bingham S, Oakes S, Welch A, et al. Glycated haemoglobin, diabetes, and mortality in men in Norfolk cohort of european prospective investigation of cancer and nutrition (EPIC-Norfolk). BMJ. 2001;322:15-8. [PMID: 11141143]

40. Blunt BA, Barrett-Connor E, Wingard DL. Evaluation of fasting plasma glucose as screening test for NIDDM in older adults. Rancho Bernardo Study. Diabetes Care. 1991;14:989-93. [PMID: 1797513]

41. Harris MI, Eastman RC, Cowie CC, Flegal KM, Eberhardt MS. Comparison of diabetes diagnostic categories in the U.S. population according to the 1997 American Diabetes Association and 1980-1985 World Health Organization diagnostic criteria. Diabetes Care. 1997;20:1859-62. [PMID: 9405907]

42. Bonora E, Calcaterra F, Lombardi S, Bonfante N, Formentini G, Bonadonna RC, et al. Plasma glucose levels throughout the day and HbA(1c) interrelationships in type 2 diabetes: implications for treatment and monitoring of metabolic control. Diabetes Care. 2001;24:2023-9. [PMID: 11723077]

43. Olefsky JM, Reaven GM. Insulin and glucose responses to identical oral glucose tolerance tests performed forty-eight hours apart. Diabetes. 1974;23:449-53. [PMID: 4830180]

44. Ollerton RL, Playle R, Ahmed K, Dunstan FD, Luzio SD, Owens DR. Day-to-day variability of fasting plasma glucose in newly diagnosed type 2 diabetic subjects. Diabetes Care. 1999;22:394-8. [PMID: 10097916]

45. Mooy JM, Grootenhuis PA, de Vries H, Kostense PJ, Popp-Snijders C, Bouter LM, et al. Intra-individual variation of glucose, specific insulin and proinsulin concentrations measured by two oral glucose tolerance tests in a general Caucasian population: the Hoorn Study. Diabetologia. 1996;39:298-305. [PMID: 8721775]

46. Rolka DB, Narayan KM, Thompson TJ, Goldman D, Lindenmayer J, Alich K, et al. Performance of recommended screening tests for undiagnosed diabetes and dysglycemia. Diabetes Care. 2001;24:1899-903. [PMID: 11679454]

47. Effect of intensive blood-glucose control with metformin on complications in overweight patients with type 2 diabetes (UKPDS 34). UK Prospective Diabetes Study (UKPDS) Group. Lancet. 1998;352:854-65. [PMID: 9742977]

48. Knatterud GL, Meinert CL, Klimt CR, Osborne RK, Martin DB. Effects of hypoglycemic agents on vascular complications in patients with adult-onset diabetes. IV. A preliminary report on phenoformin results. JAMA. 1971;217:777-84. [PMID: 4935344]

49. Knatterud GL, Klimt CR, Levin ME, Jacobson ME, Goldner MG. Effects of hypoglycemic agents on vascular complications in patients with adult-onset diabetes. VII. Mortality and selected nonfatal events with insulin treatment. JAMA. 1978;240:37-42. [PMID: 351218]

50. Azad N, Emanuele NV, Abraira C, Henderson WG, Colwell J, Levin SR, et al. The effects of intensive glycemic control on neuropathy in the VA cooperative study on type II diabetes mellitus (VA CSDM). J Diabetes Complications. 1999; 13:307-13. [PMID: 10765007]

51. Shichiri M, Kishikawa H, Ohkubo Y, Wake N. Long-term results of the Kumamoto Study on optimal diabetes control in type 2 diabetic patients. Diabetes Care. 2000;23(Suppl 2):B21-9.

52. Abraira C, Colwell J, Nuttall F, Sawin CT, Henderson W, Comstock JP, et al. Cardiovascular events and correlates in the Veterans Affairs Diabetes Feasibility Trial. Veterans Affairs Cooperative Study on Glycemic Control and Complications in Type II Diabetes. Arch Intern Med. 1997;157:181-8. [PMID: 9009975]

53. Gaede P, Vedel P, Parving HH, Pedersen O. Intensified multifactorial intervention in patients with type 2 diabetes mellitus and microalbuminuria: the Steno type 2 randomised study. Lancet. 1999;353:617-22. [PMID: 10030326]

54. Emanuele N, Klein R, Abraira C, Colwell J, Comstock J, Henderson WG, et al. Evaluations of retinopathy in the VA Cooperative Study on Glycemic Control and Complications in Type II Diabetes (VA CSDM). A feasibility study. Diabetes Care. 1996;19:1375-81. [PMID: 8941467]

55. Ohkubo Y, Kishikawa H, Araki E, Miyata T, Isami S, Motoyoshi S, et al. Intensive insulin therapy prevents the progression of diabetic microvascular complications in Japanese patients with non-insulin-dependent diabetes mellitus: a randomized prospective 6-year study. Diabetes Res Clin Pract. 1995;28:103-17. [PMID: 7587918]

56. Abraira C, Colwell JA, Nuttall FQ, Sawin CT, Nagel NJ, Comstock JP, et al. Veterans Affairs Cooperative Study on glycemic control and complications in

type II diabetes (VA CSDM). Results of the feasibility trial. Veterans Affairs Cooperative Study in Type II Diabetes. Diabetes Care. 1995;18:1113-23. [PMID: 7587846]

57. Levin SR, Coburn JW, Abraira C, Henderson WG, Colwell JA, Emanuele NV, et al. Effect of intensive glycemic control on microalbuminuria in type 2 diabetes. Veterans Affairs Cooperative Study on Glycemic Control and Complications in Type 2 Diabetes Feasibility Trial Investigators. Diabetes Care. 2000; 23:1478-85. [PMID: 11023140]

58. Ewart RM. The case against aggressive treatment of type 2 diabetes: critique of the UK prospective diabetes study. BMJ. 2001;323:854-8. [PMID: 11597972]

59. Hansson L, Zanchetti A, Carruthers SG, Dahlöf B, Elmfeldt D, Julius S, et al. Effects of intensive blood-pressure lowering and low-dose aspirin in patients with hypertension: principal results of the Hypertension Optimal Treatment (HOT) randomised trial. HOT Study Group. Lancet. 1998;351:1755-62. [PMID: 9635947]

60. Tight blood pressure control and risk of macrovascular and microvascular complications in type 2 diabetes: UKPDS 38. UK Prospective Diabetes Study Group. BMJ. 1998;317:703-13. [PMID: 9732337]

61. Estacio RO, Jeffers BW, Gifford N, Schrier RW. Effect of blood pressure control on diabetic microvascular complications in patients with hypertension and type 2 diabetes. Diabetes Care. 2000;23 Suppl 2:B54-64. [PMID: 10860192]

62. Schrier RW, Estacio RO, Esler A, Mehler P. Effects of aggressive blood pressure control in normotensive type 2 diabetic patients on albuminuria, retinopathy and strokes. Kidney Int. 2002;61:1086-97. [PMID: 11849464]

63. Efficacy of atenolol and captopril in reducing risk of macrovascular and microvascular complications in type 2 diabetes: UKPDS 39. UK Prospective Diabetes Study Group. BMJ. 1998;317:713-20. [PMID: 9732338]

64. Estacio RO, Jeffers BW, Hiatt WR, Biggerstaff SL, Gifford N, Schrier RW. The effect of nisoldipine as compared with enalapril on cardiovascular outcomes in patients with non-insulin-dependent diabetes and hypertension. N Engl J Med. 1998;338:645-52. [PMID: 9486993]

65. Pahor M, Psaty BM, Alderman MH, Applegate WB, Williamson JD, Furberg CD. Therapeutic benefits of ACE inhibitors and other antihypertensive drugs in patients with type 2 diabetes. Diabetes Care. 2000;23:888-92. [PMID: 10895836]

66. Lindholm LH, Hansson L, Ekbom T, Dahlöf B, Lanke J, Linjer E, et al. Comparison of antihypertensive treatments in preventing cardiovascular events in elderly diabetic patients: results from the Swedish Trial in Old Patients with Hypertension-2. STOP Hypertension-2 Study Group. J Hypertens. 2000;18: 1671-5. [PMID: 11081782]

67. Tatti P, Pahor M, Byington RP, Di Mauro P, Guarisco R, Strollo G, et al. Outcome results of the Fosinopril Versus Amlodipine Cardiovascular Events Randomized Trial (FACET) in patients with hypertension and NIDDM. Diabetes Care. 1998;21:597-603. [PMID: 9571349]

68. Niskanen L, Hedner T, Hansson L, Lanke J, Niklason A. Reduced cardiovascular morbidity and mortality in hypertensive diabetic patients on first-line therapy with an ACE inhibitor compared with a diuretic/beta-blocker-based treatment regimen: a subanalysis of the Captopril Prevention Project. Diabetes Care. 2001;24:2091-6. [PMID: 11723089]

69. Brown MJ, Palmer CR, Castaigne A, de Leeuw PW, Mancia G, Rosenthal T, et al. Morbidity and mortality in patients randomised to double-blind treatment with a long-acting calcium-channel blocker or diuretic in the International Nifedipine GITS study: Intervention as a Goal in Hypertension Treatment (INSIGHT). Lancet. 2000;356:366-72. [PMID: 10972368]

70. Hansson L, Hedner T, Lund-Johansen P, Kjeldsen SE, Lindholm LH, Syvertsen JO, et al. Randomised trial of effects of calcium antagonists compared with diuretics and beta-blockers on cardiovascular morbidity and mortality in hypertension: the Nordic Diltiazem (NORDIL) study. Lancet. 2000;356:359-65. [PMID: 10972367]

71. Lewis EJ, Hunsicker LG, Clarke WR, Berl T, Pohl MA, Lewis JB, et al. Renoprotective effect of the angiotensin-receptor antagonist irbesartan in patients with nephropathy due to type 2 diabetes. N Engl J Med. 2001;345:851-60. [PMID: 11565517]

72. Neal B, MacMahon S, Chapman N. Effects of ACE inhibitors, calcium antagonists, and other blood-pressure-lowering drugs: results of prospectively designed overviews of randomised trials. Blood Pressure Lowering Treatment Trialists' Collaboration. Lancet. 2000;356:1955-64. [PMID: 11130523]

73. Pahor M, Psaty BM, Alderman MH, Applegate WB, Williamson JD,

Cavazzini C, et al. Health outcomes associated with calcium antagonists compared with other first-line antihypertensive therapies: a meta-analysis of randomised controlled trials. Lancet. 2000;356:1949-54. [PMID: 11130522]

74. Lindholm LH, Ibsen H, Dahlöf B, Devereux RB, Beevers G, de Faire U, et al. Cardiovascular morbidity and mortality in patients with diabetes in the Losartan Intervention For Endpoint reduction in hypertension study (LIFE): a randomised trial against atenolol. Lancet. 2002;359:1004-10. [PMID: 11937179]

75. Dahlöf B, Devereux RB, Kjeldsen SE, Julius S, Beevers G, Faire U, et al. Cardiovascular morbidity and mortality in the Losartan Intervention For Endpoint reduction in hypertension study (LIFE): a randomised trial against atenolol. Lancet. 2002;359:995-1003. [PMID: 11937179]

76. Hansson L, Lindholm LH, Niskanen L, Lanke J, Hedner T, Niklason A, et al. Effect of angiotensin-converting-enzyme inhibition compared with conventional therapy on cardiovascular morbidity and mortality in hypertension: the Captopril Prevention Project (CAPPP) randomised trial. Lancet. 1999;353: 611-6. [PMID: 10030325]

77. Schnack C, Hoffmann W, Hopmeier P, Schernthaner G. Renal and metabolic effects of 1-year treatment with ramipril or atenolol in NIDDM patients with microalbuminuria. Diabetologia. 1996;39:1611-6. [PMID: 8960851]

78. Fogari R, Zoppi A, Corradi L, Mugellini A, Lazzari P, Preti P, et al. Long-term effects of ramipril and nitrendipine on albuminuria in hypertensive patients with type II diabetes and impaired renal function. J Hum Hypertens. 1999;13:47-53. [PMID: 9928752]

79. Effects of ramipril on cardiovascular and microvascular outcomes in people with diabetes mellitus: results of the HOPE study and MICRO-HOPE substudy. Heart Outcomes Prevention Evaluation Study Investigators. Lancet. 2000;355: 253-9. [PMID: 10675071]

80. Parving HH, Lehnert H, Bröchner-Mortensen J, Gomis R, Andersen S, Arner P, et al. The effect of irbesartan on the development of diabetic nephropathy in patients with type 2 diabetes. N Engl J Med. 2001;345:870-8. [PMID: 11565519]

81. Chan JC, Ko GT, Leung DH, Cheung RC, Cheung MY, So WY, et al. Long-term effects of angiotensin-converting enzyme inhibition and metabolic control in hypertensive type 2 diabetic patients. Kidney Int. 2000;57:590-600. [PMID: 10652036]

82. Lovell HG. Angiotensin converting enzyme inhibitors in normotensive diabetic patients with microalbuminuria. Cochrane Database Syst Rev. [PMID: 10796871]

83. Brenner BM, Cooper ME, de Zeeuw D, Keane WF, Mitch WE, Parving HH, et al. Effects of losartan on renal and cardiovascular outcomes in patients with type 2 diabetes and nephropathy. N Engl J Med. 2001;345:861-9. [PMID: 11565518]

84. Hostetter TH. Prevention of end-stage renal disease due to type 2 diabetes [Editorial]. N Engl J Med. 2001;345:910-2. [PMID: 11565525]

85. Barzilay JI, Spiekerman CF, Kuller LH, Burke GL, Bittner V, Gottdiener JS, et al. Prevalence of clinical and isolated subclinical cardiovascular disease in older adults with glucose disorders: the Cardiovascular Health Study. Diabetes Care. 2001;24:1233-9. [PMID: 11423508]

86. Resnick HE, Harris MI, Brock DB, Harris TB. American Diabetes Association diabetes diagnostic criteria, advancing age, and cardiovascular disease risk profiles: results from the Third National Health and Nutrition Examination Survey. Diabetes Care. 2000;23:176-80. [PMID: 10868827]

87. Saito I, Folsom AR, Brancati FL, Duncan BB, Chambless LE, McGovern PG. Nontraditional risk factors for coronary heart disease incidence among persons with diabetes: the Atherosclerosis Risk in Communities (ARIC) Study. Ann Intern Med. 2000;133:81-91. [PMID: 10896647]

88. Fonseca VA. Risk factors for coronary heart disease in diabetes [Editorial]. Ann Intern Med. 2000;133:154-6. [PMID: 10896642]

89. Pyörälä K, Pedersen TR, Kjekshus J, Faergeman O, Olsson AG, Thorgeirsson G. Cholesterol lowering with simvastatin improves prognosis of diabetic patients with coronary heart disease. A subgroup analysis of the Scandinavian Simvastatin Survival Study (4S). Diabetes Care. 1997;20:614-20. [PMID: 9096989]

90. Koskinen P, Mänttäri M, Manninen V, Huttunen JK, Heinonen OP, Frick MH. Coronary heart disease incidence in NIDDM patients in the Helsinki Heart Study. Diabetes Care. 1992;15:820-5. [PMID: 1516498]

91. Frick MH, Elo O, Haapa K, Heinonen OP, Heinsalmi P, Helo P, et al. Helsinki Heart Study: primary-prevention trial with gemfibrozil in middle-aged men with dyslipidemia. Safety of treatment, changes in risk factors, and incidence of coronary heart disease. N Engl J Med. 1987;317:1237-45. [PMID: 3313041]

92. Prevention of cardiovascular events and death with pravastatin in patients with coronary heart disease and a broad range of initial cholesterol levels. The Long-Term Intervention with Pravastatin in Ischaemic Disease (LIPID) Study Group. N Engl J Med. 1998;339:1349-57. [PMID: 9841303]

93. Downs JR, Clearfield M, Weis S, Whitney E, Shapiro DR, Beere PA, et al. Primary prevention of acute coronary events with lovastatin in men and women with average cholesterol levels: results of AFCAPS/TexCAPS. Air Force/Texas Coronary Atherosclerosis Prevention Study. JAMA. 1998;279:1615-22. [PMID: 9613910]

94. Randomised trial of cholesterol lowering in 4444 patients with coronary heart disease: the Scandinavian Simvastatin Survival Study (4S). Lancet. 1994;344: 1383-9. [PMID: 7968073]

95. Rubins HB, Robins SJ, Collins D, Fye CL, Anderson JW, Elam MB, et al. Gemfibrozil for the secondary prevention of coronary heart disease in men with low levels of high-density lipoprotein cholesterol. Veterans Affairs High-Density Lipoprotein Cholesterol Intervention Trial Study Group. N Engl J Med. 1999; 341:410-8. [PMID: 10438259]

96. Haffner SM, Alexander CM, Cook TJ, Boccuzzi SJ, Musliner TA, Pedersen TR, et al. Reduced coronary events in simvastatin-treated patients with coronary heart disease and diabetes or impaired fasting glucose levels: subgroup analyses in the Scandinavian Simvastatin Survival Study. Arch Intern Med. 1999;159: 2661-7. [PMID: 10597756]

97. Robins SJ, Collins D, Wittes JT, Papademetriou V, Deedwania PC, Schaefer EJ, et al. Relation of gemfibrozil treatment and lipid levels with major coronary events: VA-HIT: a randomized controlled trial. JAMA. 2001;285:1585-91. [PMID: 11268266]

98. Pignone MP, Phillips CJ, Atkins D, Teutsch SM, Mulrow CD, Lohr KN. Screening and treating adults for lipid disorders. Am J Prev Med. 2001;20:77-89. [PMID: 11306236]

99. MRC/BHF Heart Protection Study of cholesterol lowering with simvastatin in 20,536 high-risk individuals: a randomised placebo-controlled trial. Lancet. 2002;360:7-22. [PMID: 12114036]

100. Elkeles RS, Diamond JR, Poulter C, Dhanjil S, Nicolaides AN, Mahmood S, et al. Cardiovascular outcomes in type 2 diabetes. A double-blind placebo-controlled study of bezafibrate: the St. Mary's, Ealing, Northwick Park Diabetes Cardiovascular Disease Prevention (SENDCAP) Study. Diabetes Care. 1998;21: 641-8. [PMID: 9571357]

101. Goldberg RB, Mellies MJ, Sacks FM, Moyé LA, Howard BV, Howard WJ, et al. Cardiovascular events and their reduction with pravastatin in diabetic and glucose-intolerant myocardial infarction survivors with average cholesterol levels: subgroup analyses in the cholesterol and recurrent events (CARE) trial. The Care Investigators. Circulation. 1998;98:2513-9. [PMID: 9843456]

102. Colwell JA. Aspirin therapy in diabetes. Diabetes Care. 1997;20:1767-71. [PMID: 9353620]

103. Hayden M, Pignone M, Phillips C, Mulrow C. Aspirin for the primary prevention of cardiovascular events: a summary of the evidence for the U.S. Preventive Services Task Force. Ann Intern Med. 2002;136:161-72. [PMID: 11790072]

104. American Diabetes Association. Aspirin therapy in diabetes. Diabetes Care. 2001;24:S62-3.

105. Aspirin effects on mortality and morbidity in patients with diabetes mellitus. Early Treatment Diabetic Retinopathy Study report 14. ETDRS Investigators. JAMA. 1992;268:1292-300. [PMID: 1507375]

106. Collaborative overview of randomised trials of antiplatelet therapy—I: Prevention of death, myocardial infarction, and stroke by prolonged antiplatelet therapy in various categories of patients. Antiplatelet Trialists' Collaboration. BMJ. 1994;308:81-106. [PMID: 8298418]

107. Sacks FM, Tonkin AM, Craven T, Pfeffer MA, Shepherd J, Keech A, et al. Coronary heart disease in patients with low LDL-cholesterol: benefit of pravastatin in diabetics and enhanced role for HDL-cholesterol and triglycerides as risk factors. Circulation. 2002;105:1424-8. [PMID: 11914249]

108. Executive Summary of The Third Report of The National Cholesterol Education Program (NCEP) Expert Panel on Detection, Evaluation, And Treatment of High Blood Cholesterol In Adults (Adult Treatment Panel III). JAMA. 2001;285:2486-97. [PMID: 11368702]

109. McCabe CJ, Stevenson RC, Dolan AM. Evaluation of a diabetic foot screening and protection programme. Diabet Med. 1998;15:80-4. [PMID: 9472868]

110. Litzelman DK, Slemenda CW, Langefeld CD, Hays LM, Welch MA, Bild DE, et al. Reduction of lower extremity clinical abnormalities in patients with non-insulin-dependent diabetes mellitus. A randomized, controlled trial. Ann Intern Med. 1993;119:36-41. [PMID: 8498761]

111. Patout CA Jr, Birke JA, Horswell R, Williams D, Cerise FP. Effectiveness of a comprehensive diabetes lower-extremity amputation prevention program in a predominantly low-income African-American population. Diabetes Care. 2000; 23:1339-42. [PMID: 10977029]

112. Resnick HE, Valsania P, Phillips CL. Diabetes mellitus and nontraumatic lower extremity amputation in black and white Americans: the National Health and Nutrition Examination Survey Epidemiologic Follow-up Study, 1971-1992. Arch Intern Med. 1999;159:2470-5. [PMID: 10665896]

113. Haffner SM, Stern MP, Hazuda HP, Mitchell BD, Patterson JK. Cardiovascular risk factors in confirmed prediabetic individuals. Does the clock for coronary heart disease start ticking before the onset of clinical diabetes? JAMA. 1990;263:2893-8. [PMID: 2338751]

114. McPhillips JB, Barrett-Connor E, Wingard DL. Cardiovascular disease risk factors prior to the diagnosis of impaired glucose tolerance and non-insulin-dependent diabetes mellitus in a community of older adults. Am J Epidemiol. 1990;131:443-53. [PMID: 2301354]

115. Harris MI, Eastman RC. Is there a glycemic threshold for mortality risk? [Editorial] Diabetes Care. 1998;21:331-3. [PMID: 9540010]

116. Dyson PA, Hammersley MS, Morris RJ, Holman RR, Turner RC. The Fasting Hyperglycaemia Study: II. Randomized controlled trial of reinforced healthy-living advice in subjects with increased but not diabetic fasting plasma glucose. Metabolism. 1997;46:50-5. [PMID: 9439560]

117. Pan XR, Li GW, Hu YH, Wang JX, Yang WY, An ZX, et al. Effects of diet and exercise in preventing NIDDM in people with impaired glucose tolerance. The Da Qing IGT and Diabetes Study. Diabetes Care. 1997;20:537-44. [PMID: 9096977]

118. Chiasson JL, Josse RG, Gomis R, Hanefeld M, Karasik A, Laakso M, et al. Acarbose for prevention of type 2 diabetes mellitus: the STOP-NIDDM randomised trial. Lancet. 2002;359:2072-7. [PMID: 12086760]

119. Knowler WC, Barrett-Connor E, Fowler SE, Hamman RF, Lachin JM, Walker EA, et al. Reduction in the incidence of type 2 diabetes with lifestyle intervention or metformin. N Engl J Med. 2002;346:393-403. [PMID: 11832527]

120. Tuomilehto J, Lindström J, Eriksson JG, Valle TT, Hämäläinen H, Ilanne-Parikka P, et al. Prevention of type 2 diabetes mellitus by changes in lifestyle among subjects with impaired glucose tolerance. N Engl J Med. 2001; 344:1343-50. [PMID: 11333990]

121. The Diabetes Prevention Program. Design and methods for a clinical trial in the prevention of type 2 diabetes. Diabetes Care. 1999;22:623-34. [PMID: 10189543]

122. Edelman D, Olsen MK, Dudley TK, Harris AC, Oddone EZ. Impact of diabetes screening on quality of life. Diabetes Care. 2002;25:1022-6. [PMID: 12032109]

123. Warram JH, Sigal RJ, Martin BC, Krolewski AS, Soeldner JS. Natural history of impaired glucose tolerance: follow-up at Joslin Clinic. Diabet Med. 1996;13:S40-5. [PMID: 8894480]

124. Yudkin JS, Alberti KG, McLarty DG, Swai AB. Impaired glucose tolerance. BMJ. 1990;301:397-402. [PMID: 2282392]

125. Balkau B, Eschwège E. Repeatability of the oral glucose tolerance test for the diagnosis of impaired glucose tolerance and diabetes mellitus [Letter]. Diabetologia. 1991;34:201-2. [PMID: 1884894]

126. Eriksson KF, Lindgärde F. Impaired glucose tolerance in a middle-aged male urban population: a new approach for identifying high-risk cases. Diabetologia. 1990;33:526-31. [PMID: 2253828]

127. Swai AB, McLarty DG, Kitange HM, Kilima PM, Masuki G, Mtinangi BI, et al. Study in Tanzania of impaired glucose tolerance. Methodological myth? Diabetes. 1991;40:516-20. [PMID: 2010053]

128. Bourn DM, Williams SM, Mann JI. Distinguishing between persistent and transient impaired glucose tolerance using a prediction model. Diabet Med. 1992;9:744-8. [PMID: 1395468]

129. Burke JP, Haffner SM, Gaskill SP, Williams KL, Stern MP. Reversion from type 2 diabetes to nondiabetic status. Influence of the 1997 American Diabetes Association criteria. Diabetes Care. 1998;21:1266-70. [PMID: 9702431]

130. Eschwège E, Charles MA, Simon D, Thibult N, Balkau B. Reproducibility of the diagnosis of diabetes over a 30-month follow-up: the Paris Prospective Study. Diabetes Care. 2001;24:1941-4. [PMID: 11679461]

131. Israili ZH, Hall WD. Cough and angioneurotic edema associated with angiotensin-converting enzyme inhibitor therapy. A review of the literature and pathophysiology. Ann Intern Med. 1992;117:234-42. [PMID: 1616218]

132. Bradford RH, Shear CL, Chremos AN, Dujovne CA, Franklin FA, Grillo RB, et al. Expanded Clinical Evaluation of Lovastatin (EXCEL) study results: two-year efficacy and safety follow-up. Am J Cardiol. 1994;74:667-73. [PMID: 7942524]

133. Pierce LR, Wysowski DK, Gross TP. Myopathy and rhabdomyolysis associated with lovastatin-gemfibrozil combination therapy. JAMA. 1990;264: 71-5. [PMID: 2355431]

134. Quality of life in type 2 diabetic patients is affected by complications but not by intensive policies to improve blood glucose or blood pressure control (UKPDS 37). U.K. Prospective Diabetes Study Group. Diabetes Care. 1999;22:1125-36. [PMID: 10388978]

135. Testa MA, Simonson DC. Health economic benefits and quality of life during improved glycemic control in patients with type 2 diabetes mellitus: a randomized, controlled, double-blind trial. JAMA. 1998;280:1490-6. [PMID: 9809729]

136. Testa MA, Simonson DC, Turner RR. Valuing quality of life and improvements in glycemic control in people with type 2 diabetes. Diabetes Care. 1998;21 Suppl 3:C44-52. [PMID: 9850489]

137. Carter JS, Pugh JA, Monterrosa A. Non-insulin-dependent diabetes mellitus in minorities in the United States. Ann Intern Med. 1996;125:221-32. [PMID: 8686981]

138. Karter AJ, Ferrara A, Liu JY, Moffet HH, Ackerson LM, Selby JV. Ethnic disparities in diabetic complications in an insured population. JAMA. 2002;287: 2519-27. [PMID: 12020332]

APPENDIX
Methods

The Research Triangle Institute–University of North Carolina Evidence-based Practice Center, together with members of the USPSTF, sought to clarify issues concerning screening adults for diabetes by performing a systematic review of the relevant scientific literature on this topic.
Analytic Framework

The systematic evidence review examined the evidence for screening for diabetes, comparing systematic screening with no screening. **Appendix Figure 1** presents the analytic framework that we used to guide our literature search. The analytic framework describes the logical chain that evidence must support to link screening to improved health outcomes. Each arrow in the analytic framework represents a key question. We searched systematically for evidence concerning each key question in the analytic framework.

The analytic framework begins on the left side of the figure with a sample at risk for undiagnosed diabetes and moves to the right. The first key question (represented by the overarching arrow) examines direct evidence that screening improves health outcomes. Because no such studies were found, we continued to examine the indirect evidence in the following key questions, represented as linkages in the analytic framework.

Key question 2 examines the yield of screening, involving both the accuracy and reliability of various screening tests as well as the prevalence of undiagnosed diabetes in the population. Farther to the right in the analytic framework, the third key question examines the efficacy of various treatments to prevent diabetic complications, including tight glycemic control, cardiovascular risk reduction, foot care, or enhanced counseling for lifestyle changes. It is important to note that the critical issue here is the efficacy of the treatment among persons who would be detected by screening. Some studies examine treatment for persons with new clinically detected diabetes; these are useful only insofar as they allow extrapolation to the efficacy of treatment at screening detection. In addition, key question 3 actually implies that the issue of interest is the *added* efficacy of initiating treatment after screening detection as opposed to initiation after clinical detection. An additional treatment (key question 4) is lifestyle intervention programs for persons with impaired fasting glucose or impaired glucose tolerance. These interventions may reduce the intermediate outcome of developing diabetes, but the critical question is the extent to which they improve health outcomes.

In between the treatment arrows and health outcomes are a variety of "intermediate outcomes," such as retinopathy and albuminuria. Although changes in these outcomes may herald later improved health outcomes, they may or

Appendix Figure 1. **Analytic framework for screening for type 2 diabetes.**

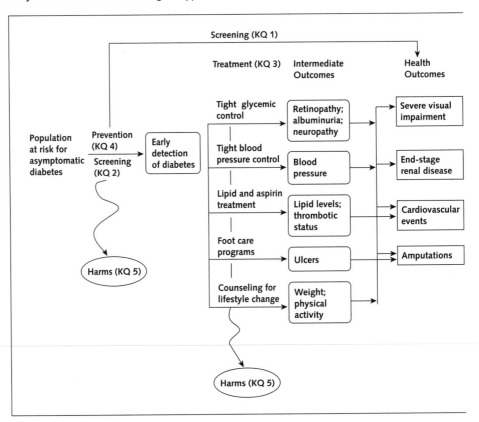

KQ = key question.

Appendix Table 1. Eligibility Criteria, Search Strategy, and Results of Searches*

Key Question	Eligibility Criteria	Articles Identified for Abstract Review	Articles Meeting Criteria
		n	
All	Published 1 January 1994 through 30 July 2002 English language MEDLINE, Cochrane Human subjects		
1. Efficacy of screening (direct evidence)	RCT of screening	130	0
2. Accuracy and reliability of screening tests	Population relevant to primary care Screening test offered to all Screening test compared with a valid reference standard, including all positive tests and at least a sample of negatives	487	7
3. Efficacy of knowledge of diabetes status for optimizing the following treatments: Tight glycemic control Tight blood pressure control; type of drug Lipid and aspirin treatment Foot care programs Counseling for lifestyle change	RCT Follow-up ≥2 years ≥75% of patients followed Health outcomes	436 426 191 48 6	5 13 8 2 0
4. Lifestyle intervention for people with impaired fasting glucose or impaired glucose tolerance	RCT Intervention at impaired fasting glucose or impaired glucose tolerance stage Valid measure of development of diabetes	39	8
5. Harms of screening and treatment	Use of valid measurement instrument Follow-up for ≥12 months during treatment Comparison with similar untreated or unscreened control group	57	6

* RCT = randomized, controlled trial.

may not be sufficient in themselves to allow estimation of the magnitude of health benefit with reasonable certainty.

At the far right in the analytic framework are the health outcomes—the outcomes that people can experience and care about. These include the major diabetic complications: severe visual impairment, ESRD, lower-extremity amputation, and cardiovascular events. In the end, the indirect evidence must allow a reasonable estimation of the magnitude of benefit in these outcomes attributable to screening. At the bottom of the analytic framework is linkage and key question 5, the issue of the harms of screening (for example, labeling) or harms of treatment (for example, side effects).

Key Questions

Key question 1: Is there direct evidence from an RCT of screening that screening for diabetes improves health outcomes?

Key question 2: What is the yield of screening, both in terms of the accuracy and reliability of screening tests and the prevalence of undiagnosed diabetes in the population?

Key question 3: What is the added efficacy of initiating treatments (tight glycemic control, tight blood pressure control, lipid and aspirin treatment, foot care programs, counseling for lifestyle change) at screening detection com-

pared with clinical detection in improving health outcomes?

Key question 4: What is the efficacy of lifestyle intervention for people with impaired fasting glucose or impaired glucose tolerance in improving health outcomes?

Key question 5: What are the harms of screening or treatment?

Eligibility Criteria for Admissible Evidence

The Evidence-based Practice Center staff and USP-STF liaisons developed eligibility criteria for selecting the evidence relevant to answer the key questions (**Appendix Table 1**). For key question 1, we required a well-conducted RCT of screening of adequate size and length to estimate health outcomes with reasonable accuracy. For key question 2, we required cross-sectional or cohort studies in which screening tests were performed on a primary care or general unselected sample and compared with an acceptable reference standard. For key question 3, we accepted RCTs of treatments with health outcomes that provided information about disease duration and comorbid conditions in persons with diabetes. For key question 4, we accepted RCTs of persons with impaired fasting glucose or impaired glucose tolerance treated with lifestyle or other interventions in which diabetes incidence or development of diabetic complications was an outcome. For key ques-

Appendix Table 2. **Search Strategies***

Key Question	Search Strategy
1. Is there direct evidence from an RCT of screening that screening for diabetes improves health outcomes?	*Noninsulin-dependent diabetes* *Mass screening* *RCT*
2. What is the yield of screening?	*Noninsulin-dependent diabetes* *Prevalence, incidence* *Fasting glucose* *Random glucose* *Postload glucose* *Glucose tolerance test* *Mass screening* *Hemoglobin A$_{1c}$* *Glycosylated hemoglobin* *Diagnosis* *Sensitivity/specificity* *Predictive value* *Reproducibility* *Screening programs*
3. What is the added efficacy of initiating the treatments below at screening detection compared with clinical detection in improving health outcomes? Tight glycemic control Tight blood pressure control Lipid and aspirin treatment Foot care programs Counseling for lifestyle change	*Noninsulin-dependent diabetes* *Insulin* *Glycemic control* *Antihypertensives* *ACE inhibitors* *Calcium-channel blockers* *Statins* *Aspirin* *Counseling* *Smoking* *Tobacco* *Weight change* *Physical activity* *Oral hypoglycemics* *Foot care programs* *Therapeutics* *Treatment*
4. What is the efficacy of lifestyle intervention for people with impaired fasting glucose or impaired glucose tolerance in improving health outcomes?	*Noninsulin-dependent diabetes* *RCT* *Primary prevention* *Impaired glucose tolerance/ impaired fasting glucose*
5. What are the harms of screening or treatment?	*Therapeutics* *Treatment* *Noninsulin-dependent diabetes* *Mass screening* *Labeling* *Hypoglycemia* *Adverse effects* *Side effects* *Quality of life* *False positive* *False negative* *Predictive value*

* ACE = angiotensin-converting enzyme; RCT = randomized, controlled trial.

Appendix Figure 2. **Selection of articles based on key question 1.**

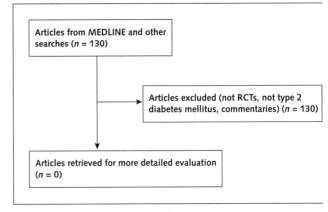

RCT = randomized, controlled trial.

Literature Search Strategy, Results, and Review of Abstracts and Articles

The analytic framework and key questions guided our literature searches. We examined the critical literature described in the previous review of this topic by the USPSTF (published in 1996) and used our eligibility criteria to develop search terms. We used the search terms to search MEDLINE and the Cochrane Library for English-language articles that met inclusion criteria and were published between 1 January 1994 and 30 July 2002. We also examined the bibliographies of pertinent articles and contacted experts for other references. When we found that a key question could best be answered by older literature, we also examined these studies. The search strategies are given

Appendix Figure 3. **Selection of articles based on key question 2.**

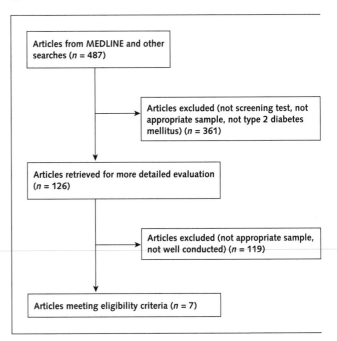

tion 5, we required RCTs of screened (or treated) versus nonscreened (or nontreated) samples. When we could not find such studies, we also examined cohort studies of screening-detected diabetic persons for evidence of quality of life or psychosocial harms.

Appendix Figure 4. Selection of articles based on key question 3.

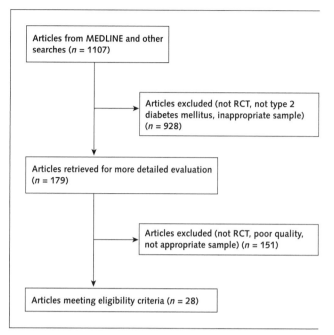

RCT = randomized, controlled trial.

Appendix Figure 6. Selection of articles based on key question 5.

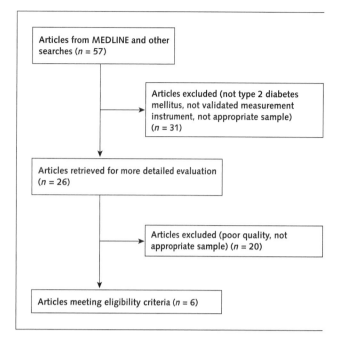

in **Appendix Table 2.** All searches started with the term *noninsulin dependent diabetes*, and other terms were added as appropriate.

The first author and at least one other coauthor or trained assistant reviewed all abstracts to find those that

Appendix Figure 5. Selection of articles based on key question 4.

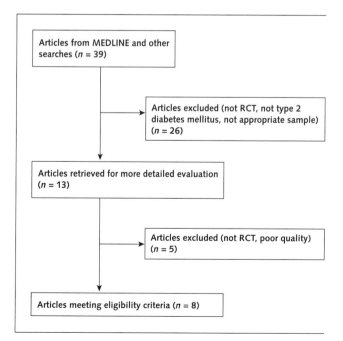

RCT = randomized, controlled trial.

met eligibility criteria. When either reviewer thought that an abstract might meet criteria, the article was copied for full review. The first author and at least one other coauthor or trained assistant reviewed each full article. Those that met eligibility criteria after full review and, when necessary, discussion, were abstracted. **Appendix Figures 2** through **6** illustrate our selection process for each key question. We critically appraised each study using criteria developed by the USPSTF Methods Work Group. If we found an article that met criteria but had methodologically fatal flaws that invalidated its findings, it was excluded from further review. Abstracted articles that met eligibility criteria and had no fatal flaws were entered into predesigned evidence tables (see Appendix B in the systematic evidence review "Screening Adults for Type 2 Diabetes," available at www.ahrq.preventiveservices.gov).

Development of the Systematic Evidence Review and Review of the Evidence Article

The authors presented an initial work plan, including a provisional analytic framework and key questions, to the entire Task Force. Interim reports were presented at subsequent meetings. The Task Force discussed and made important contributions to the review on several occasions. The two Task Force liaisons participated in every phase of the review, including several conference calls to discuss critical parts of the evidence.

A draft systematic evidence review was presented to the Task Force and then sent for broad peer review. The peer review included individual experts in the field, representatives of relevant professional organizations, and representatives of appropriate federal agencies. We made revisions to the evidence review as appropriate after receiving peer review comments. The Task Force reviewed all information and voted on a recommendation. We then finalized the systematic evidence review for publication by the Agency for Healthcare Research and Quality and separately adapted it for journal publication.

Current Author Addresses: Dr. Harris: Sheps Center for Health Services Research, 725 Airport Road, CB #7590, Chapel Hill, NC 27599-2949.

Dr. Donahue: University of North Carolina, CB #7595 Manning, Chapel Hill, NC 27599.

Dr. Rathore: Yale University School of Medicine, PO Box 208025, New Haven, CT 06520-8025.

Dr. Frame: Tri-County Family Medicine, Box 112, Cohocton, NY 14826.

Dr. Woolf: Virginia Commonwealth University, 3712 Charles Stewart Drive, Fairfax, VA 22033.

Dr. Lohr: Research Triangle Institute, 3040 Cornwallis Road, Research Triangle Park, NC 27709.

Key Points

Postmenopausal osteoporosis

❏ There are no studies of the effectiveness of screening on preventing fractures. All studies have studied intermediate outcomes such as bone density (at different sites) and risk factor assessments (with different definitions of risk factors).

❏ Dual-energy X-ray densitometry of the femoral neck is the best predictor of hip fracture and is comparable to forearm measurements for predicting fractures at other sites.

❏ Based on the increasing risk of osteoporosis in women over age 65, routine screening in that population is reasonable. For women aged 60 to 64, screening may be triggered by the presence of risk factors. Low body weight is the single best predictor of low bone density.

❏ Screening intervals of 5 years may be reasonable for younger (<65 years) postmenopausal women; 2-year intervals may be reasonable for older (≥65 years) women.

Screening for Postmenopausal Osteoporosis: A Review of the Evidence for the U.S. Preventive Services Task Force

Heidi D. Nelson, MD, MPH; Mark Helfand, MD, MPH; Steven H. Woolf, MD, MPH; and Janet D. Allan, PhD, RN

Background: Although osteoporotic fractures present an enormous health burden, it is not clear whether screening to identify high-risk persons is appropriate.

Purpose: To examine evidence on the benefits and harms of screening postmenopausal women for osteoporosis.

Data Sources: MEDLINE (1966 to May 2001), HealthSTAR (1975 to May 2001), and Cochrane databases; reference lists; and experts.

Study Selection: English-language abstracts that included original data about postmenopausal women and osteoporosis and addressed the effectiveness of risk factor assessment, bone density tests, or treatment were included.

Data Extraction: Selected information about patient population, interventions, clinical end points, and study design were extracted, and a set of criteria was applied to evaluate study quality.

Data Synthesis: No trials of the effectiveness of screening have been published. Instruments developed to assess clinical risk factors for low bone density or fractures have moderate to high sensitivity and low specificity. Among different bone density tests measured at various sites, bone density measured at the femoral neck by dual-energy x-ray absorptiometry is the best predictor of hip fracture. Women with low bone density have approximately a 40% to 50% reduction in fracture risk when treated with bisphosphonates.

Conclusions: Population screening would be based on evidence that the risk for osteoporosis and fractures increases with age, that the short-term risk for fracture can be estimated by bone density tests and risk factors, and that fracture risk can be reduced with treatment. The role of risk factor assessment and different bone density techniques, frequency of screening, and identification of subgroups for which screening is most effective remain unclear.

Half of all postmenopausal women will have an osteoporosis-related fracture during their lives, including one quarter who will develop a vertebral deformity (1) and 15% who will suffer a hip fracture (2). Hip fractures are associated with high mortality rates and loss of independence (3, 4). Although many vertebral fractures are detected only incidentally on radiography, some cause severe pain, leading to 150 000 hospital admissions per year in persons older than 65 years of age, 161 000 physician office visits, and more than 5 million days of restricted activity in those 45 years of age or older (5).

Low bone density has been used to predict risk for fractures as well as to diagnose osteoporosis. Osteoporosis has been defined as "a systemic skeletal disease characterized by low bone mass and microarchitectural deterioration of bone tissue, leading to enhanced bone fragility and a consequent increase in fracture risk" (6, 7). This definition emphasizes that, in addition to bone mass, the structure of bone is an important factor in the pathogenesis of fractures.

A World Health Organization working group (8) proposed that osteoporosis should be diagnosed in epidemiologic studies when bone mineral density is 2.5 SDs or more below the mean for healthy young adult women at the spine, hip, or wrist (corresponding to a T-score ≤ -2.5) or when patients have a history of atraumatic fracture (9). By the World Health Organization definition, up to 70% of women older than 80 years of age have osteoporosis (10). Age is also an important factor in the relationship between bone density and the absolute risk for fracture. Older women have a much higher fracture rate than younger women with the same bone density because of increasing risk from other factors, such as bone quality and tendency to fall (11).

Despite the high prevalence of osteoporosis and the effect of fractures on mortality, independence, and quality of life, it is not clear whether it is appropriate to screen asymptomatic postmenopausal women. Recent systematic reviews and guidelines disagree about which women should be screened and when (12–20). This disagreement reflects, in part, gaps in the evidence. For example, most guidelines recommend using risk factors to select patients for bone density testing, but because of inadequate data there is no consensus on which risk factors to use. As part of the U.S. Preventive Services Task Force update of its 1996 recommendation (21), we examined evidence on the benefits and harms of screening postmenopausal women for osteoporosis. Specifically, we addressed the role of risk factors in identifying high-risk women, techniques of bone density testing to identify fracture risks, effectiveness of treatment in reducing fracture risk, and harms of screening and treatment.

METHODS

Additional methods used for this review, including determination of the quality of studies (22), are detailed in **Appendix Tables 1, 2,** and **3** (available at www.annals.org) and in a separate report (23). The analytic framework and key questions are detailed in the **Appendix Figure** (available at www.annals.org). Relevant studies were identified from multiple searches of MEDLINE (1966 to May

2001), HealthSTAR (1975 to May 2001), and Cochrane databases; reference lists of systematic reviews; and experts. We also sent letters to manufacturers of bone density devices requesting additional information about the performance of their instruments, but we received no new data.

Two reviewers read each abstract to determine its eligibility. We included English-language abstracts that contained original data about postmenopausal women and osteoporosis and addressed screening or the effectiveness of risk factor assessment, bone density testing, or treatment. We considered screening to be the process of assessing postmenopausal women without known osteoporosis for risk of osteoporotic fractures by identification of risk factors, including low bone density. Postmenopausal women were those who had experienced surgical or natural menopause, regardless of age. Women with preexisting atraumatic fractures were not considered in the screening population because they had confirmed osteoporosis according to the World Health Organization definition.

For studies of prediction, we selected articles that reported the relationship between risk factor assessment methods or bone density tests and bone density, bone loss, or fractures. We reviewed studies of medications used for treatment and present results for bisphosphonates. We focused on randomized, controlled trials of therapies reporting radiographically verified, nontraumatic fracture outcomes because fractures are a stronger measure of effectiveness than bone density. We excluded studies of primary prevention of osteoporosis, such as the role of nutrition, calcium consumption, and physical activity. We also excluded secondary causes of osteoporosis, such as corticosteroid use and certain chronic diseases, and studies that did not provide sufficient information to allow determination of the method for selecting patients and for analyzing data. Investigators read the full-text versions of the retrieved papers and reapplied the initial eligibility criteria. To assess the internal validity of individual studies, we applied a set of criteria developed by the third U.S. Preventive Services Task Force (**Appendix Table 1**, available at www.annals.org) (22).

In this paper, we highlight studies that are applicable to current practice standards, have high-quality internal validity ratings, and are most generalizable to the U.S. population of postmenopausal women under consideration for screening. We created an outcomes table to summarize the number of hip and vertebral fractures prevented based on age-specific prevalence rates and treatment effects obtained from results of the reviewed studies. We conducted a sensitivity analysis to determine the influence of risk factors on the number needed to screen.

This research was funded by the Agency for Healthcare Research and Quality under a contract to support the work of the U.S. Preventive Services Task Force. Agency staff and Task Force members participated in the initial design of the study and reviewed interim analyses and the final manuscript. Additional reports were distributed for review to content experts and revised accordingly before preparation of this manuscript (23, 24). The authors are responsible for the content of the manuscript and the decision to submit it for publication.

RESULTS

Studies of Screening

We identified no studies about the effectiveness of screening in reducing osteoporotic fractures. Without direct evidence from screening studies, recommendations about screening need to rely on evidence that risk factor assessment or bone density testing can adequately identify women who could ultimately benefit from treatment.

Risk Factor Assessment

Hundreds of studies report associations between risk factors and low bone density and fractures in postmenopausal women (24). The most comprehensive study of risk factors in a U.S. population is the Study of Osteoporotic Fractures, a good-quality prospective study of 9516 women 65 years of age and older (25). In this study, 14 clinical risk factors were identified as significant predictors of hip fracture in multivariable models (age; maternal hip fracture; no weight gain; height; poor self-rated health; hyperthyroidism; current use of benzodiazepines, anticonvulsants, or caffeine; not walking for exercise; lack of ambulation; inability to rise from a chair; poor scores on two measures of vision; high resting pulse; and any fracture since 50 years of age). The relative risk for hip fracture per decrease of 1 SD in calcaneal bone density was 1.6 (95% CI, 1.3 to 1.9). This was comparable to the magnitude of the relative risks of most of the other significant predictors in the model, which ranged from 1.2 to 2.0. Women with at least 5 of the 14 risk factors had increased rates of hip fractures compared with those who had 0 to 2 risk factors at all levels of calcaneal bone density.

To determine which risk factors could be important in women younger than 65 years of age, we reviewed eight observational studies of risk factors and fractures of various types conducted in populations in which at least 50% of participants were younger than 65 years of age. **Table 1** lists risk factors that were statistically significant predictors for fractures in multivariable models (26–33). These results could not be quantitatively combined because risk factors were defined differently in each study.

Results of risk factor studies have been used to assess risk in individuals. We identified 10 cross-sectional studies that described methods of determining risk for low bone density for individual women based on selected clinical risk factors (**Table 2**) (34–43). The most common methodologic limitations of these studies are lack of validation and lack of generalizability because of small numbers of patients or nonrepresentative patients. We also identified 8 studies of clinical risk factors to determine fracture risk (**Table 2**) (44–51). None of these studies received a good rating for internal validity. Four studies evaluated hip frac-

Table 1. Risk Factors for Fractures in Women 50–65 Years of Age

Risk Factor	Relative Risk for Fracture (95% CI)	Reference
Age		
Per 2 y	1.11 (1.01–1.21)	26
Per 5 y	1.94 (1.55–2.42)	27
Body mass index		
Per increase of 10 kg/m²	0.58 (0.36–0.92)	27
≥25.6 kg/m²	wrist, 0.7 (0.5–0.9); ankle, 1.6 (1.0–2.4)	26
≥28.6 kg/m²	wrist, 0.5 (0.4–0.7); ankle, 2.0 (1.3–3.1)	26
Low	1.1 (1.0–1.2)	29
Height (per 0.1 m)	1.58 (1.18–2.12)	27
Mother with fracture	1.27 (1.16–1.40)	30
Grandmother with hip fracture	3.70 (1.55–8.85)	31
Hormone replacement therapy		
Current use	0.82 (0.74–0.91)	30
Per 5 y of use	0.5 (0.2–0.9)	28
>2 y of use	0.44 (0.22–0.89)	32
Long history of use	0.70 (0.50–0.96)	33
African American ethnicity	0.54 (0.41–0.72)	30
Diabetes mellitus	9.17 (3.38–24.92)	27
Chronic conditions	1.3 (1.1–1.5)	26
Disability pension	3.79 (2.15–6.68)	27
Long-term work disability	1.3 (1.1–1.6)	26
Self-rated health (fair or poor)	1.79 (1.52–2.11)	30
Moderate daily physical activity	0.61 (0.37–0.99)	32
Alcohol		
≥100 g/wk	1.70 (1.08–2.67)	33
Regular use	1.4 (1.3–4.4)	29
1 to 6 drinks/wk	0.85 (0.75–0.96)	30
Smoking		
Current	1.5 (1.3–1.5); 1.14 (1.00–1.30)	26, 30
Former	1.09 (1.00–1.19)	30
≥11 cigarettes/d	3.0 (1.9–4.6)	26
Unmarried	2.16 (1.28–3.64)	27
College education or higher	1.26 (1.16–1.38)	30
Age at menopause	0.94 (0.88–0.99)	32
Time since menopause		30
10–19 y	1.18 (1.01–1.38)	
20–29 y	1.31 (1.12–1.54)	
30 y	1.51 (1.26–1.81)	
Oophorectomy before age 45	3.64 (1.01–13.04)	33
≥5 children	2.5 (1.1–6.7)	29

ture outcomes, two evaluated vertebral fractures, and two evaluated all types of fractures. These studies described the association of risk factors with fractures known to have occurred already (four case–control studies) or how well they would predict fractures in the future (four prospective cohort studies).

A recent study compared the performance of five clinical decision rules for bone density testing among 2365 postmenopausal women 45 years of age or older who were enrolled in a community-based study of osteoporosis in Canada (52). These rules included guidelines from the National Osteoporosis Foundation (53); the Simple Calculated Osteoporosis Risk Estimation (SCORE) rule (age, weight, ethnicity, estrogen use, presence of rheumatoid arthritis, history of fractures) (41); the Osteoporosis Risk Assessment Instrument (ORAI) (age, weight, current use of hormone replacement therapy) (43); the Age, Body Size, No Estrogen rule (54); and body weight criterion (weight < 70 kg) (38). None of the decision rules had good discriminant performance. In this study, SCORE and ORAI had the highest area under the receiver-operating

characteristic curves (0.80 and 0.79, respectively [sensitivity, 99.6% and 97.5%; specificity, 17.9% and 27.8%, respectively]). Details of how to use SCORE and ORAI are given in **Table 2.**

Bone Density Tests

Several technologies are available to measure bone density (55–58), although correlations among different bone density devices are low (0.35 to 0.60) (59–79). Dual-energy x-ray absorptiometry is considered the gold standard because it is the most extensively validated test against fracture outcomes. When used in the same patients, dual-energy x-ray absorptiometry machines from different manufacturers differ in the proportion of patients diagnosed as having osteoporosis by 6% to 15% (80–85). Published studies consistently show that the probability of receiving a diagnosis of osteoporosis depends on the choice of test and site (86–90). One analytic study, for example, found that 6% of women older than 60 years of age would receive a diagnosis of osteoporosis if dual-energy x-ray absorptiometry of the total hip were used as the only test, compared

Table 2. **Studies of Risk Factor Assessment***

Study, Year (Reference)	Design	Participants, n	Validated	Risk Factors Included	Outcome
Bone density outcomes					
Slemenda et al., 1990 (34)	Cross-sectional	124	No	Age, height, weight, calcium intake, caffeine intake, alcohol and tobacco use, urinary markers of bone turnover	Correct classification of high or low BMD (lowest third of participants)
Falch et al., 1992 (35)	Cross-sectional	73	Yes	Low body weight, reduced renal phosphate reabsorption, smoking	Bone loss
Ribot et al., 1992 (36)	Cross-sectional	1565	No	Weight, menopause, duration of menopause	Vertebral BMD < −2 SD
Elliot et al., 1993 (37)	Cross-sectional	320	Yes	Spine BMD: age, weight, smoking status, age at menarche; femoral neck BMD: age, weight, family history, activity, smoking status	Low lumbar spine and femoral neck BMD (lowest third of age-matched normal range)
Michaëlsson et al., 1996 (38)	Cross-sectional	175	No	Weight > 70 kg	Femoral neck BMD < −2.5 SD
Verhaar et al., 1998 (39)	Cross-sectional	61	No	Arm span–height difference of ≥3 cm; arm span–height difference, age < or > 70 y, and whether arm span was < or >160 cm	BMD ≤−2.5 SD and vertebral fracture
Ballard et al., 1998 (40)	Cross-sectional	1158	No	Age, age at menopause, height, weight, gravidity, parity, current use of steroids, current use of HRT	Osteoporosis of femoral neck, spine, or both
Lydick et al., 1998 (41)	Cross-sectional	1279	Yes	SCORE = age (3 × first digit of age in years), weight (−1 × weight in pounds/10 and truncated to integer), ethnicity (5 if not black), estrogen use (1 if never used), rheumatoid arthritis (4 if present), history of fractures (4 for each fracture after age 45 y of wrist, hip, or rib, to a maximum of 12)	Femoral neck BMD ≤−2 SD
Goemaere et al., 1999 (42)	Cross-sectional	300	No	18-item questionnaire of risk factors for osteoporosis (ethnicity; height loss; age; weight; smoking, coffee, alcohol, dairy product use; activity; family history; existence of comorbid conditions; history of wrist fracture; menopause before age 45 y; corticosteroid use)	Lumbar spine, femoral neck, and hip BMD
Cadarette et al., 2000 (43)	Cross-sectional	926	Yes	ORAI = age (15 points if ≥75 y, 9 if 65–74 y, 5 if 55–64 y), weight (9 if <60 kg, 3 if 60–69.9 kg), current use of HRT (2 if not currently using)	Hip or lumbar spine BMD ≤−2.5 SD
Fracture outcomes					
Kleerekoper et al., 1989 (44)	Case–control	663	No	Model 1: total months of lactation, family history of osteoporosis, years postmenopause, weight Model 2: breastfed, surgical menopause, age at menarche, age, smoking status	Vertebral fractures
van Hemert et al., 1990 (45)	Cohort	1014	No	Age, metacarpal cortical area, relative cortical area, BMI, height, diameter of forearm, diameter of knee, age at menarche, age at menopause, smoking, number of children, period of lactation	Osteoporotic fractures
Cooper et al., 1991 (46)	Case–control	1012	No	Age, height, vertebral fracture after age 45 y, age at last menstrual period, number of children, ever use of oral corticosteroids	Vertebral fractures
Wolinsky and Fitzgerald, 1994 (47)	Cohort	368	No	White ethnicity, female sex, living in southern United States, age, hospitalization in the previous year, previous fall, body mass	Hip fractures
Johnell et al., 1995 (48)	Case–control	5618	No	Late menarche, poor mental score, low BMI, low level of physical activity, little exposure to sunlight, and low consumption of calcium and tea	Hip fractures
Ranstam et al., 1996 (49)	Case–control	7474	No	Mental–functional risk score: knowledge of the day of week, knowledge of age, ability to wash, ability to dress	Hip fractures
Tromp et al., 1998 (50)	Cohort	1469	No	Female sex, living alone, past fractures, inactivity, height, use of analgesics	Probability of fractures
Burger et al., 1999 (51)	Cohort	5208	No	Model with BMD: age, sex, height, use of a walking aid, current smoking, BMD of femoral neck Model without BMD: age, sex, height, use of a walking aid, current smoking, weight	Hip fractures

* BMD = bone mineral density; BMI = body mass index; HRT = hormone replacement therapy; NPV = negative predictive value; PPV = positive predictive value; ORAI = Osteoporosis Risk Assessment Instrument; ROC = receiver-operating characteristic (≥0.80 usually indicates effectiveness); SCORE = Simple Calculated Osteoporosis Risk Estimation.

† Based on criteria developed by the U.S. Preventive Services Task Force (22).

with 14% with dual-energy x-ray absorptiometry of the lumbar spine, 3% with quantitative ultrasonography, and 50% with quantitative computed tomography (87).

The likelihood of receiving a diagnosis of osteoporosis also depends on the number of sites tested. Testing in the forearm, hip, spine, or heel generally identifies different

Table 2—**Continued**

Performance	Quality Rating†
Midshaft radius: 68% low, 77% high Lumbar spine: 61% low, 45% high Femoral neck: 66% low, 53% high	Poor
Sensitivity, 36%; specificity, 89%; PPV, 74%	Poor
Sensitivity, 73%; specificity, 66%	Fair
Lumbar spine: sensitivity, 86%; specificity, 32% Femoral neck: sensitivity, 89%; specificity, 25%	Fair
Sensitivity, 94%; specificity, 36%; PPV, 21%; NPV, 97%	Fair
Arm span only: sensitivity, 58%; specificity, 56% Arm span, age, arm span length: sensitivity, 81%; specificity, 64% ROC area, 0.73	Poor Fair
Sensitivity, 89%; specificity, 50%; ROC area, 0.81 using a score of ≥6	Good
Lumbar spine: ROC area, 0.66 Femoral neck: ROC area, 0.69 Hip: ROC area, 0.76	Fair
Sensitivity, 95%; specificity, 41%, using a score of ≥9	Good
Model 1: mean ROC area ± SE, 0.55 ± 0.07; sensitivity, 56%; specificity, 54% Model 2: mean ROC area ± SE, 0.51 ± 0.042; sensitivity, 63% specificity, 39%	Fair
Sensitivity, 48%; specificity, 82%	Fair
Sensitivity, 51%; specificity, 69%	Fair
ROC area, 0.71; sensitivity, 64.7%; specificity, 65.7%	Fair
Sensitivity, 55%; specificity, 65%	Fair
A less than perfect score had a sensitivity of 46% and a specificity of 79%	Fair
No predictors, 0%; 4 predictors, 12.9%	Fair
Model with BMD: ROC area, 0.88; sensitivity, 70%; specificity, 84% Model without BMD: ROC area, 0.83; sensitivity, 70%; specificity, 83%	Fair

results at any site are associated to some degree with fractures at other sites, a physician may not be able to assess whether a patient with a low T-score on a hand or forearm test has substantial bone loss at other sites.

A meta-analysis assessed 23 publications from 11 separate prospective cohort studies published before 1996 (91). Nearly all of the data were from women in their late 60s or older. No studies of ultrasonography were included. The meta-analysis indicated that dual-energy x-ray absorptiometry at the femoral neck predicted hip fracture better than measurements at other sites and was comparable to forearm measurements for predicting fractures at other sites (92–94). For bone density measurements at the femoral neck, the pooled relative risk per decrease of 1 SD in bone density was 2.6 (CI, 2.0 to 3.5). In direct comparisons, heel ultrasonography was slightly worse than but comparable to dual-energy x-ray absorptiometry of the hip in women older than 65 years of age (**Table 3**) (92, 94–100). For both tests, a result in the osteoporotic range is associated with an increased short-term probability of hip fracture. No data compare dual-energy x-ray absorptiometry and ultrasonography for prediction of fracture in women younger than 65 years of age.

The National Osteoporosis Risk Assessment study (30) recently evaluated the performance of peripheral densitometry in predicting fractures. This prospective study of ambulatory postmenopausal women 50 years of age or older with no previous osteoporosis diagnoses recruited 200 160 participants from 4236 primary care practices in 34 U.S. states. Women received baseline T-scores by measuring bone density at the heel (single-energy x-ray absorptiometry or quantitative ultrasonography), forearm (peripheral dual-energy x-ray absorptiometry), or finger (peripheral dual-energy x-ray absorptiometry). After 12 months of follow-up, women with T-scores less than or equal to −2.5 had an adjusted risk for all types of fractures that was 2.74 (CI, 2.40 to 3.13) times higher than women with normal baseline bone density. Results varied by type of test and site; those identified as osteoporotic by dual-energy x-ray absorptiometry had higher fracture rates. Tests were not compared with dual-energy x-ray absorptiometry of the femoral neck, and the study did not describe how tests performed by age group or risk category.

Treatment

The U.S. Food and Drug Administration has approved hormone replacement therapy, bisphosphonates, raloxifene, and calcitonin for osteoporosis prevention or treatment, or both. Our review of estrogen and selective estrogen receptor modulators is presented elsewhere (101).

A recent meta-analysis (102) of 11 randomized trials (103–113) enrolling 12 855 women found that at least 5 mg of alendronate per day reduced vertebral fractures in 8 trials (relative risk, 0.52 [CI, 0.43 to 0.65]). Alendronate also reduced forearm fractures in 6 trials involving 3723 participants (dosage, ≥10 mg/d; weighted relative risk,

groups of patients. For example, a physician cannot definitively say that a patient does not have osteoporosis on the basis of a forearm test alone. Conversely, although test

Table 3. **Prospective Studies of Dual-Energy X-Ray Absorptiometry and Ultrasonography That Reported Hip Fractures***

Cohort (Reference)	Sample	Age (Range)	Follow-up	Participants	Probability of Hip Fracture†	DEXA of the Hip		QUS of the Heel	
						Low Risk	High Risk	Low Risk	High Risk
			y	*n*					
Study of Osteoporotic Fractures (92, 94–96)	Community-dwelling white women from 4 areas in the United States who were recruited from lists	≥65	1.8–2.9	5236	0.009	0.005	0.023	0.006	0.018
		65–79	2.9					0.006	0.23
		≥80	2.9						
		65–69	1.8	2371	0.003	0.0028	0.005		
		70–74	1.8	3013	0.0076	0.005	0.016		
		75–79	1.8	1728	0.007	0.003	0.019		
		80–84	1.8	731	0.018	0.007	0.049		
		≥85	1.8	291	0.024	0.014	0.028		
Epidemiologie de L'Osteoporose (97–100)	Women from 5 cities in France who were recruited from voting lists and health insurance companies	≥75	2	5656	0.02	0.033	0.008	0.012	0.029
		<80	2	3982	0.013	0.002	0.025		
		≥80	2	3616	0.028	0.006	0.04		

* DEXA = dual-energy x-ray absorptiometry; QUS = quantitative ultrasonography.
† Probability of hip fracture if bone density was classified as high or low risk.

0.48 [CI, 0.29 to 0.78]), hip fractures in 11 trials involving 11 808 participants (dosage, ≥5 mg/d; weighted relative risk, 0.63 [CI, 0.43 to 0.92]), and other nonvertebral fractures in 6 trials involving 3723 participants (dosage, 10 to 40 mg/d; weighted relative risk, 0.51 [CI, 0.38 to 0.69]). These trials included follow-up data ranging from 1 to 4 years; effect sizes for longer periods of use are not known. We evaluated data from these trials to determine whether women who have a similar overall risk for fracture but different bone densities derive similar benefit from treatment. This question is clinically important because accepted criteria for initiating treatment are lacking.

The Fracture Intervention Trial (FIT) of alendronate was conducted with two groups of participants and provides some information about levels of risk. One group (FIT-I) included a higher-risk sample of 2027 women who had T-scores of −1.6 or lower and preexisting vertebral fractures (104). The 3-year risk for hip fracture was 2.2% in the placebo group and 1.1% in the alendronate group (relative hazard, 0.49 [CI, 0.23 to 0.99]), and the 3-year risk for any clinical fracture was 18.2% in the placebo group and 13.6% in the alendronate group (relative hazard, 0.72 [CI, 0.58 to 0.90]). A second study from FIT (FIT-II) included a lower-risk sample of 4432 women who also had T-scores of −1.6 or lower but did not have preexisting vertebral fractures (114). The 4-year incidences of hip fracture (1.1%) and any clinical fractures (14.1%) in the placebo group were lower than those observed in the FIT-1 placebo group. In FIT-II, only the subgroup of treated patients who had T-scores lower than −2.5 (*n* = 1627) had a significant risk reduction for all clinical fractures, from 19.6% to 13.1% (relative risk, 0.64 [CI, 0.50 to 0.82]). No reduction in risk for fractures was seen in patients who had T-scores between −1.6 and −2.5.

The results from FIT suggest that women with more risk factors for fracture relating to bone structure and integrity, such as age, very low bone density, or preexisting vertebral fractures, derive the greatest absolute benefit from treatment. However, FIT did not examine other nonskeletal risk factors, such as psychomotor impairment, poor gait, and other factors that increase the risk for falling. The effect of some of these risk factors on the benefit of treatment was examined in a randomized trial of another bisphosphonate, risedronate (115). Risedronate had no effect on hip fracture rates among women 80 years of age or older who had one or more risk factors for falls but who did not necessarily have low bone density. In the same report, in women 70 to 79 years of age with severe osteoporosis (T-score < −3), risedronate reduced hip fractures by 40% (relative risk, 0.6 [CI, 0.4 to 0.9]; number needed to treat for benefit, 77).

Trial results are not applicable to a screening program unless the trials included patients who would be identified by screening the general population. We examined recruitment and eligibility characteristics of the 10 published randomized trials of alendronate to assess whether selection biases or other biases might have affected their generalizability (**Table 4**) (103–112). Overall, the trials included relatively healthy women with low bone density who were not using estrogen. Except for participants in two trials involving women who had recently gone through menopause and were not osteoporotic, most participants were older than 65 years of age.

The FIT-II is the largest study and provided the most detailed description of recruitment and results (107). In FIT-II, researchers recruited the sample of 4432 women by mailing a query to more than 1 million women selected from the general population in 11 cities. Women who had medical problems (for example, dyspepsia) or who used estrogen were excluded. Fifty-four thousand women (approximately 5.4%) responded by telephone; of these, 26 137 (52%) had a screening visit. A higher than expected proportion of these (65%) had sufficiently low bone density to enroll in the study. Of this 65%, 57% were classified as "ineligible, did not wish to continue, or screened after recruitment to this arm." It is not clear from this description how many patients did not meet the eligibility criteria. In addition, an unspecified number of patients (up to 28 000) were found to be ineligible at the initial stage of recruitment. The demographic characteristics of eligible and screened but excluded participants were not reported. None of the other randomized trials disclosed any details of how their samples were recruited or how many respondents were found to be ineligible before randomization.

In other clinical areas, the results of industry-sponsored trials were significantly more favorable to newer therapies than trials funded by nonprofit organizations (116, 117). Because all 11 trials of alendronate were funded wholly or in part by the manufacturer, we were unable to assess the influence of sponsorship on effect size. If effectiveness of treatments is less than estimated in these trials, the efficiency of screening to identify candidates for treatment will be reduced and the number needed to screen for benefit will increase.

Harms

Several potential harms are associated with screening and treatment. A test result indicating osteoporosis could produce anxiety and perceived vulnerability (118) that may be unwarranted. On a quality-of-life questionnaire, women with osteoporosis voiced significantly more fears than women who had normal bone density (119). Some women may be falsely reassured if abnormal results from last year's dual-energy x-ray absorptiometry of the hip appear "improved" on this year's normal calcaneal ultrasonogram. The potential time, effort, expense, and radiation exposure of repeated scans over a lifetime have not yet been determined.

Potential harms may also arise from inaccuracies and misinterpretations of bone density tests. The variation among techniques, along with the lack of methods to integrate bone density results with clinical predictors, makes it difficult for clinicians to provide accurate information to patients about test results. In one study, physicians found densitometry reports confusing and were not confident that their interpretations of T-scores were accurate (120). False-positive results could lead to inappropriate treatment, and false-negative results could lead to missed treatment opportunities.

Harms of treatment depend on the medication used. Overall, gastrointestinal side effects occur in approximately 25% of patients taking alendronate, but in controlled trials these rates were usually not significantly higher than those for placebo. High rates of serious gastrointestinal side effects have been observed among Medicare enrollees taking

Table 4. **Randomized, Controlled Trials of Alendronate with Fracture Outcomes***

Study, Year (Reference)	Duration	Age	Sample	Exclusion Criteria†	Participants Lost to Follow-up	Quality Rating‡
		y			*n/n (%)*	
Adami et al., 1995 (103)	2	48–76	9 Italian centers; T-score < −2 (0.67 g/cm²); 5% vertebral fractures	Narrow	32/211 (15.2)	Fair to good
Black et al., 1996 (104)	3	55–81	11 U.S. cities; BMD <0.68 g/cm²; no previous vertebral fractures	Broad (medical illness, dyspepsia)	81/2027 (4)	Good
Bone et al., 1997 (105)	2	>60	15 U.S. sites; BMD <0.84 g/cm²; average of 20 y since menopause; 30.7% vertebral fractures	Broad (medical illness, NSAIDs, GI drugs)	19/359 (5.3)	Fair to good
Chesnut et al., 1995 (106)	2	42–75 (avg. 63)	7 centers; spine BMD <0.88 g/cm²; average hip BMD, 0.7 g/cm²; ≥5 y since menopause	Broad	26/157 (16.6)	Fair
Cummings et al., 1998 (107)	4	55–81	11 U.S. cities; BMD <0.68 g/cm² (average, 0.59 g/cm²); no previous vertebral fractures	Broad (medical illness, dyspepsia)	179/4432 (4)	Good
Greenspan et al., 1998 (108)	2.5	>65	1 Boston center; no BMD entry criteria	Narrow ("good health")	33/120 (27.5)	Fair
Hosking et al., 1998 (109)	4	45–59	4 centers; BMD >0.8 g/cm²; <10% prevalent vertebral fractures	Narrow ("good health")	287/1499 (19.1)	Fair
Liberman et al., 1995 (110)	3	45–80	2 multicenter trials; T-score <−2.5; 21% prevalent vertebral fractures	Narrow ("good health")	170/994 (17.1)	Good
McClung et al., 1998 (111)	3	40–59	15 centers; T-score <−2; 6–36 mo since menopause; no previous vertebral fractures	Narrow ("good health," estrogen use)	(31 at 3 y)	Fair
Pols et al., 1999 (112)	1	40–82 (mean 63)	153 centers; T-score <−2.8	Narrow ("good health")	211/1908 (11.1)	Fair

* BMD = bone mineral density; GI = gastrointestinal; NSAID = nonsteroidal anti-inflammatory drug.
† In general, "narrow" criteria excluded estrogen users and patients with illnesses affecting bone metabolism.
‡ Based on criteria developed by the U.S. Preventive Services Task Force (22).

Table 5. Screening for Osteoporosis in 10 000 Postmenopausal Women: Hip and Vertebral Fracture Outcomes by 5-Year Age Intervals*

Variable	Age Group					
	50–54 y	55–59 y	60–64 y	65–69 y	70–74 y	75–79 y
Base-case assumptions†						
Prevalence of osteoporosis	0.0305	0.0445	0.065	0.120	0.2025	0.285
Relative risk for hip fracture with treatment	0.63	0.63	0.63	0.63	0.63	0.63
Relative risk for vertebral fracture with treatment	0.52	0.52	0.52	0.52	0.52	0.52
Adherence to treatment	0.7	0.7	0.7	0.7	0.7	0.7
Results, *n*						
Identified as high risk (osteoporotic)	305	445	650	1200	2025	2850
Hip fractures prevented	1	2	5	14	39	70
NNS to prevent 1 hip fracture	7446	4338	1856	731	254	143
NNT to prevent 1 hip fracture	227	193	121	88	51	41
Vertebral fractures prevented	5	7	22	40	95	134
NNS to prevent 1 vertebral fracture	1952	1338	458	248	105	75
NNT to prevent 1 vertebral fracture	60	60	30	30	21	21

* NNS = number needed to screen for benefit; NNT = number needed to treat.
† Estimates for assumptions include age-specific prevalence rates for osteoporosis and probabilities of fractures; relative risk of 0.63 for hip fractures and 0.52 for vertebral fractures with treatment; treatment adherence of 0.7 (see text). Formulas for calculations are described in Appendix Table 2.

alendronate (121). The long-term adverse effects of alendronate are unknown.

Costs of screening vary with technique, and average 2000 Medicare reimbursement rates were $133 for dual-energy x-ray absorptiometry and $34 for ultrasonography (122). Abnormal results on ultrasonography may require confirmatory dual-energy x-ray absorptiometry before treatment because clinical trials are based on entry criteria using dual-energy x-ray absorptiometry. Most women would require repeated tests over several years before receiving a diagnosis of osteoporosis and leaving the screening pool. Treatment costs also vary; alendronate currently costs approximately $3 per daily dose.

Screening Strategies

To estimate the effect of screening 10 000 postmenopausal women for osteoporosis on reducing hip and vertebral fractures, we created an outcomes table based on assumptions from the reviewed studies (**Table 5**). These estimates include age-specific prevalence rates expressed in 5-year age intervals (123) and treatment effects based on trial results (risk reduction, 37% for hip fracture and 50% for vertebral fracture) (102, 104, 115, 124). We estimated an adherence rate of 70% based on reports of adherence and side effects from treatment trials, assuming less optimal adherence in the general population.

When the assumptions in **Table 5** are used, if 10 000 women 65 to 69 years of age underwent bone densitometry (dual-energy x-ray absorptiometry of the femoral neck), 1200 would be identified as high risk (T-score ≤ −2.5). If these women were offered treatment that resulted in a 37% reduction in hip fracture risk and a 50% reduction in vertebral fracture risk and 70% adhered to therapy, then 14 hip fractures and 40 vertebral fractures would be prevented over a 5-year period. The number of women in this age group needed to screen to prevent one hip fracture in 5 years would be 731, and the number of women with low

bone density needed to treat for benefit would be 88. The number needed to screen to prevent one vertebral fracture would be 248, and the number needed to treat for benefit would be 30. Treatment has significant costs and potential harms; when the number needed to screen for benefit is high, the balance of benefits and harms may become unfavorable. These numbers become more favorable in older persons because the prevalence of osteoporosis increases steadily with age.

There is interest in whether risk assessment can be used to select patients for bone densitometry, which is costly. Our literature review indicated that the prevalence of osteoporosis, the predictability of densitometry, and the effectiveness of treatment might be lower for younger than for older postmenopausal women. To determine whether it is useful to consider clinical risk factors when screening younger postmenopausal women, we also included risk estimates for clinical risk factors in a sensitivity analysis. Our review of observational studies with younger postmenopausal women indicated that three consistent predictors of fracture are increasing age, low weight or body mass index, and nonuse of hormone replacement therapy (defined by current use, ever use, or certain durations of use). These three variables are also used in ORAI to identify women with low bone density (43) and were the variables most strongly associated with low bone density in a study enrolling mostly younger postmenopausal women in the United States (125). On the basis of these studies, we estimated that one of these risk factors increases the probability of having osteoporosis by up to 100% and increases the risk for fracture by 70% (relative risk, 1.7).

For younger age groups, the presence of clinical risk factors influences outcomes. For example, only five hip fractures are prevented over 5 years when all women 60 to 64 years of age are screened; however, nine hip fractures are prevented if women have a factor that increases fracture risk by 70%. For women 60 to 64 years of age who have such a risk factor, the number needed to screen is 1092 and the number needed to treat for benefit is 72 to prevent 1 hip fracture. These numbers approach those of women 65 to 69 years of age (**Figure**).

DISCUSSION

Although many studies have been published about osteoporosis in postmenopausal women, no trials have evaluated the effectiveness of screening; therefore, no direct evidence that screening improves outcomes is available. Instruments developed to assess clinical risk factors for low bone density or fractures generally have moderate to high sensitivity and low specificity. Many have not been validated, and none have been widely tested in a practice setting. Among different bone density tests measured at various sites, bone density measured by dual-energy x-ray absorptiometry at the femoral neck is the best predictor of hip fracture and is comparable to forearm measurements for predicting fractures at other sites. Heel ultrasonography and other peripheral bone density tests, however, can also predict short-term fracture risk. Bisphosphonates decrease fracture risk by approximately 40% to 50% in women with low bone density.

Support for population screening would be based on evidence that the prevalences of osteoporosis and fractures increase with age, that the short-term risk for fracture can be estimated by bone density tests and risk factors, and that the fracture risk among women with low bone density can be significantly reduced with treatment. We applied these data to generate an outcomes table of screening strategies that provides estimates of the numbers of women needed to screen and treat to prevent fractures. Age-based screening is supported by prevalence data, that is, the number needed to screen to prevent fractures decreases sharply as age and prevalence increase. Use of risk factors, particularly increasing age, low weight, and nonuse of estrogen replacement, to screen younger women may identify additional high-risk women and provide absolute benefit similar to that yielded by screening older women without risk factors. These findings relate to screening asymptomatic women only and do not apply to women considered for testing because of preexisting or new fractures or the presence of secondary causes of osteoporosis.

Our approach has several limitations, however, and results from a well-designed trial of screening strategies should supersede our estimations, which are based on indirect evidence. The estimates in the outcomes table are limited by assumptions that are arguable or highly variable by patient and setting. Our assumptions of treatment effect and adherence are especially optimistic and reflect results of clinical trials, not clinical practice. We chose a 5-year time horizon based on the short-term predictability of bone density tests as well as on results of short-term treatment trials. Long-term outcomes may provide a more ac-

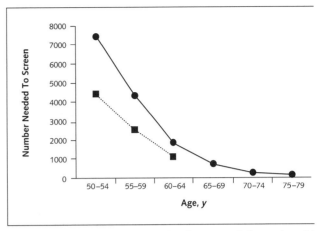

Figure. **Number needed to screen to prevent one hip fracture in 5 years.**

The dotted line indicates women with at least one risk factor; the solid line indicates women without risk factors.

curate estimate of benefits. Also, we cannot exclude the possibility that harms outweigh benefits, particularly since the long-term effects of bisphosphonates are not yet known.

The evidence on which we based our conclusions is also limited. Overall, evidence is stronger for women older than 65 years of age than for younger women because more research has been done in older age groups. Bone loss in the perimenopausal and early postmenopausal years is important to long-term bone health, but few published studies address screening and treatment for younger postmenopausal women. Fracture risk is determined not only by bone density but also by bone characteristics that are difficult to measure in a clinical setting, such as bone structure and morphologic characteristics. No bone density studies or treatment trials include large numbers of nonwhite women, and it may be difficult to provide ethnicity-specific screening recommendations in the absence of more evidence.

The role of clinical risk factors is still unclear. Although many risk factors are associated with osteoporosis and fractures, how to use them to select women to test or treat is uncertain. The risk factors identified by our literature review and used in the outcomes table are only best estimates. Other risk factors may prove to be equally predictive when used for screening purposes. Further validation of existing risk assessment instruments or development of new ones would be useful. Few studies have evaluated the effect of altering modifiable risk factors, such as smoking cessation, strength and balance training, and visual correction. These interventions may prove to be as effective as drug therapy in preventing fractures and may also be important effect modifiers that would alter the effectiveness of treatments.

Peripheral bone density tests have not been extensively studied for screening. Results from the National Osteoporosis Risk Assessment Study (30) indicate that peripheral tests can predict short-term fracture rates in a primary care population that would be targeted for screening. Most treatment trials use dual-energy x-ray absorptiometry of the hip as an entry criterion, and results may not apply to women whose diagnosis is determined by other tests. A sequential approach, in which women with low values on a peripheral test are subsequently tested by dual-energy x-ray absorptiometry of the hip to determine treatment needs, may be useful, although this approach has not been evaluated. Further research is needed to define the appropriate use of these technologies.

How frequently to screen has also not been specifically studied, but data are needed to determine optimal screening intervals. Estimations can be made based on the age-specific prevalence of osteoporosis and the precision of bone density tests. Less frequent testing for younger postmenopausal women when prevalence is lower (for example, 5-year intervals) and more frequent testing for older women (for example, 2-year intervals) might be reasonable, but further research is needed. Screening intervals of less than 2 years seem unwarranted because the precision error of densitometry would likely exceed the estimated bone loss in such a brief period (126). After a woman is screened and determined to have osteoporosis, future screening with bone density testing would be unnecessary.

Osteoporotic fractures present an enormous health burden on an expanding elderly population. Further research to more accurately determine the benefits and harms of screening is of paramount importance.

From the Oregon Health & Science University and Veterans Affairs Medical Center, Portland, Oregon; Virginia Commonwealth University, Fairfax, Virginia; and University of Maryland, Baltimore, Baltimore, Maryland.

Disclaimer: The authors of this article are responsible for its contents, including any clinical or treatment recommendations. No statement in this article should be construed as an official position of the U.S. Agency for Healthcare Research and Quality or the U.S. Department of Health and Human Services.

Acknowledgments: The authors thank Peggy Nygren, MA; Nancy Carney, PhD; Kathryn Pyle Krages, AMLS, MA; Benjamin Chan, MS; and the reviewers of the full evidence report for their contributions to this project.

Grant Support: This study was conducted by the Oregon Health & Science University Evidence-based Practice Center under contract to the Agency for Healthcare Research and Quality, Rockville, Maryland (contract no. 290-97-0018, task order nos. 2 and 4).

Requests for Single Reprints: Reprints are available from the Agency for Healthcare Research and Quality Web site (www.ahrq.gov/clinic /uspstffix.htm) or the Agency for Healthcare Research and Quality Publications Clearinghouse (800-358-9295).

Current author addresses, the Appendix Tables, and the Appendix Figure are available at www.annals.org.

References

1. Melton LJ 3rd, Kan SH, Frye MA, Wahner HW, O'Fallon WM, Riggs BL. Epidemiology of vertebral fractures in women. Am J Epidemiol. 1989;129:1000-11. [PMID: 2784934]

2. Barrett JA, Baron JA, Karagas MR, Beach ML. Fracture risk in the U.S. Medicare population. J Clin Epidemiol. 1999;52:243-9. [PMID: 10210242]

3. White BL, Fisher WD, Laurin CA. Rate of mortality for elderly patients after fracture of the hip in the 1980's. J Bone Joint Surg Am. 1987;69:1335-40. [PMID: 3440792]

4. Cauley JA, Thompson DE, Ensrud KC, Scott JC, Black D. Risk of mortality following clinical fractures. Osteoporos Int. 2000;11:556-61. [PMID: 11069188]

5. Melton LJ 3rd. Epidemiology of spinal osteoporosis. Spine. 1997;22:2S-11S. [PMID: 9431638]

6. Consensus development conference: prophylaxis and treatment of osteoporosis. Am J Med. 1991;90:107-10. [PMID: 1986575]

7. Consensus development conference: diagnosis, prophylaxis, and treatment of osteoporosis. Am J Med. 1993;94:646-50. [PMID: 8506892]

8. Assessment of Fracture Risk and Its Application to Screening for Postmenopausal Osteoporosis. World Health Organization. WHO Technical Report Series 843. Geneva: World Health Organization; 1994.

9. Kanis JA. Assessment of fracture risk and its application to screening for postmenopausal osteoporosis: synopsis of a WHO report. WHO Study Group. Osteoporos Int. 1994;4:368-81. [PMID: 7696835]

10. Melton LJ 3rd. How many women have osteoporosis now? J Bone Miner Res. 1995;10:175-7. [PMID: 7754796]

11. Heaney RP. Bone mass, bone loss, and osteoporosis prophylaxis. [Editorial] Ann Intern Med. 1998;128:313-4. [PMID: 9471936]

12. Bone density measurement—a systematic review. A report from SBU, the Swedish Council on Technology Assessment in Health Care. J Intern Med Suppl. 1997;739:1-60. [PMID: 9104441].

13. Hailey D, Sampietro-Colom L, Marshall D. INAHTA project on the effectiveness of bone density measurement and associated treatments for prevention of fractures. Statement of findings. Edmonton, Alberta, Canada: Alberta Heritage Foundation for Medical Research; 1996.

14. Green CJ, Bassett K, Foerster V. Bone mineral density testing: does the evidence support its selective use in well women? British Columbia, Canada: British Columbia Office of Health Technology Assessment; 1997. Report no. 97:2T.

15. Osteoporosis: review of the evidence for prevention, diagnosis and treatment and cost-effectiveness analysis. National Osteoporosis Foundation. Osteoporos Int. 1998;8(Suppl 4):S7-S80. [PMID: 10197173]

16. Homik J, Hailey D. Quantitative ultrasound for bone density measurement. Edmonton, Alberta, Canada: Alberta Heritage Foundation for Medical Research; 1998. Health Technology Assessment 11.

17. Homik J, Hailey D. Selective testing with bone density measurement. Edmonton, Alberta, Canada: Alberta Heritage Foundation for Medical Research; 1999. Health Technology Brief 4.

18. Osteoporosis: clinical guidelines for prevention and treatment. Royal College of Physicians. London: Royal College of Physicians of London; 1999.

19. Ultrasonography of the heel for diagnostic osteoporosis and selecting patients for pharmacologic treatment. Blue Cross Blue Shield Association. Chicago: Blue Cross Blue Shield Assoc; 1999.

20. Siebzehner MI. Consensus statement on prevention and treatment of osteoporosis. Israel Medical Association Journal. 2000;2:397-401.

21. Guide to Clinical Preventive Services:. Report of the U.S. Preventive Services Task Force. 2nd ed. U.S. Preventive Services Task Force. Baltimore: Williams & Wilkins; 1996.

22. Harris RP, Helfand M, Woolf SH, Lohr KN, Mulrow CD, Teutsch SM, et al. Current methods of the US Preventive Services Task Force: a review of the process. Am J Prev Med. 2001;20:21-35. [PMID: 11306229]

23. Nelson H, Helfand M, Woolf S, Allan J. Screening for Postmenopausal Osteoporosis: A Systematic Review. Rockville, MD: Agency for Healthcare Research and Quality; 2002.

24. Nelson H, Morris CD, Kraemer D, Mahon S, Carney N, Nygren P, et al. Osteoporosis in Postmenopausal Women: Diagnosis and Monitoring, Rockville, MD: Agency for Healthcare Research and Quality; 2002.

25. **Cummings SR, Nevitt MC, Browner WS, Stone K, Fox KM, Ensrud KE, et al.** Risk factors for hip fracture in white women. Study of Osteoporotic Fractures Research Group. N Engl J Med. 1995;332:767-73. [PMID: 7862179]

26. **Honkanen R, Tuppurainen M, Kröger H, Alhava E, Saarikoski S.** Relationships between risk factors and fractures differ by type of fracture: a population-based study of 12,192 perimenopausal women. Osteoporos Int. 1998;8:25-31. [PMID: 9692074]

27. **Meyer HE, Tverdal A, Falch JA.** Risk factors for hip fracture in middle-aged Norwegian women and men. Am J Epidemiol. 1993;137:1203-11. [PMID: 8322761]

28. **Kreiger N, Kelsey JL, Holford TR, O'Connor T.** An epidemiologic study of hip fracture in postmenopausal women. Am J Epidemiol. 1982;116:141-8. [PMID: 7102649]

29. **Fujiwara S, Kasagi F, Yamada M, Kodama K.** Risk factors for hip fracture in a Japanese cohort. J Bone Miner Res. 1997;12:998-1004. [PMID: 9199997]

30. **Siris ES, Miller PD, Barrett-Connor E, Faulkner KG, Wehren LE, Abbott TA, et al.** Identification and fracture outcomes of undiagnosed low bone mineral density in postmenopausal women: results from the National Osteoporosis Risk Assessment. JAMA. 2001;286:2815-22. [PMID: 11735756]

31. **Torgerson DJ, Campbell MK, Thomas RE, Reid DM.** Prediction of perimenopausal fractures by bone mineral density and other risk factors. J Bone Miner Res. 1996;11:293-7. [PMID: 8822354]

32. **Mallmin H, Ljunghall S, Persson I, Bergström R.** Risk factors for fractures of the distal forearm: a population-based case-control study. Osteoporos Int. 1994;4:298-304. [PMID: 7696821]

33. **Tuppurainen M, Kröger H, Honkanen R, Puntila E, Huopio J, Saarikoski S, et al.** Risks of perimenopausal fractures—a prospective population-based study. Acta Obstet Gynecol Scand. 1995;74:624-8. [PMID: 7660769]

34. **Slemenda CW, Hui SL, Longcope C, Wellman H, Johnston CC Jr.** Predictors of bone mass in perimenopausal women. A prospective study of clinical data using photon absorptiometry. Ann Intern Med. 1990;112:96-101. [PMID: 2294827]

35. **Falch JA, Sandvik L, Van Beresteijn EC.** Development and evaluation of an index to predict early postmenopausal bone loss. Bone. 1992;13:337-41. [PMID: 1389575]

36. **Ribot C, Pouilles JM, Bonneu M, Tremollieres F.** Assessment of the risk of post-menopausal osteoporosis using clinical factors. Clin Endocrinol (Oxf). 1992; 36:225-8. [PMID: 1563075]

37. **Elliot JR, Gilchrist NL, Wells JE, Ayling E, Turner J, Sainsbury R.** Historical assessment of risk factors in screening for osteopenia in a normal Caucasian population. Aust N Z J Med. 1993;23:458-62. [PMID: 8297274]

38. **Michaëlsson K, Bergström R, Mallmin H, Holmberg L, Wolk A, Ljunghall S.** Screening for osteopenia and osteoporosis: selection by body composition. Osteoporos Int. 1996;6:120-6. [PMID: 8704349]

39. **Verhaar HJ, Koele JJ, Neijzen T, Dessens JA, Duursma SA.** Are arm span measurements useful in the prediction of osteoporosis in postmenopausal women? Osteoporos Int. 1998;8:174-6. [PMID: 9666942]

40. **Ballard PA, Purdie DW, Langton CM, Steel SA, Mussurakis S.** Prevalence of osteoporosis and related risk factors in UK women in the seventh decade: osteoporosis case finding by clinical referral criteria or predictive model? Osteoporos Int. 1998;8:535-9. [PMID: 10326057]

41. **Lydick E, Cook K, Turpin J, Melton M, Stine R, Byrnes C.** Development and validation of a simple questionnaire to facilitate identification of women likely to have low bone density. Am J Manag Care. 1998;4:37-48. [PMID: 10179905]

42. **Goemaere S, Zegels B, Toye K, Cremer S, Demuynck R, Daems M, et al.** Limited clinical utility of a self-evaluating risk assessment scale for postmenopausal osteoporosis: lack of predictive value of lifestyle-related factors. Calcif Tissue Int. 1999;65:354-8. [PMID: 10541759]

43. **Cadarette SM, Jaglal SB, Kreiger N, McIsaac WJ, Darlington GA, Tu JV.** Development and validation of the Osteoporosis Risk Assessment Instrument to facilitate selection of women for bone densitometry. CMAJ. 2000;162:1289-94. [PMID: 10813010]

44. **Kleerekoper M, Peterson E, Nelson D, Tilley B, Phillips E, Schork MA, et al.** Identification of women at risk for developing postmenopausal osteoporosis with vertebral fractures: role of history and single photon absorptiometry. Bone Miner. 1989;7:171-86. [PMID: 2804452]

45. **van Hemert AM, Vandenbroucke JP, Birkenhäger JC, Valkenburg HA.** Prediction of osteoporotic fractures in the general population by a fracture risk score. A 9-year follow-up among middle-aged women. Am J Epidemiol. 1990; 132:123-35. [PMID: 2192546]

46. **Cooper C, Shah S, Hand DJ, Adams J, Compston J, Davie M, et al.** Screening for vertebral osteoporosis using individual risk factors. The Multicentre Vertebral Fracture Study Group. Osteoporos Int. 1991;2:48-53. [PMID: 1790421]

47. **Wolinsky FD, Fitzgerald JF.** The risk of hip fracture among noninstitutionalized older adults. J Gerontol. 1994;49:S165-75. [PMID: 8014400]

48. **Johnell O, Gullberg B, Kanis JA, Allander E, Elffors L, Dequeker J, et al.** Risk factors for hip fracture in European women: the MEDOS Study. Mediterranean Osteoporosis Study. J Bone Miner Res. 1995;10:1802-15. [PMID: 8592959]

49. **Ranstam J, Elffors L, Kanis JA.** A mental-functional risk score for prediction of hip fracture. Age Ageing. 1996;25:439-42. [PMID: 9003879]

50. **Tromp AM, Smit JH, Deeg DJ, Bouter LM, Lips P.** Predictors for falls and fractures in the Longitudinal Aging Study Amsterdam. J Bone Miner Res. 1998; 13:1932-9. [PMID: 9844112]

51. **Burger H, de Laet CE, Weel AE, Hofman A, Pols HA.** Added value of bone mineral density in hip fracture risk scores. Bone. 1999;25:369-74. [PMID: 10495142]

52. **Cadarette SM, Jaglal SB, Murray TM, McIsaac WJ, Joseph L, Brown JP, et al.** Evaluation of decision rules for referring women for bone densitometry by dual-energy x-ray absorptiometry. JAMA. 2001;286:57-63. [PMID: 11434827]

53. Physician's Guide to Prevention and Treatment of Osteoporosis. National Osteoporosis Foundation. Washington, DC: Excerpta Medica; 1999.

54. **Weinstein L, Ullery B.** Identification of at-risk women for osteoporosis screening. Am J Obstet Gynecol. 2000;183:547-9. [PMID: 10992172]

55. **Blake GM, Glüer CC, Fogelman I.** Bone densitometry: current status and future prospects. Br J Radiol. 1997;70 Spec No:S177-86. [PMID: 9534732]

56. **Blake GM, Fogelman I.** Applications of bone densitometry for osteoporosis. Endocrinol Metab Clin North Am. 1998;27:267-88. [PMID: 9669138]

57. **Genant HK, Engelke K, Fuerst T, Glüer CC, Grampp S, Harris ST, et al.** Noninvasive assessment of bone mineral and structure: state of the art. J Bone Miner Res. 1996;11:707-30. [PMID: 8725168]

58. **Jergas M, Genant HK.** Spinal and femoral DXA for the assessment of spinal osteoporosis. Calcif Tissue Int. 1997;61:351-7. [PMID: 9351874]

59. **Agren M, Karellas A, Leahey D, Marks S, Baran D.** Ultrasound attenuation of the calcaneus: a sensitive and specific discriminator of osteopenia in postmenopausal women. Calcif Tissue Int. 1991;48:240-4. [PMID: 2059875]

60. **Alenfeld FE, Wüster C, Funck C, Pereira-Lima JF, Fritz T, Meeder PJ, et al.** Ultrasound measurements at the proximal phalanges in healthy women and patients with hip fractures. Osteoporos Int. 1998;8:393-8. [PMID: 9850344]

61. **Cunningham JL, Fordham JN, Hewitt TA, Speed CA.** Ultrasound velocity and attenuation at different skeletal sites compared with bone mineral density measured using dual energy X-ray absorptiometry. Br J Radiol. 1996;69:25-32. [PMID: 8785618]

62. **Faulkner KG, McClung MR, Coleman LJ, Kingston-Sandahl E.** Quantitative ultrasound of the heel: correlation with densitometric measurements at different skeletal sites. Osteoporos Int. 1994;4:42-7. [PMID: 8148571]

63. **Formica CA, Nieves JW, Cosman F, Garrett P, Lindsay R.** Comparative assessment of bone mineral measurements using dual X-ray absorptiometry and peripheral quantitative computed tomography. Osteoporos Int. 1998;8:460-7. [PMID: 9850355]

64. **Graafmans WC, Van Lingen A, Ooms ME, Bezemer PD, Lips P.** Ultrasound measurements in the calcaneus: precision and its relation with bone mineral density of the heel, hip, and lumbar spine. Bone. 1996;19:97-100. [PMID: 8853851]

65. **Grampp S, Jergas M, Lang P, Steiner E, Fuerst T, Glüer CC, et al.** Quantitative CT assessment of the lumbar spine and radius in patients with osteoporosis. AJR Am J Roentgenol. 1996;167:133-40. [PMID: 8659357]

66. **Greenspan SL, Bouxsein ML, Melton ME, Kolodny AH, Clair JH, Delucca PT, et al.** Precision and discriminatory ability of calcaneal bone assessment technologies. J Bone Miner Res. 1997;12:1303-13. [PMID: 9258762]

67. **Langton CM, Ballard PA, Bennett DK, Purdie DW.** A comparison of the sensitivity and specificity of calcaneal ultrasound measurements with clinical cri-

teria for bone densitometry (DEXA) referral. Clin Rheumatol. 1997;16:117-8. [PMID: 9132320]

68. Laval-Jeanet AM, Bergot C, Williams M, Davidson K, Laval-Jeanet M. Dual-energy X-ray absorptiometry of the calcaneus: comparison with vertebral dual-energy X-ray absorptiometry and quantitative computed tomography. Calcif Tissue Int. 1995;56:14-8. [PMID: 7796340]

69. Martin JC, Reid DM. Appendicular measurements in screening women for low axial bone mineral density. Br J Radiol. 1996;69:234-40. [PMID: 8800867]

70. Massie A, Reid DM, Porter RW. Screening for osteoporosis: comparison between dual energy X-ray absorptiometry and broadband ultrasound attenuation in 1000 perimenopausal women. Osteoporos Int. 1993;3:107-10. [PMID: 8453190]

71. Naganathan V, March L, Hunter D, Pocock NA, Markovey J, Sambrook PN. Quantitative heel ultrasound as a predictor for osteoporosis. Med J Aust. 1999;171:297-300. [PMID: 10560444]

72. Pocock NA, Noakes KA, Howard GM, Nguyen TV, Kelly PJ, Sambrook PN, et al. Screening for osteoporosis: what is the role of heel ultrasound? Med J Aust. 1996;164:367-70. [PMID: 8606664]

73. Rosenthall L, Tenenhouse A, Caminis J. A correlative study of ultrasound calcaneal and dual-energy X-ray absorptiometry bone measurements of the lumbar spine and femur in 1000 women. Eur J Nucl Med. 1995;22:402-6. [PMID: 7641747]

74. Roux C, Lemonnier E, Kolta S, Charpentier E, Dougados M, Amor B, et al. [Ultrasound attenuation in calcaneus and bone density]. Rev Rhum Ed Fr. 1993;60:897-906. [PMID: 8012315]

75. Salamone LM, Krall EA, Harris S, Dawson-Hughes B. Comparison of broadband ultrasound attenuation to single X-ray absorptiometry measurements at the calcaneus in postmenopausal women. Calcif Tissue Int. 1994;54:87-90. [PMID: 8012876]

76. Schott AM, Weill-Engerer S, Hans D, Duboeuf F, Delmas PD, Meunier PJ. Ultrasound discriminates patients with hip fracture equally well as dual energy X-ray absorptiometry and independently of bone mineral density. J Bone Miner Res. 1995;10:243-9. [PMID: 7754803]

77. Tromp AM, Smit JH, Deeg DJ, Lips P. Quantitative ultrasound measurements of the tibia and calcaneus in comparison with DXA measurements at various skeletal sites. Osteoporos Int. 1999;9:230-5. [PMID: 10450412]

78. Turner CH, Peacock M, Timmerman L, Neal JM, Johnson CC Jr. Calcaneal ultrasonic measurements discriminate hip fracture independently of bone mass. Osteoporos Int. 1995;5:130-5. [PMID: 7599449]

79. Young H, Howey S, Purdie DW. Broadband ultrasound attenuation compared with dual-energy X-ray absorptiometry in screening for postmenopausal low bone density. Osteoporos Int. 1993;3:160-4. [PMID: 8481593]

80. Ahmed AI, Blake GM, Rymer JM, Fogelman I. Screening for osteopenia and osteoporosis: do the accepted normal ranges lead to overdiagnosis? Osteoporos Int. 1997;7:432-8. [PMID: 9425500]

81. Petley GW, Cotton AM, Murrills AJ, Taylor PA, Cooper C, Cawley MI, et al. Reference ranges of bone mineral density for women in southern England: the impact of local data on the diagnosis of osteoporosis. Br J Radiol. 1996;69:655-60. [PMID: 8696703]

82. Chen Z, Maricic M, Lund P, Tesser J, Gluck O. How the new Hologic hip normal reference values affect the densitometric diagnosis of osteoporosis. Osteoporos Int. 1998;8:423-7. [PMID: 9850349]

83. Simmons A, Barrington S, O'Doherty MJ, Coakley AJ. Dual energy X-ray absorptiometry normal reference range use within the UK and the effect of different normal ranges on the assessment of bone density. Br J Radiol. 1995;68:903-9. [PMID: 7551789]

84. Lunt M, Felsenberg D, Reeve J, Benevolenskaya L, Cannata J, Dequeker J, et al. Bone density variation and its effects on risk of vertebral deformity in men and women studied in thirteen European centers: the EVOS Study. J Bone Miner Res. 1997;12:1883-94. [PMID: 9383693]

85. Laskey MA, Crisp AJ, Cole TJ, Compston JE. Comparison of the effect of different reference data on Lunar DPX and Hologic QDR-1000 dual-energy X-ray absorptiometers. Br J Radiol. 1992;65:1124-9. [PMID: 1286422]

86. Arlot ME, Sornay-Rendu E, Garnero P, Vey-Marty B, Delmas PD. Apparent pre- and postmenopausal bone loss evaluated by DXA at different skeletal sites in women: the OFELY cohort. J Bone Miner Res. 1997;12:683-90. [PMID: 9101381]

87. Faulkner KG, von Stetten E, Miller P. Discordance in patient classification using T-scores. J Clin Densitom. 1999;2:343-50. [PMID: 10548828]

88. Grampp S, Henk CB, Fuerst TP, Lu Y, Bader TR, Kainberger F, et al. Diagnostic agreement of quantitative sonography of the calcaneus with dual X-ray absorptiometry of the spine and femur. AJR Am J Roentgenol. 1999;173:329-34. [PMID: 10430129]

89. Kröger H, Lunt M, Reeve J, Dequeker J, Adams JE, Birkenhager JC, et al. Bone density reduction in various measurement sites in men and women with osteoporotic fractures of spine and hip: the European quantitation of osteoporosis study. Calcif Tissue Int. 1999;64:191-9. [PMID: 10024374]

90. Varney LF, Parker RA, Vincelette A, Greenspan SL. Classification of osteoporosis and osteopenia in postmenopausal women is dependent on site-specific analysis. J Clin Densitom. 1999;2:275-83. [PMID: 10548823]

91. Marshall D, Johnell O, Wedel H. Meta-analysis of how well measures of bone mineral density predict occurrence of osteoporotic fractures. BMJ. 1996;312:1254-9. [PMID: 8634613]

92. Cummings SR, Black DM, Nevitt MC, Browner W, Cauley J, Ensrud K, et al. Bone density at various sites for prediction of hip fractures. The Study of Osteoporotic Fractures Research Group. Lancet. 1993;341:72-5. [PMID: 8093403]

93. Melton LJ 3rd, Atkinson EJ, O'Fallon WM, Wahner HW, Riggs BL. Long-term fracture prediction by bone mineral assessed at different skeletal sites. J Bone Miner Res. 1993;8:1227-33. [PMID: 8256660]

94. Black DM, Cummings SR, Genant HK, Nevitt MC, Palermo L, Browner W. Axial and appendicular bone density predict fractures in older women. J Bone Miner Res. 1992;7:633-8. [PMID: 1414481]

95. Bauer DC, Glüer CC, Cauley JA, Vogt TM, Ensrud KE, Genant HK, et al. Broadband ultrasound attenuation predicts fractures strongly and independently of densitometry in older women. A prospective study. Study of Osteoporotic Fractures Research Group. Arch Intern Med. 1997;157:629-34. [PMID: 9080917]

96. Nevitt MC, Johnell O, Black DM, Ensrud K, Genant HK, Cummings SR. Bone mineral density predicts non-spine fractures in very elderly women. Study of Osteoporotic Fractures Research Group. Osteoporos Int. 1994;4:325-31. [PMID: 7696827]

97. Duboeuf F, Hans D, Schott AM, Kotzki PO, Favier F, Marcelli C, et al. Different morphometric and densitometric parameters predict cervical and trochanteric hip fracture: the EPIDOS Study. J Bone Miner Res. 1997;12:1895-902. [PMID: 9383694]

98. Garnero P, Dargent-Molina P, Hans D, Schott AM, Bréart G, Meunier PJ, et al. Do markers of bone resorption add to bone mineral density and ultrasonographic heel measurement for the prediction of hip fracture in elderly women? The EPIDOS prospective study. Osteoporos Int. 1998;8:563-9. [PMID: 10326062]

99. Hans D, Dargent-Molina P, Schott AM, Sebert JL, Cormier C, Kotzki PO, et al. Ultrasonographic heel measurements to predict hip fracture in elderly women: the EPIDOS prospective study. Lancet. 1996;348:511-4. [PMID: 8757153]

100. Schott AM, Cormier C, Hans D, Favier F, Hausherr E, Dargent-Molina P, et al. How hip and whole-body bone mineral density predict hip fracture in elderly women: the EPIDOS Prospective Study. Osteoporos Int. 1998;8:247-54. [PMID: 9797909]

101. Nelson H. Hormone Replacement Therapy and Osteoporosis: Systematic Evidence Review. Rockville, MD: Agency for Healthcare Research and Quality; 2002.

102. Cranney A, Wells G, Willan A, Griffith L, Zytaruk N, Robinson V, et al. Meta-analysis of alendronate for the treatment of postmenopausal women. Endocr Rev. 2002;23:517-23.

103. Adami S, Passeri M, Ortolani S, Broggini M, Carratelli L, Caruso I, et al. Effects of oral alendronate and intranasal salmon calcitonin on bone mass and biochemical markers of bone turnover in postmenopausal women with osteoporosis. Bone. 1995;17:383-90. [PMID: 8573412]

104. Black DM, Cummings SR, Karpf DB, Cauley JA, Thompson DE, Nevitt MC, et al. Randomised trial of effect of alendronate on risk of fracture in women with existing vertebral fractures. Fracture Intervention Trial Research Group. Lancet. 1996;348:1535-41. [PMID: 8950879]

105. Bone HG, Downs RW Jr, Tucci JR, Harris ST, Weinstein RS, Licata AA, et al. Dose-response relationships for alendronate treatment in osteoporotic el-

derly women. Alendronate Elderly Osteoporosis Study Centers. J Clin Endocrinol Metab. 1997;82:265-74. [PMID: 8989272]

106. Chesnut CH 3rd, McClung MR, Ensrud KE, Bell NH, Genant HK, Harris ST, et al. Alendronate treatment of the postmenopausal osteoporotic woman: effect of multiple dosages on bone mass and bone remodeling. Am J Med. 1995;99:144-52. [PMID: 7625419]

107. Cummings SR, Black DM, Thompson DE, Applegate WB, Barrett-Connor E, Musliner TA, et al. Effect of alendronate on risk of fracture in women with low bone density but without vertebral fractures: results from the Fracture Intervention Trial. JAMA. 1998;280:2077-82. [PMID: 9875874]

108. Greenspan SL, Parker RA, Ferguson L, Rosen HN, Maitland-Ramsey L, Karpf DB. Early changes in biochemical markers of bone turnover predict the long-term response to alendronate therapy in representative elderly women: a randomized clinical trial. J Bone Miner Res. 1998;13:1431-8. [PMID: 9738515]

109. Hosking D, Chilvers CE, Christiansen C, Ravn P, Wasnich R, Ross P, et al. Prevention of bone loss with alendronate in postmenopausal women under 60 years of age. Early Postmenopausal Intervention Cohort Study Group. N Engl J Med. 1998;338:485-92. [PMID: 9443925]

110. Liberman UA, Weiss SR, Bröll J, Minne HW, Quan H, Bell NH, et al. Effect of oral alendronate on bone mineral density and the incidence of fractures in postmenopausal osteoporosis. The Alendronate Phase III Osteoporosis Treatment Study Group. N Engl J Med. 1995;333:1437-43. [PMID: 7477143]

111. McClung M, Clemmesen B, Daifotis A, Gilchrist NL, Eisman J, Weinstein RS, et al. Alendronate prevents postmenopausal bone loss in women without osteoporosis. A double-blind, randomized, controlled trial. Alendronate Osteoporosis Prevention Study Group. Ann Intern Med. 1998;128:253-61. [PMID: 9471927]

112. Pols HA, Felsenberg D, Hanley DA, Stepán J, Muñoz-Torres M, Wilkin TJ, et al. Multinational, placebo-controlled, randomized trial of the effects of alendronate on bone density and fracture risk in postmenopausal women with low bone mass: results of the FOSIT study. Foxamax International Trial Study Group. Osteoporos Int. 1999;9:461-8. [PMID: 10550467]

113. Bonnick S, Rosen C, Mako B, DeLucca P, Byrnes C, Melton M. Alendronate vs. calcium for treatment of osteoporosis in postmenopausal women [Abstract]. Bone. 1998;23(5S):S476.

114. Cummings SR, Black DM, Thompson DE, Applegate WB, Barrett-Connor E, Musliner TA, et al. Effect of alendronate on risk of fracture in women with low bone density but without vertebral fractures: results from the Fracture Intervention Trial. JAMA. 1998;280:2077-82. [PMID: 9875874]

115. McClung MR, Geusens P, Miller PD, Zippel H, Bensen WG, Roux C, et al. Effect of risedronate on the risk of hip fracture in elderly women. Hip Intervention Program Study Group. N Engl J Med. 2001;344:333-40. [PMID: 11172164]

116. Johansen HK, Gotzsche PC. Problems in the design and reporting of trials of antifungal agents encountered during meta-analysis. JAMA. 1999;282:1752-9. [PMID: 10568648]

117. Djulbegovic B, Lacevic M, Cantor A, Fields KK, Bennett CL, Adams JR, et al. The uncertainty principle and industry-sponsored research. Lancet. 2000; 356:635-8. [PMID: 10968436]

118. Rimes KA, Salkovskis PM, Shipman AJ. Psychological and behavioural effects of bone density screening for osteoporosis. Psychology and Health. 1999; 14:585-608.

119. Lyles KW, Gold DT, Shipp KM, Pieper CF, Martinez S, Mulhausen PL. Association of osteoporotic vertebral compression fractures with impaired functional status. Am J Med. 1993;94:595-601. [PMID: 8506884]

120. Stock JL, Waud CE, Coderre JA, Overdorf JH, Janikas JS, Heiniluoma KM, et al. Clinical reporting to primary care physicians leads to increased use and understanding of bone densitometry and affects the management of osteoporosis. A randomized trial. Ann Intern Med. 1998;128:996-9. [PMID: 9625686]

121. Ettinger B, Pressman A, Schein J. Clinic visits and hospital admissions for care of acid-related upper gastrointestinal disorders in women using alendronate for osteoporosis. Am J Manag Care. 1998;4:1377-82. [PMID: 10338731]

122. National Physician Fee Schedule Payment Amount File. Baltimore, MD: Health Care Financing Administration; 2000.

123. Melton LJ 3rd, Chrischilles EA, Cooper C, Lane AW, Riggs BL. Perspective. How many women have osteoporosis? J Bone Miner Res. 1992;7:1005-10. [PMID: 1414493]

124. Reginster J, Minne HW, Sorensen OH, Hooper M, Roux C, Brandi ML, et al. Randomized trial of the effects of risedronate on vertebral fractures in women with established postmenopausal osteoporosis. Vertebral Efficacy with Risedronate Therapy (VERT) Study Group. Osteoporos Int. 2000;11:83-91. [PMID: 10663363]

125. Weinstein L, Ullery B, Bourguignon C. A simple system to determine who needs osteoporosis screening. Obstet Gynecol. 1999;93:757-60. [PMID: 10912981]

126. Health Technology Assessment. Number 6: Bone Densitometry: Patients with Asymptomatic Hyperparathyroidism. Agency for Health Care Policy and Research, U.S. Department of Health and Human Services. Rockville, MD: Agency for Health Care Policy and Research; 1995. AHRQ publication no. 96-0004.

Current Author Addresses: Drs. Nelson and Helfand: Oregon Health & Science University, Mail Code BICC 504, 3181 SW Sam Jackson Park Road, Portland, OR 97201.
Dr. Woolf: Virginia Commonwealth University, Department of Family Practice, 3712 Charles Stewart Drive, Fairfax, VA 22033.

Dr. Allan: School of Nursing, the University of Maryland Baltimore, 655 West Lombard, Room 725, Baltimore, MD 21201.

Appendix Table 1. **Summary of Evidence Quality**

Key Questions	Evidence Code*	Quality of Evidence†	
		Internal Validity	External Validity
Does screening using risk factor assessment or bone density testing reduce fractures?	None		
Does risk factor assessment accurately identify women who may benefit from bone density testing?	II-2	Poor to good: small studies, risk assessment instruments often not validated	Poor to fair: no instruments used widely for screening purposes, although some were developed from community-based studies
Do bone density measurements accurately identify women who may benefit from treatment?	II-2	Fair to good: studies indicate the short-term predictability for fracture	Fair: not known how well results of studies translate to practice
What are the harms of screening?	II-2, III	Poor to fair: small studies, descriptive	Poor: small studies, selected participants
Does treatment reduce the risk of fractures in women identified by screening?	I	Good: bisphosphonate trials indicate fracture prevention	Poor to fair: may be differences between trial participants and primary care patients
What are the harms of treatment?	I, II-2	Poor to good: long-term effects of newer agents not known	Poor to fair: difficult to know how risks affect individual patients

* Evidence codes are based on study design categories (22): I = randomized, controlled trials; II-1 = controlled trials without randomization; II-2 = cohort or case–control analytic studies; II-3 = multiple time series, dramatic uncontrolled experiments; III = opinions of respected authorities, descriptive studies.
† Based on criteria developed by the U.S. Preventive Services Task Force (22).

Appendix Table 2. **Formulas for Calculations in Outcomes Table**

Number of hip fractures in untreated women with osteoporosis
   No risk factors: (5-year probability of hip fracture in women with osteoporosis) × (prevalence of osteoporosis) × N
   At least one risk factor: 1.7 × (5-year probability of hip fracture in women with osteoporosis) × (prevalence of osteoporosis) × N

Number of hip fractures in treated women with osteoporosis
   No risk factors: (RR for hip fracture from treatment trials) × (0.7 adherence) × (number of hip fractures in untreated women with osteoporosis) + (1 − 0.7 adherence) × (number of hip fractures in untreated women with osteoporosis)
   At least one risk factor: (relative risk for hip fracture from treatment trials) × (0.7 adherence) × (number of hip fractures in untreated women with osteoporosis with ≥1 risk factor) + (1 − 0.7 compliance) × (number of hip fractures in untreated women with osteoporosis with ≥1 risk factor)

Number needed to screen for benefit
   N/(number of hip fractures without treatment − number with treatment)

Number needed to treat
   Number of women with osteoporosis/(number of hip fractures without treatment − number with treatment)

Appendix Table 3. **Criteria for Grading the Internal Validity of Individual Studies***

Randomized, controlled trials
   Adequate randomization, including concealment and equal distribution of potential confounders among groups
   Maintenance of comparable groups (includes attrition, crossovers, adherence, contamination)
   Important differential loss to follow-up or overall high loss to follow-up
   Equal, reliable, and valid measurements (includes masking of outcome assessment)
   Clear definition of interventions
   Important outcomes considered
   Intention-to-treat analysis
Case–control studies
   Accurate ascertainment of cases
   Nonbiased selection of case-patients and controls with exclusion criteria applied equally to both
   High response rate
   Diagnostic testing procedures applied equally to each group
   Measurement of exposure accurate and applied equally to each group
   Appropriate attention to potential confounding variables
Cohort studies
   Consideration of potential confounders with restriction or measurement for adjustment in the analysis; consideration of inception cohorts
   Maintenance of comparable groups (includes attrition, crossovers, adherence, contamination)
   Important differential loss to follow-up or overall high loss to follow-up
   Equal, reliable, and valid measurements (includes masking of outcome assessment)
   Clear definition of interventions
   Important outcomes considered
   Adjustment for potential confounders in analysis
Diagnostic accuracy studies
   Screening test relevant, available for primary care, adequately described
   Uses a credible reference standard, performed regardless of test results
   Reference standard interpreted independently of screening test
   Handles indeterminate results in a reasonable manner
   Spectrum of patients included in study
   Adequate sample size
   Administration of reliable screening test

* The Methods Work Group for the U.S. Preventive Services Task Force developed a set of criteria to determine how well individual studies were conducted (internal validity) (22). The Task Force defined a three-category rating of "good," "fair," and "poor," based on these criteria. In general, a good study is one that meets all criteria well. A fair study is one that does not meet, or it is not clear that it meets, at least one criterion but has no known important limitation that could invalidate its results. A poor study has important limitations. These specifications are not meant to be rigid rules but rather are intended to be general guidelines; individual exceptions, when explicitly explained and justified, can be made.

Appendix Figure. **Analytic framework.**

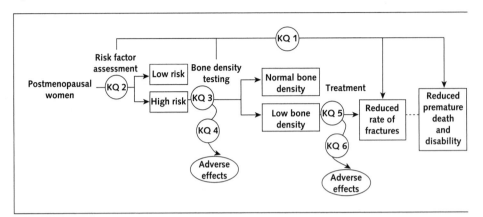

The analytic framework is a schematic outline used to define the population, preventive service, diagnostic or therapeutic interventions, and intermediate and health outcomes considered in the review. The arrows represent key questions that the evidence must answer, and demonstrate the chain of logic that evidence must support, to link the preventive service to improved health outcomes. KQ = key question. KQ 1: Does screening using risk factor assessment or bone density testing reduce fractures? KQ 2: Does risk factor assessment accurately identify women who may benefit from bone density testing? KQ 3: Do bone density measurements accurately identify women who may benefit from treatment? KQ 4: What are the harms of screening? KQ 5: Does treatment reduce the risk of fractures in women identified by screening? KQ 6: What are the harms of treatment?

Postmenopausal hormone replacement therapy and primary prevention of cardiovascular disease

❏ Evidence for the benefits of postmenopausal HRT (combined estrogens plus progestins) includes: good evidence for increased bone mineral density, fair-to-good evidence for reduced risk of fractures, and fair evidence for reduced risk of colorectal cancer.

❏ Evidence for the harms of postmenopausal HRT (combined estrogens plus progestins) includes: good evidence for increased risk of breast cancer and thromboembolism, fair-to-good evidence for increased risk of coronary artery disease, and fair evidence for increased risk of stroke and cholecystits.

❏ Based on these results from the Women's Health Initiative (WHI), the harms of postmenopausal HRT (combined estrogens plus progestins) are likely to exceed the benefits of chronic disease prevention in most patients.

❏ Results from the WHI study of unopposed estrogen in women with hysterectomies are pending.

Postmenopausal Hormone Replacement Therapy and the Primary Prevention of Cardiovascular Disease

Linda L. Humphrey, MD, MPH; Benjamin K.S. Chan, MS; and Harold C. Sox, MD

Purpose: To evaluate the value of hormone replacement therapy (HRT) in the primary prevention of cardiovascular disease (CVD) and coronary artery disease (CAD).

Data Sources: MEDLINE and Cochrane databases were searched for all primary prevention studies reporting CVD or CAD incidence, mortality, or both in association with HRT; reference lists, letters, editorials, and reviews were also reviewed.

Data Extraction: All studies were reviewed, abstracted, and rated for quality.

Study Selection: Only studies of good or fair quality, according to U.S. Preventive Services Task Force (USPSTF) criteria, were included in the detailed review and meta-analysis.

Data Synthesis: The summary relative risk with any HRT use was 0.75 (95% credible interval [CrI], 0.42 to 1.23) for CVD mortality and 0.74 (CrI, 0.36 to 1.45) for CAD mortality. The summary relative risk with any use was 1.28 (CrI, 0.86 to 2.00) for

CVD incidence and 0.87 (CrI, 0.62 to 1.21) for CAD incidence. Further analysis of studies adjusting for socioeconomic status, as well as other major CAD risk factors, showed a summary relative risk of 1.07 (CrI, 0.79 to 1.48) for CAD incidence associated with any HRT use. Similar results were found when the analysis was stratified by studies adjusting for alcohol consumption, exercise, or both, in addition to other major risk factors, suggesting confounding by these factors.

Conclusions: This meta-analysis differs from previous meta-analyses by evaluating potential explanatory variables of the relationship between HRT, CVD, and CAD. The adjusted meta-analysis is consistent with recent randomized trials that have shown no benefit in the secondary or primary prevention of CVD events. A valid answer to the role of HRT in the primary prevention of CVD will best come from randomized, controlled trials.

Postmenopausal hormone replacement therapy (HRT) is one of the most commonly prescribed drug regimens in the United States. This pattern of use reflects a large number of postmenopausal women, many of whom choose to take HRT to treat symptoms of menopause. Also contributing to the high prevalence of use has been significant publicity aimed at physicians and women regarding the effect of HRT on intermediate biological outcomes, such as lipid levels (1) and bone density, and its potential effect in decreasing cardiovascular disease (CVD) as well as several other serious diseases, such as Alzheimer disease and colon cancer.

Cardiovascular disease, primarily coronary artery disease (CAD), is the leading cause of death among women in the United States. Many observational studies and analyses have suggested that HRT protects against CVD. However, in the past 4 years, three secondary prevention trials (2–4) and, most relevantly, the Women's Health Initiative (WHI) primary prevention study (5) have shown no benefit or increased rates of CVD events among women randomly assigned to HRT. These results were surprising to many because of the benefit shown in many observational studies and because estrogen use is associated with many effects that could have favorable effects on CVD, including lower low-density lipoprotein cholesterol levels (6), lower lipoprotein(a) levels (7), and increased high-density lipoprotein cholesterol levels (8). However, HRT is also associated with potentially unfavorable effects, including increased levels of triglycerides (6), factor VII, and C-reactive protein (8) and decreased levels of antithrombin III (6).

Given the mix of intermediate biological outcomes,

limitations of observational data, and recent trial results, we conducted this systematic review and meta-analysis to examine the value of HRT for the primary prevention of CVD. We were particularly interested in whether bias might explain discordant results between recent trials and the observational literature. Our review is one of several that will serve as background for the Third U.S. Preventive Services Task Force (USPSTF) recommendations on HRT and the prevention of chronic diseases.

METHODS

We searched the topic of HRT and CVD and CAD in the MEDLINE and Cochrane databases from 1966 to December 2000. We also used bibliographies of original research and other publications to identify studies for review. Criteria for inclusion in the systematic review were evaluation of HRT and the primary prevention of CVD, CAD, or both among postmenopausal women and availability of an English-language abstract for review. We included randomized, controlled trials, and cohort and case–control studies if they evaluated CVD or CAD incidence or mortality. We did not review cross-sectional studies because they are limited by prevalence bias. Two investigators reviewed all abstracts to identify papers for full-text review.

We abstracted study data and created evidence tables organized by study type. Definitions of current, past, recent, never, and ever use were taken directly from the individual studies (**Appendix Tables 1** and **2**, available at www.annals.org). Hormone use was classified in each study as unopposed estrogen replacement therapy or estrogen

Table 1. U.S. Preventive Services Task Force Categories for Rating Internal Validity of Studies*

Case–control studies
  Accurate ascertainment of cases
  Nonbiased selection of cases and controls, with exclusion criteria applied
    equally to both
  Response rate
  Testing or outcomes procedures applied equally to each group
  Measurement of exposure accurate and applied equally to each group
  Appropriate attention to potential confounding variables
Cohort studies
  Initial assembly of comparable groups
  Maintenance of comparable groups
  Level of follow-up (differential and overall)
  Equal, reliable, and valid measurements of exposures and outcomes
  Masking of outcome
  All important outcomes considered
  Adjustment for potential confounders

* Adapted from reference 9.

plus progesterone "combined therapy" when it was specified, which was infrequent. When the type of estrogen or progesterone therapy was not specified, the exposure was categorized as HRT.

Definitions of CVD and CAD events were taken directly from the reviewed studies. Most often, CVD mortality was defined by International Classification of Disease codes or World Health Organization criteria or included any death resulting from any type of CVD or CVD-related procedure, including stroke, CAD, sudden cardiac death, congestive heart failure, peripheral vascular disease, coronary artery bypass graft surgery, or percutaneous transluminal coronary angioplasty. Coronary artery disease is a subset of CVD. For the purposes of this review, CAD deaths included all fatal myocardial infarctions, sudden cardiac deaths, or both attributed to CAD; CAD events included myocardial infarction, coronary artery bypass graft surgery, percutaneous transluminal coronary angioplasty, and, in some studies, angina. In an effort to measure a global effect on CVD, as well as a more specific effect on CAD, we evaluated CVD and CAD separately when the data allowed.

Two investigators independently rated the quality of each study based on criteria created by the Third USPSTF

(9); discrepancies were adjudicated by a third reviewer. These criteria are shown in **Table 1. Appendix Tables 1** and **2**, available at www.annals.org, show each study's rating by quality. In ranking the quality of observational studies, we gave significant weight to adequate control of potential CVD risk factors because of known differences in risk profiles among women who use HRT and those who do not (10, 11).

After reviewing and rating the studies, we limited our formal review and meta-analyses to only studies rated as fair or good quality and included randomized, controlled trials; population-based, case–control studies; and cohort studies with internal controls and at least 3 years of follow-up. In studies with multiple publications from the same cohort or population, only data from the most recent publication were included in the meta-analyses, with reference in the text to older publications if they presented unique findings. To evaluate each study's control of confounding variables that might explain their results, for each outcome and each study providing data relevant to the outcome, we listed potential CVD risk factors included in the multivariable models determining relative risk. These included age, diabetes, hypertension, smoking, lipid levels, family history, exercise, socioeconomic status, education level, alcohol use, body mass index, and others. Definitions for the presence or absence of these factors, as well as their assessment, are taken directly from the included studies.

This research was funded by the U.S. Agency for Healthcare Research and Quality under a contract to support the work of the USPSTF. Agency for Healthcare Research and Quality staff and USPSTF members participated in the initial design of the study and reviewed interim analyses and the final manuscript. Since our report was prepared for the Third USPSTF, it was distributed for review to 15 content experts and revised accordingly before preparation of this manuscript.

For each outcome, a meta-analytic model was fitted, stratifying by HRT exposure status: current, past, and ever (if the study did not report results for current and past use separately). The model also allowed for a global effect of HRT to be estimated; this is referred to as the effect of any

Table 2. Meta-Analysis Summary Table

Variable	Relative Risk according to Measure of Hormone Replacement Therapy (95% Credible Interval)*			
	Current	Past	Ever	Any*
Mortality				
Total cardiovascular disease	0.64 (0.44–0.93)	0.79 (0.52–1.09)	0.81 (0.58–1.13)	0.75 (0.42–1.23)
Coronary artery disease	0.62 (0.40–0.90)	0.76 (0.53–1.02)	0.81 (0.37–1.60)	0.74 (0.36–1.45)
Incidence				
Total cardiovascular disease	1.27 (0.80–2.00)	1.26 (0.79–2.08)	1.35 (0.92–2.00)	1.28 (0.86–2.00)
Coronary artery disease	0.80 (0.68–0.95)	0.89 (0.75–1.05)	0.91 (0.67–1.33)	0.88 (0.64–1.21)
Summary estimate†	0.97 (0.82–1.16)	1.07 (0.90–1.27)	1.11 (0.84–1.53)	1.04 (0.79–1.44)

* "Current," "past," and "ever" use are categories used in the individual studies. "Any use" is a category created for this meta-analysis combining data from studies evaluating ever and never use of HRT with data from studies evaluating current, past, or never use (current + past + ever use).
† Includes only studies with adjustments for socioeconomic status as assessed by social class (12, 13), education (14, 15), and income (14).

Figure 1. **Relative risk or odds ratio for cardiovascular disease mortality.**

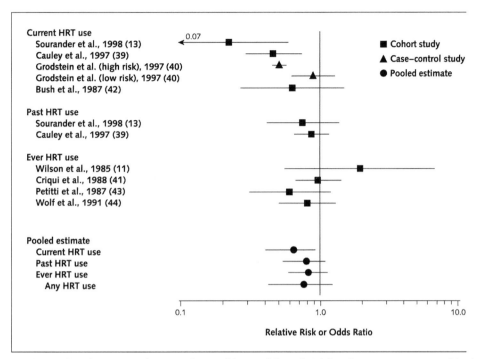

Error bars represent 95% CIs. HRT = hormone replacement therapy. "Current," "past," and "ever" use are categories used in the individual studies. "Any use" is a category created for this meta-analysis combining data from studies evaluating ever and never use of HRT with data from studies evaluating current, past, or never use (current + past + ever use).

HRT exposure (current, ever, or past). Our primary analysis compared event rates in patients with "any HRT use" (current, past, or ever use) to those who had "never" used HRT. We also compared event rates in "current," "past," or "ever" HRT use groups to "never" use to further evaluate variable findings among the studies. Results by category of use are shown in **Table 2.** All relative risk estimates are compared with never use. Estimation was made by using the Bayesian data analytic framework, in which the analogue to the confidence interval is the credible interval (CrI) (16). Further details of the meta-analysis are given in the Appendix (available at www.annals.org).

RESULTS

Scope of Literature

The MEDLINE search identified 3035 abstracts of papers evaluating primary prevention published between 1966 and December 2000. From them, 24 cohort studies; 18 case–control studies; one very small randomized, controlled trial; and one meta-analysis were reviewed. After the quality of the studies was rated, 20 observational studies; one randomized, controlled trial conducted among institutionalized women; and 1 meta-analysis that combined data from 23 randomized, controlled trials of HRT for outcomes other than CVD (such as bone density or lipid levels) were included in our meta-analyses. Data from studies graded as poor quality were not included in the meta-analyses. Our search results are shown in the **Appendix Figure** (available at www.annals.org).

We reviewed 18 case–control studies and rated 6 as poor quality, generally because of very small size, poor evaluation of CVD risk factors, or potential bias in selection of controls (17–22). We excluded 1 study (23) because data were provided in an updated study. Five of the excluded studies did not report risk estimates, 2 suggested decreased risk, and 1 suggested increased risk (**Appendix Table 3,** available at www.annals.org). The major difference between studies rated as good or fair quality was in adjustment for CVD risk factors.

Twenty-four cohort studies were reviewed for inclusion in the meta-analyses, and 11 were excluded because of poor quality (24–34), usually because they had little or no adjustment for CVD risk factors, they used external controls, or the entire cohort was exposed to HRT. Four studies were excluded because the data were updated (35–37) or published in another form (38). Qualitatively, fair-quality studies had relative risks similar to those of good-quality studies (range, 0.21 to 1.94). However, all of the poor-quality cohort studies had relative risks or standardized mortality ratios significantly below 1 (range, 0.27 to 0.79) (**Appendix Table 3**).

Cardiovascular and Coronary Artery Disease Mortality

All of the studies contributing to our mortality analyses were prospective cohort studies, except for a nested case–control study from the Nurses' Health Cohort. There was little variation among the cohort studies and this study; therefore, these studies were combined. Similarly, when stratified by study quality (fair or good) in the meta-

Figure 2. Relative risk or odds ratio for coronary artery disease mortality.

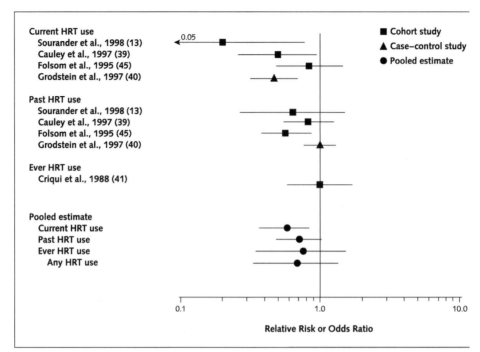

Error bars represent 95% CIs. HRT = hormone replacement therapy. "Current," "past," and "ever" use are categories used in the individual studies. "Any use" is a category created for this meta-analysis combining data from studies evaluating ever and never use of HRT with data from studies evaluating current, past, or never use (current + past + ever use).

analyses, the findings were similar and the results were combined. More details about the studies are presented in **Appendix Tables 4** and **5**, available at www.annals.org.

Among 8 observational studies evaluating CVD mortality, 3 (13, 39, 40) showed lower risk among women using HRT (**Figure 1**). One study (11) reported an in-

crease in CVD deaths among ever users of HRT (relative risk, 1.94), which was not statistically significant. The reasons for different results among the studies are unclear. Each study adjusted for different sets of confounders, but review of their assessment does not help in understanding the different results. In addition, differences in the studies'

Figure 3. Relative risk or odds ratio for cardiovascular disease incidence.

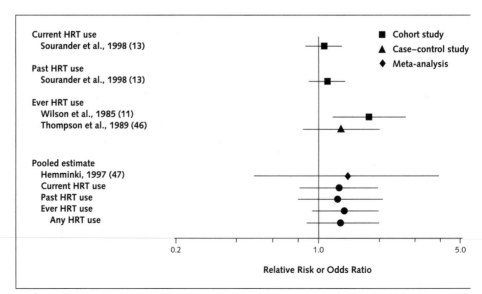

Error bars represent 95% CIs. Reference 47 is pooled data from a previously published meta-analysis. HRT = hormone replacement therapy. "Current," "past," and "ever" use are categories used in the individual studies. "Any use" is a category created for this meta-analysis combining data from studies evaluating ever and never use of HRT with data from studies evaluating current, past, or never use (current + past + ever use).

Figure 4. **Relative risk or odds ratio for coronary artery disease incidence.**

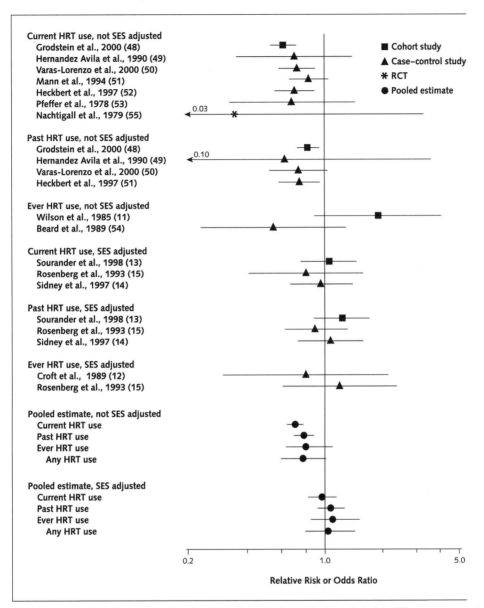

Error bars represent 95% CIs. HRT = hormone replacement therapy; RCT = randomized, controlled trial; SES = socioeconomic status. "Current," "past," and "ever" use are categories used in the individual studies. "Any use" is a category created for this meta-analysis combining data from studies evaluating ever and never use of HRT with data from studies evaluating current, past, or never use (current + past + ever use). Adjustments for SES were adjustments as assessed by social class (12, 13), education (14, 15), and income.

quality or in the methods by which HRT use was assessed do not explain the different results.

In our meta-analysis evaluating CVD mortality, the global measure of HRT exposure, "any use," was associated with a summary relative risk of 0.75 (CrI, 0.42 to 1.23) (**Table 2** and **Figure 1**). Five studies specifically evaluated the risk for CAD death (13, 39–42). In our meta-analysis of HRT and CAD mortality, "any use" had a summary relative risk of 0.74 (CrI, 0.36 to 1.45) (**Table 2** and **Figure 2**).

Cardiovascular Disease Incidence

Two cohort studies, one case–control study, and the data from the meta-analysis described earlier contributed to our meta-analysis of CVD incidence. Since only four stud-

ies (11, 13, 46, 47) contributed to this analysis and the effect sizes were in the same direction (range, 1.07 to 1.76), the data were pooled. In our meta-analysis, "any use" of HRT was associated with a summary relative risk of 1.28 (CrI, 0.86 to 2.00) for CVD incidence. Results were similar when a previous meta-analysis (47) was used as the prior distribution (**Table 2** and **Figure 3**). More details about the studies are presented in **Appendix Table 6**, available at www.annals.org.

Coronary Artery Disease Incidence

The association between HRT use and CAD incidence was evaluated in 3 cohort studies (11, 13, 48); 9 case–control studies (12, 14, 15, 49–54); and one small randomized, controlled trial (55). Relative risks ranged from 0.33 to 1.90. Because of the marked range of results, we conducted analyses stratifying by study type and identified little difference in our summary estimates. Therefore, the case–control and cohort studies were combined. Since only 1 trial of HRT in primary prevention has formally published data, we included it in our summary estimate. Past use of HRT was evaluated in 6 studies (13–15, 48, 49, 52), and combined therapy was evaluated in 4 studies (15, 48, 51, 55); these findings varied (**Figure 4**).

Table 3 indicates that many studies had point estimates below 1.0 (52). This suggests benefit, although only four studies had statistically significant results. The reasons for disparity among the five good-quality studies are uncertain but may be related to variable assessment of confounders, as shown in **Table 3**. **Appendix Tables 1** and **2** show that all studies included in this systematic review assessed and defined HRT use differently. However, these tables do not show a pattern that helps further explain disparate findings among studies evaluating CAD incidence.

Results of the meta-analysis evaluating the association between CAD incidence and HRT use varied by exposure status (**Table 2**). For CAD incidence, "any use" was associated with a relative risk of 0.88 (CrI, 0.64 to 1.21). To further explore the differences found among the studies evaluating CAD incidence, we conducted sensitivity analyses stratified by several confounding variables. First, we compared the summary relative risks among the studies with statistical adjustment for socioeconomic status or education with those that did not adjust. Among the studies adjusting for these factors, there was no association between any measure of HRT use and CAD events, with relative risks ranging from 0.97 to 1.11 (**Table 2**). However, the summary relative risks among studies that did not adjust for socioeconomic status were reduced with current exposure (relative risk, 0.71 [CrI, 0.64 to 0.78]) and past exposure (relative risk, 0.78 [CrI, 0.69 to 0.87]) (**Figure 4**). Similar results were found when the analysis stratified studies that adjusted for alcohol consumption, exercise, or both, suggesting confounding by these factors. Further stratification did not show any differences between results of case–control and cohort studies or between results of fair- and good-quality studies.

Table 3. **Coronary Artery Disease Incidence and Hormone Replacement Therapy***

Study (Reference), Year	Quality	Design	Patients, *n*	Hormone Type	Hormone Exposure Status	Relative Risk or Odds Ratio (95% CI)
Pfeffer (53), 1978	Fair	Case–control	274	HRT	Ever	0.86 (0.54–1.37)
				HRT	Current	0.68 (0.32–1.42)
Natchigall et al. (55), 1979†	Fair	RCT	168	CHRT	10 years	0.33 (NS)
Wilson et al. (11), 1985	Good	Cohort	1234	HRT	Ever	1.9‡
Croft and Hannaford (12), 1989	Fair	Case–control	158	HRT	Ever	0.8 (0.3–1.8)
Beard et al. (54), 1989	Fair	Case–control	133	HRT	Ever	0.55 (0.24–1.30)
Hernandez Avila et al. (49), 1990	Fair	Nested case–control from cohort study	120	HRT	Current	0.7 (0.4–1.4)
					Past	0.6 (0.1–2.1)
Rosenberg et al. (15), 1993	Good	Case–control	858	ERT	Ever	0.9 (0.7–1.2)
				CHRT	Ever	1.2 (0.6–2.4)
				ERT	Past	0.9 (0.7–1.3)
				ERT	Recent	0.8 (0.4–1.3)
Mann et al. (51), 1994	Fair	Case–control	1521	HRT	Recent	0.83 (0.66–1.03)
				CHRT	Recent	0.68 (0.47–0.97)
				ERT	Recent	0.93 (0.47–1.86)
Grodstein et al. (48), 2000	Good	Cohort	59 337	ERT	Current	0.60 (0.43–0.83)
				CHRT	Current	0.39 (0.19–0.78)
				HRT	Current	0.60 (0.47–0.76)
				HRT	Past	0.85 (0.71–1.01)
Heckbert et al. (52), 1997†	Fair	Case–control	850	HRT	Ever	0.72 (0.59–0.88)
				HRT	Current	0.7 (0.55–0.89)
				HRT	Past	0.74 (0.57–0.96)
Sidney et al. (14), 1997	Good	Case–control	438	HRT	Current	0.96 (0.66–1.40)
				HRT	Past	1.07 (0.72–1.58)
Sourander et al. (13), 1998	Fair	Cohort	7944	HRT	Current	1.05 (0.76–1.46)
					Past	1.23 (0.88–1.71)
Varas-Lorenzo et al. (50), 2000	Good	Case–control	1031	HRT	Current/recent	0.72 (0.59–0.88)
					Past	0.73 (0.51–1.03)

* All studies were adjusted for age and hypertension unless otherwise indicated. BMI = body mass index; CHRT = combined hormone replacement therapy; ERT = estrogen replacement therapy; HDL = high-density lipoprotein; HRT = hormone replacement therapy; LDL = low-density lipoprotein; NS = not significant; RCT = randomized, controlled trial.
† Not adjusted for hypertension.
‡ *P* <0.01.

DISCUSSION

Earlier data on HRT and the primary prevention of CVD showing benefit to users are not supported by newer studies or by our analysis. The major points from our review and meta-analyses are as follows. First, no significant association was identified between past, ever, or any use of HRT and CVD or CAD death. Second, HRT use did not reduce CVD incidence and, in fact, suggests a small increase in risk. Third, HRT showed no benefit in preventing CAD among the studies that adjusted for major CAD risk factors and socioeconomic status or education and showed reduced risk among studies that did not adjust for these factors, suggesting confounding.

We approached this review differently than other researchers (56–58). First, in an effort to measure a global effect on CVD, as well as a more specific effect on CAD, we evaluated CVD and CAD separately when the data allowed. Second, we conducted separate analyses of incidence and mortality for each outcome. Third, we limited our detailed review and meta-analyses to studies of good or fair quality based on preestablished criteria. Finally, in an effort to better explain variable findings, we evaluated risks in our meta-analyses using different measures of exposure (current, past, ever), as well as a global measure (any use).

Other meta-analyses have had different findings. A meta-analysis in 1991 (56) that included 6 case–control studies, 16 cohort studies, and 3 angiography studies found a relative risk of 0.56 (CI, 0.50 to 0.61) for CAD events (incidence and mortality). A 1992 meta-analysis of HRT and CAD calculated a relative risk of 0.65 (CI, 0.59 to 0.71) for CAD events and of 0.63 (CI, 0.55 to 0.72) for CAD death when comparing ever use with nonuse (57). A more recent meta-analysis calculated a summary risk estimate for CAD of 0.70 (CI, 0.65 to 0.75) for HRT use (58). Each of these meta-analyses included studies that we rated as poor quality and excluded from our analysis. As discussed earlier, poor-quality studies tended to suggest greater protection against CVD and CAD in association with HRT use. In addition, previous meta-analyses included angiography studies that involved symptomatic women and cross-sectional design, which has many shortcomings. These meta-analyses also differ from ours because they combine mortality and incidence relative risks for HRT. These differences may explain why our review, un-

Table 3—**Continued**

	Cardiovascular Disease Risk Factors Included in Multivariable Models				
Diabetes Mellitus	Cholesterol	Smoking	Alcohol	Socioeconomic Status or Education	Other
	Yes	Yes	Yes		LDL/HDL cholesterol, BMI
	Yes			Yes	Oral contraceptive use, hysterectomy
Yes		Yes			Menopausal status, type, year
Yes					Antiarrhythmic drug therapy
Yes	Yes	Yes	Yes	Yes	BMI exercise, coffee, angina, myocardial infarction before 60 y of age, age/type menopause, physician visits
Yes	Yes				Hysterectomy, surgical menopause
Yes	Yes	Yes			BMI, family history, oral contraceptive use, parity, menarche
Yes		Yes			Year, angina
Yes		Yes	Yes	Yes	Exercise, coronary artery disease, race, facility
Yes		Yes		Yes	Exercise
Yes		Yes			LDL/HDL cholesterol, BMI, family history, aspirin use, surgical menopause

like previous analyses, suggests no overall benefit from HRT in preventing CVD or CAD.

One of the difficulties in assessing the literature on HRT and CVD is the large span of years represented in the observational studies, during which dramatic changes in clinical practice and CVD knowledge occurred. There have also been significant secular changes in the use of estrogen, including type, administration, and dose, as well as the relatively recent practice of adding progesterone to estrogen therapy. Complicating this evaluation is that many studies measured estrogen use at only one point in time, asked women if they had "ever" used HRT, or combined past use with non-use, allowing substantial room for misclassification. Such misclassification would dilute any potential association between HRT and CVD (**Appendix Tables 1 and 2**). The importance of characterizing HRT use is illustrated in the Framingham study, where a change in how HRT use was assessed (single vs. multiple assessments) changed the direction of relative risk estimates for total mortality among younger postmenopausal women (11).

One of the most important findings of our review and analysis is how different evaluation and statistical control of CAD risk factors affect summary estimates. This is highlighted in our meta-analysis, which showed markedly different relative risks depending on the inclusion or exclusion of socioeconomic status or education as predictor variables in a study's multivariable analysis. These findings suggest confounding, which is important because lower socioeconomic status is a strong risk factor for CVD and CAD, as well as for most other poor outcomes (59). In addition, women using HRT tend to have higher socioeconomic status, which may explain their better outcomes (60). Similarly, none of the studies with adjustment for alcohol use or exercise, both known to be more common in women who use HRT, showed benefit with HRT use.

Several biases complicate the interpretation of our results, as well as those of others. The first consideration is selection bias, particularly healthy-user bias. Women who use HRT tend to be more affluent, leaner, and more educated; tend to exercise more often; and tend to drink more alcohol (11, 61). Women who take HRT also have different health characteristics before menopause (10, 11, 62). Researchers can adjust for these protective factors analytically when measuring them; what cannot be adjusted for statistically, however, are lifestyle, environmental exposures, and genetic characteristics that are not measured or may not yet be identified as important etiologically in CVD. This is particularly an issue in CVD, where 50% of CVD incidence is unexplained by traditional risk factors (63).

Women prescribed HRT have access to health care and are therefore more likely to be receiving treatment for other CVD–CAD risk factors, such as high cholesterol levels or high blood pressure, which would lower their risk (60). In contrast to reduced mortality in association with current HRT use, there is a consistent although not statistically significant increase in rates of CVD associated with any HRT exposure. Several possibilities may explain this finding. Women receiving HRT have access to health care and may be more likely to receive diagnoses of CVD, such as myocardial infarction, peripheral vascular disease, stroke, or transient ischemic attack. In addition, after receiving these diagnoses, they may undergo more aggressive risk factor modification or medical management, which may partially explain reduced mortality in the setting of average or slightly increased incidence. Finally, several sources suggest that women using HRT have higher rates of ischemic stroke, which would increase rates of CVD events (48, 64, 65).

Selection for healthy users is also a consequence of secular trends in estrogen use (66). Many studies of estrogen use were conducted when physicians were concerned about the risk for HRT and CVD, based on the Coronary Drug Project findings among men and myocardial infarction rates in women taking oral contraceptives (66). In addition, for many of the years represented in these studies, hypertension, diabetes, and CAD were considered contraindications to HRT (58).

A more subtle bias, which may be apparent to practicing physicians, is a tendency to offer and prescribe HRT to women who are perceived as being in better overall "health," even in the absence of defined CVD or CAD risk factors. Supporting this contention are empirical data showing that women with medical or psychiatric problems are less likely to receive HRT or treatment of other unrelated problems (67). This type of selection bias is more difficult to measure and could lead to systematic overestimates of the benefit of HRT in CVD.

Another aspect of healthy user bias is that women often discontinue HRT when they become ill (68). This tendency would bias studies that evaluate recent or current use by underestimating use in ill patients. Such underestimation would result in reduced relative risk estimates associated with current or recent exposure, suggesting a protective effect of HRT. This bias may have occurred in studies where only current or recent users have reduced risk for CVD or CAD. It is even more strongly suggested in studies where past users have higher rates of CVD than nonusers or current users, suggesting that they may have stopped HRT because of CVD- or CAD-related illness (32). Healthy user bias may particularly affect mortality associations because most deaths occur among women with comorbid conditions that led them or their clinician to stop HRT, making hormone use, particularly current use, appear protective against CVD death. This is suggested in our meta-analyses evaluating CVD and CAD mortality, where only current use of HRT was associated with decreased risk and "any use" of HRT (past, current, or ever) showed no association. Supporting the concept of healthy user bias among women using HRT are several studies showing reduced all-cause mortality, as well as reduced mortality from accidents and homicides, among women who take HRT. These findings may reflect multiple benefits but more likely indicate systematic differences among users and nonusers (42, 43).

Another consideration in evaluating the relationship between HRT and CVD is the issue of adherence bias. Women who take HRT, especially for long periods, are by definition adherent to therapy. In randomized, controlled trials, good adherence to placebo has been shown to decrease CAD events by 30% to 60%, suggesting that good adherence is a marker for other healthy behaviors (43, 69–71). Adherence bias itself may explain much of the benefit seen in observational studies of HRT and CVD.

In the past 4 years, data from two randomized, controlled trials of HRT in the secondary prevention of CAD have been published (2, 3), and one trial of HRT in primary prevention has released information to the public (5). These findings are important because randomization is the only way to deal with the inherent biases in observational studies and to ensure equal distribution of known and unknown CVD risk factors. The Heart and Estrogen/progestin Replacement Study (HERS), which examined secondary prevention, showed a 52% increased risk for myocardial infarction during the first year of use and suggested increased CAD deaths in the first 3 years of use (72). The Estrogen Replacement and Atherosclerosis Trial of secondary prevention showed no benefit from HRT in reducing angiographic CAD progression (73). Finally, early results from the WHI randomized, controlled trial of HRT and primary prevention, involving 27 348 postmenopausal U.S. women, have shown increased rates of stroke, CAD, and blood clots among women randomly assigned to HRT compared with those receiving placebo (5). These findings have persisted into the third year of the study (5, 73).

How can the results of these trials of secondary prevention, and especially the WHI study of primary prevention, be explained, given the results from many previous observational studies suggesting benefit? As discussed earlier, it is likely that selection and adherence bias play a major role in the findings from the observational studies. What is especially surprising in two of these studies, however, is the suggestion of harm in the first 2 to 3 years (5, 72). For years, it has been thought that the most likely biological explanation for some of the observed reduction in CVD risk among HRT users was an improvement in lipid levels. However, the fact that two randomized, controlled studies have shown that women had higher CVD risks in the first 2 to 3 years of the study, one in the setting of more favorable lipid profiles (72), suggests that other important biological effects occur in women who take HRT. For example, HRT plays a complex role in clotting, thrombolysis, and inflammation, which must be considered because CVD and CAD events are partially mediated through these processes. Biological changes associated with HRT may result in a shift in balance toward increased blood clotting, inflammation, or both. This shift may be a more immediate or acute effect of estrogen and is consistent with the observation of increased risk during the early years of estrogen use. An important interaction or synergism between the multiple, relatively prevalent hypercoagulable states and HRT may also account for early increased risk, as suggested in several recent studies (74–76). More studies are needed in this area.

With the publication of the HERS results and the preliminary reporting of increased event rates in the first 3 years of the WHI, one of the most pressing questions facing investigators and clinicians is whether this early increase in events is later offset by a reduction, perhaps related to improved lipid profiles or other physiologic changes. Among the studies of primary prevention included in our meta-analyses, only one large, high-quality, case–control study (15) suggests an early increased risk for CAD events (relative risk for myocardial infarction was 1.5 during the first year) that decreases with time. Four other studies evaluating estrogen use in the secondary prevention of CAD also suggest an increase in early CVD events in association with estrogen, which later decreases (77–80). In addition, increased rates of clotting in the first 2 years of HRT use are supported by a recent meta-analysis of thrombosis and HRT (81). Finally, a recent study of HRT use in the secondary prevention of stroke showed a marked increase in stroke risk during the first 6 months of use (relative risk, 2.3) that decreased to 1.1 after 33 months of use (4). Thus, several forms of evidence suggest increased rates of cardiovascular, coronary, and thrombotic events in the first 2 to 3 years of HRT use.

In summary, on the basis of this review and meta-analysis, and after extrapolation from two trials of secondary prevention, there is good reason to question the results of observational studies supporting the use of HRT in the primary prevention of CVD and CAD. Because of the limitations of observational studies, randomized, controlled trials are the best way to evaluate the relationship between HRT and CVD or CAD. We hope that such trials will yield better information in the near future. Until such information is available, the primary prevention of CVD and CAD in women should focus on proven strategies to reduce CVD and CAD risk. On the basis of current evidence, we do not advise consideration of CVD prevention when discussing HRT use with women.

Addendum: One week before this article went to press, the WHI reported the results of a randomized trial comparing estrogen plus progesterone with placebo (82). The data safety monitoring board halted the study because the risk for breast cancer exceeded a prespecified level. The report included CVD outcomes that are highly pertinent to this review of the cardiovascular effects of HRT. This addendum summarizes the WHI cardiovascular outcomes.

The study recruited 50- to 79-year-old postmenopausal women by direct letter solicitation and a study-awareness media campaign and randomly assigned 16 608 of them to take 0.625 mg of conjugated equine estrogens plus 2.5 mg of progesterone acetate in a single tablet or an identical placebo. Follow-up was by semiannual structured interview and self-administered questionnaire with annual in-clinic visits. Cardiovascular outcomes included coronary heart disease (CHD) (defined as acute myocardial infarction, silent myocardial infarction, or coronary heart disease death), as determined at each study center by a blinded adjudicator who used prespecified diagnostic criteria. The authors expressed the primary outcomes as hazard ratios (HRs) with two types of 95% CIs. Nominal CIs corresponded to the results of a simple trial with one outcome; adjusted CIs corrected for many end point determinations over time and were wider than nominal CIs. The authors based their conclusions on the nominal CIs (shown here).

After a mean of 5.2 years of follow-up, the annual rate of CHD was 37 per 10 000 women in the HRT group and 30 per 10 000 women in the placebo group (HR, 1.29 [CI, 1.02 to 1.63]). The annual stroke rate was 29 per 10 000 women in the HRT group and 21 per 10 000 women in the placebo group (HR, 1.41 [CI, 1.07 to 1.85]). The rates of coronary artery bypass grafting and percutaneous transluminal coronary angioplasty were 42 and 41 per 10 000 women in the HRT and placebo groups, respectively. The curves showing the cumulative hazard of CHD diverged shortly after randomization and showed no signs of converging at any time after follow-up. Annual rates of cardiovascular death were 15 per 10 000 women in the HRT group and 13 per 10 000 women in the placebo group.

A subgroup analysis of women who met the entry criteria of the HERS study (68) (previous myocardial infarction or revascularization) had the same results as the women who had no previous CHD. The increased risk for CHD was present in all strata (age, ethnicity, antecedent CHD risk). Limitations of the study included a very high rate of discontinuing HRT (which should have biased the results toward no effect of HRT). The study could not apportion the increased disease risk between estrogen and progesterone.

The WHI results underscore the main conclusion of our review and meta-analyses: Reducing CVD or CHD is not a valid reason for using HRT. Indeed, the WHI confirms the unexpected finding of the HERS study by showing that HRT increases the risk for CHD. According to the WHI results, 10 000 women would suffer an additional 7 CHD events per year if they took HRT. Women at higher baseline risk for CHD are likely to suffer even more events if they take HRT.

APPENDIX: BAYESIAN STATISTICAL MODEL

Four outcomes were analyzed separately: the incidence and mortality of CVD and CAD. Studies contributed multiple data points if they reported separate results for current and past users of HRT. Such studies almost never reported results for the combined group of "ever" HRT users. The results from studies that did not distinguish current users from past users were categorized

under "ever" users. The measure of "any use" was created for this meta-analysis and includes data from studies measuring only "ever" use with data from studies measuring "current," "past," or "never" use. Any use equals ever + current + past use and is a global measure of use. All studies reported relative risk estimates using either odds ratios or hazard ratios. Adjusted relative risks were used because they represent the original authors' best estimate of the relative risk. The logarithm of the relative risk (logRR) is used as the data point for the effect size since it is assumed to be normally distributed. Standard errors for logRR were calculated from reported CIs or P values.

The mean logRR for study or data point i is defined as μ_i, which has the general form $\mu_i = \beta_0 + \beta_1 x_{i,1} + \ldots + \beta_j x_{i,j}$, where the $x_{i,j}$ are indicator variables for study-level factors. In the presence of no study-level covariates, $\mu_i = \beta_0$. Study-level factors examined in the analysis include study design (cohort; case–control; and randomized, controlled trial); HRT exposure type (unopposed estrogen, combined therapy, and unspecified HRT); study quality (fair and good); HRT exposure status (current, past, and ever use); and whether the study adjusted for socioeconomic status, alcohol use, exercise, or cholesterol level.

Since studies measure and report HRT use differently, we wanted to preserve stratification by exposure status. However, we also wanted to allow for the estimation of a global measure of relative risk associated with any HRT exposure and for variation between status categories. To do this, we created the category of "any HRT use" by specifying a hierarchical model. Under this model, $\mu_i = \beta_{current} x_{i,current} + \beta_{past} x_{i,past} + \beta_{ever} x_{i,ever} + \beta_1 x_{i,1} + \ldots + \beta_j x_{i,j}$, and $x_{i,current}$, $x_{i,past}$, $x_{i,ever}$ are indicator variables for whether the data point i corresponds to the exposure category. $\beta_{current}$, β_{past}, and β_{ever} are assumed to have normal distribution with a common mean, μ_{anyHRT}, and variance, σ^2_{anyHRT}. The global effect of any exposure is represented by μ_{anyHRT}. Variance among exposure categories is represented by σ^2_{anyHRT}. The model allows for further stratification by adding terms to μ_i.

The logarithm of the relative risk is assumed to have the following distribution: $\log RR_i \sim \text{Normal}(\mu_i + z_i \sqrt{\tau^2}, s^2_i)$, where $z_i \sim \text{Normal}(0,1)$ and s_i is the standard error calculated from reported CIs or P values. τ^2 represents between-study variance and z_i represents the deviation between the logRR of the individual study or data point and the population. Under a fixed-effects model, $\tau^2 = 0$; under a random-effects model, $\tau^2 > 0$. The model is estimated by using a Bayesian data analytic framework ADDIN ENRfu (16). The data were analyzed by using WinBUGS (MRC Biostatistics Unit, Cambridge, United Kingdom) (83), which uses Gibbs sampling to simulate posterior probability distributions. Noninformative (proper) prior probability distributions were used. Specifically, Normal(0, 10^6) prior distributions were used for β_j, $\beta_{current}$, β_{past}, and β_{ever}, and inverse γ (0,001, 0.001) prior distributions were used for τ^2 and σ^2_{anyHRT}. Five separate Markov chains with various initial values were used to generate draws from posterior distributions. Point estimates (mean) and 95% credible intervals (2.5 and 97.5 percentiles) were derived from the subsequent 5 × 2000 draws after reasonable convergence of the five chains was attained.

Appendix Figure. Search methods and results.

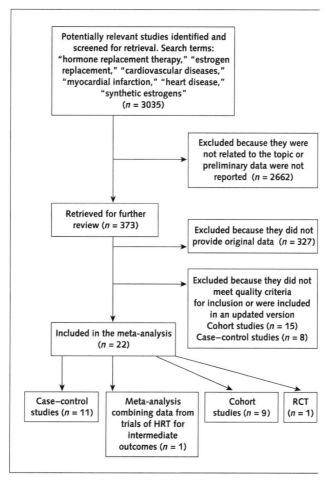

HRT = hormone replacement therapy; RCT = randomized, controlled trial.

Appendix Table 1. Characterization of Hormone Replacement Therapy Use in Case–Control Studies: Assessment and Definitions*

Study (Reference), Year	Quality	Assessment of HRT Use	Definition of HRT Use
Pfeffer (53), 1978	Fair	File of estrogen prescriptions 1964–1974	Ever, current, and never use not defined. Continuous use = not interrupted over 30 d
Thompson et al. (46), 1989	Fair	Medical record review	Use = receiving ≥2 prescriptions
Croft and Hannaford (12), 1989	Fair	Medical record review	Use/nonuse not defined
Beard et al. (54), 1989	Fair	Medical record review	Current, ever, former use not specified
Hernandez Avila et al. (49), 1990	Fair	Pharmacy record review	Current use = using 12 mo after receiving prescription, recent use = used 12–23 mo after last prescription, nonuse = no use ever or >23 mo since last use
Rosenberg et al. (15), 1993	Good	Personal or telephone interview	Use = >1 mo, nonuse = <1 mo
Mann et al. (51), 1994	Fair	Computer records	Current use = record of HRT prescription in 6 mo before index date
Grodstein et al. (40), 1997	Good	Baseline questionnaires beginning 1976 and updated biennially to 1992	Hormone use defined according to questionnaire before patient's death or disease leading to death. Current and past use not defined
Heckbert et al. (52), 1997	Fair	Pharmacy database	Ever use = 2 prescriptions, current use = filled enough to reach index date
Sidney et al. (14), 1997	Good	Personal interview	Lifetime HRT use assessed, both current and past; current and past not specifically defined
Varas-Lorenzo et al. (50), 2000	Good	National formulary	Nonuse = no prescription ever, current/recent use = use within 6 mo of the index date, past use = women stopping therapy 6 mo before index date

* HRT = hormone replacement therapy.

Appendix Table 2. **Characterization of Hormone Replacement Therapy Use in Cohort Studies: Assessment, Prevalence, and Definitions***

Study (Reference), Year	Quality	Ever Use of HRT, %	Assessment of HRT Use	Definition of HRT Use
Wilson et al. (11), 1985	Good		Biennial questionnaire over 10 y	Ever use = one report of use, nonuse not defined
Bush et al. (42), 1987	Good	26	Personal interview	Use = use within 2 wk of second visit
Petitti et al. (43), 1987	Fair	NR	Questionnaire with annual updates through 1977	Never/ever use not defined
Criqui et al. (41), 1988	Fair	39	One questionnaire in 1972, repeated 9 y later	Current use/nonuse not defined but characterized with both questionnaires
Wolf et al. (44), 1991	Fair	21	Questionnaires between 1982–1984, 2 y apart	Ever or nonuse not defined
Folsom et al. (45), 1995	Good	38	Questionnaire 1985	Former, current, ever use not defined
Grodstein et al. (48), 2000	Good	51	Questionnaires beginning 1976 and updated biennially	Current and ever use not defined
Cauley et al. (39), 1997	Good	36	Questionnaire at baseline with one update in 1991	Never use = <1 y, current use = >1 y, former use = past use of <1 y
Sourander et al. (13), 1998	Fair	22	Baseline questionnaire in 1987 and three biennial follow-up questionnaires	Current use = use at baseline, former use = use before baseline, never use = no use before or after baseline

* HRT = hormone replacement therapy.

Appendix Table 3. **Reasons for Poor Quality Rating and Exclusion from Meta-Analyses***

Study (Reference), Year	Effect Size	Reasons for Poor Rating and Exclusion				
		No or Poor Control of Confounding	Nonrepresentative Cohort or Cases	Outcomes Poorly Defined	Exposure Poorly Characterized	Bias in Control Selection
Cohort						
Byrd et al. (24), 1977	SMR, 13/35	Yes	Yes	Yes	Yes	
McMahon (25), 1978	RR, 0.4	Yes				
Hammond et al. (26), 1979	0.2 (estimated)	Yes	Yes		Yes	
Henderson et al. (27), 1986	RR, 0.54	Yes				
Hunt et al. (28), 1990	RR, 0.40/0.41	Yes	Yes	Yes		
Henderson et al. (29), 1991	RR, 0.60–0.79	Yes				
Falkeborn et al. (30), 1992	RR, 0.73	Yes	Yes			
Lafferty and Fiske (31), 1994	RR, 0.34	Yes	Yes			
Sturgeon et al. (32), 1995	RR, 0.3	Yes				
Ettinger et al. (33), 1996	RR, 0.4/0.27	Yes	Yes			
Schairer et al. (34), 1997	SMR, 0.69	Yes	Yes			
Case–control						
Talbot et al. (17), 1977	Not reported	Yes	Yes			
Jick et al. (19), 1978	OR, 7.5	Yes	Yes		Yes	Yes
Adam et al. (18), 1981	Not reported	Yes	Yes			Yes
Ross et al. (21), 1981	0.43/0.57	Yes				Yes
Szklo et al. (22), 1984	Not reported	Yes				
La Vecchia et al. (20), 1987	Not reported	Yes				

* OR = odds ratio; RR = relative risk; SMR = standardized mortality ratio.

Appendix Table 4. **Cardiovascular Disease Mortality and Hormone Replacement Therapy***

Study (Reference), Year	Quality	Design	Patients, *n*	Hormone Exposure Status	Relative Risk (95% CI)
Wilson et al. (11), 1985	Good	Cohort	1234	Ever	1.94 (NS)
Petitti et al. (43), 1987	Fair	Cohort	6093	Ever	0.60 (0.3–1.1)
Bush et al. (42), 1987	Good	Cohort	2270	Current	0.63†
Criqui et al. (41), 1988	Fair	Cohort	1868	Ever	0.96 (0.65–1.43)
Wolf et al. (44), 1991	Fair	Cohort	1944	Ever	0.66 (0.48–0.90)
Cauley et al. (39), 1997	Good	Cohort	9704	Current	0.46 (0.29–0.73)
				Past	0.86 (0.65–1.15)
Grodstein et al. (40), 1997	Good	Nested case–control	3637	Current high CVD risk	0.51 (0.45–0.57)
				Current low CVD risk	0.89 (0.62–1.28)
Sourander et al. (13), 1998	Fair	Cohort	7944	Current	0.21 (0.08–0.59)
				Past	0.75 (0.41–1.37)

* All studies were adjusted for age and hypertension. HDL = high-density lipoprotein; HRT = hormone replacement therapy; LDL = low-density lipoprotein; NS = not stated.
† *P* > 0.2.

Appendix Table 5. **Coronary Artery Disease Mortality and Hormone Replacement Therapy***

Study (Reference), Year	Quality	Design	Patients, *n*	Hormone Exposure Status	Relative Risk (95% CI)
Criqui et al. (41), 1988	Fair	Cohort	1868	Ever	0.99 (0.59–1.67)
Folsom et al. (45), 1995	Good	Cohort	41 000	Current	0.82 (0.47–1.43)
				Past	0.57 (0.38–0.85)
Grodstein et al. (40), 1997	Good	Nested case–control	3637	Current	0.47 (0.32–0.69)
				Past	0.99 (0.75–1.30)
Cauley et al. (39), 1997	Good	Cohort	9704	Current	0.49 (0.26–0.93)
				Past	0.82 (0.55–1.23)
Sourander et al. (13), 1998	Fair	Cohort	7944	Current	0.19 (0.05–0.77)
				Past	0.64 (0.27–1.47)

* All studies were adjusted for age, hypertension, diabetes mellitus, and body mass index. HDL = high-density lipoprotein; HRT = hormone replacement therapy; LDL = low-density lipoprotein.

Appendix Table 6. **Cardiovascular Disease Incidence and Hormone Replacement Therapy***

Study (Reference), Year	Quality	Design	Patients, *n*	Hormone Type	Hormone Exposure Status	Relative Risk (95% CI)
Wilson et al. (11), 1985	Fair	Cohort	1234	HRT	Ever	1.76†
Thompson et al. (46), 1989	Good	Case–control	603	HRT	Ever	1.29 (0.82–2.00)
				ERT	Ever	1.09 (0.65–1.82)
				CHRT	Ever	1.16 (0.43–3.12)
Hemminki and McPherson (47), 1997	Good	Meta-analysis		HRT	Short term	1.39 (0.48–3.95)
Sourander et al. (13), 1998	Fair	Cohort	7944	HRT	Current	1.07 (0.86–1.32)
					Past	1.11 (0.89–1.39)

* All studies except Hemminki and McPherson (47) were adjusted for age, hypertension, and smoking; no studies were adjusted for exercise. CHRT = combined hormone replacement therapy; ERT = estrogen replacement therapy; HDL = high-density lipoprotein; HRT = hormone replacement therapy; LDL = low-density lipoprotein.
† *P* < 0.01.

Appendix Table 4—**Continued**

		Cardiovascular Disease Risk Factors Included in Multivariable Models					
Diabetes Mellitus	Cholesterol Level	LDL/HDL Cholesterol Level	Smoking	Body Mass Index	Alcohol	Socioeconomic Status and Education	Other
		Yes	Yes	Yes	Yes		
			Yes	Yes	Yes	Yes	Marital status
		Yes	Yes	Yes			
Yes	Yes		Yes	Yes		Yes	Glucose level
	Yes		Yes	Yes		Yes	Previous myocardial infarction
Yes			Yes	Yes	Yes	Yes	Surgical menopause, health status, clinic, stroke, exercise
Yes	Yes		Yes	Yes			Age at menopause, type of menopause, oral contraceptive use, family history
Yes			Yes	Yes		Yes	Coronary artery disease, congestive heart failure

Appendix Table 5—**Continued**

	Cardiovascular Disease Risk Factors Included in Multivariable Models					
Cholesterol	LDL/HDL Cholesterol Level	Smoking	Alcohol	Socioeconomic Status and Education	Exercise	Other
Yes		Yes		Yes		Glucose level
			Yes		Yes	Waist-to-hip ratio, marital status
Yes		Yes				Family history, age at menopause, type of menopause, oral contraceptive use
		Yes	Yes	Yes	Yes	Surgical menopause, clinic, stroke, health status
		Yes		Yes		Coronary artery disease, congestive heart failure

Appendix Table 6—**Continued**

	Cardiovascular Disease Risk Factors Included in Multivariable Models					
Diabetes Mellitus	Cholesterol Level	LDL/HDL Cholesterol Level	Body Mass Index	Alcohol	Socioeconomic Status and Education	Other
	Yes	Yes	Yes	Yes		
Yes						Family history, marital status, myocardial infarction, stroke, deep venous thrombosis
Yes			Yes		Yes	

From Veterans Affairs Medical Center and Oregon Health & Science University, Portland, Oregon; and American College of Physicians–American Society of Internal Medicine, Philadelphia, Pennsylvania.

Note: This manuscript is based on a longer systematic evidence review that was reviewed by outside experts and representatives of professional societies. A complete list of peer reviewers is available in the complete report, which can be accessed online at www.ahrq.gov/clinic/uspstfix.htm.

Disclaimer: Review of this material does not imply agreement with or endorsement of the conclusions of this article, which are solely those of the authors. No statement in this article should be construed as official policy of the Agency for Healthcare Research and Quality.

As a coauthor, Dr. Sox did not participate in the review process or in the decision to accept the manuscript for publication.

Acknowledgments: The authors thank Steven Teutsch, MD, MPH; Janet Allan, PhD, RN; and David Atkins, MD, MPH, from the U.S. Preventive Services Task Force and Mark Helfand, MD, MS; Heidi Nelson, MD, MPH; and Gary Miranda, MA, from the Oregon Health & Science University Evidence-based Practice Center for their helpful comments on earlier versions of this review. They also thank Susan Wingenfeld and Jim Wallace for assistance in manuscript preparation.

Grant Support: This study was conducted by the Oregon Health & Science University Evidence-based Practice Center under contract to the Agency for Healthcare Research and Quality (contract no. 290-97-0018, task order no. 2), Rockville, Maryland.

Requests for Single Reprints: Reprints are available from the AHRQ Web site at www.preventiveservices.ahrq.gov and in print through the AHRQ Publications Clearinghouse.

Current author addresses, the Appendix, the Appendix Tables, and the Appendix Figure are available at www.annals.org.

Current Author Addresses: Dr. Humphrey and Mr. Chan: Oregon Health & Science University, Mail Code BICC 504, 3181 SW Sam Jackson Park Road, Portland, OR 97201.
Dr. Sox: American College of Physicians–American Society of Internal Medicine, 190 N. Independence Mall West, Philadelphia, PA 19106.

References

1. National Cholesterol Education Program. Second Report of the Expert Panel on Detection, Evaluation, and Treatment of High Blood Cholesterol in Adults (Adult Treatment Panel II). Circulation. 1994;89:1333-445. [PMID: 8124825]

2. **Grady D, Applegate W, Bush T, Furberg C, Riggs B, Hulley SB.** Heart and Estrogen/progestin Replacement Study (HERS): design, methods, and baseline characteristics. Control Clin Trials. 1998;19:314-35. [PMID: 9683309]

3. **Herrington DM, Reboussin DM, Brosnihan KB, Sharp PC, Shumaker SA, Snyder TE, et al.** Effects of estrogen replacement on the progression of coronary-artery atherosclerosis. N Engl J Med. 2000;343:522-9. [PMID: 10954759]

4. **Viscoli CM, Brass LM, Kernan WN, Sarrel PM, Suissa S, Horwitz RI.** A clinical trial of estrogen-replacement therapy after ischemic stroke. N Engl J Med. 2001;345:1243-9. [PMID: 11680444]

5. **Lenfant C.** Statement from Claude Lenfant, MD, NHLBI Director, on preliminary trends in the Women's Health Initiative. National Heart, Lung, and Blood Institute. 3 April 2000.

6. Effects of estrogen or estrogen/progestin regimens on heart disease risk factors in postmenopausal women. The Postmenopausal Estrogen/Progestin Interventions (PEPI) Trial. The Writing Group for the PEPI Trial. JAMA. 1995;273:199-208. [PMID: 7807658]

7. **Shlipak MG, Simon JA, Vittinghoff E, Lin F, Barrett-Connor E, Knopp RH, et al.** Estrogen and progestin, lipoprotein(a), and the risk of recurrent coronary heart disease events after menopause. JAMA. 2000;283:1845-52. [PMID: 10770146]

8. **Cushman M, Legault C, Barrett-Connor E, Stefanick ML, Kessler C, Judd HL, et al.** Effect of postmenopausal hormones on inflammation-sensitive proteins: the Postmenopausal Estrogen/Progestin Interventions (PEPI) Study. Circulation. 1999;100:717-22. [PMID: 10449693]

9. **Harris RP, Helfand M, Woolf SH, Lohr KN, Mulrow CD, Teutsch SM, et al.** Current methods of the US Preventive Services Task Force: a review of the process. Am J Prev Med. 2001;20:21-35. [PMID: 11306229]

10. **Matthews KA, Kuller LH, Wing RR, Meilahn EN, Plantinga P.** Prior to use of estrogen replacement therapy, are users healthier than nonusers? Am J Epidemiol. 1996;143:971-8. [PMID: 8629615]

11. **Wilson PW, Garrison RJ, Castelli WP.** Postmenopausal estrogen use, cigarette smoking, and cardiovascular morbidity in women over 50. The Framingham Study. N Engl J Med. 1985;313:1038-43. [PMID: 2995808]

12. **Croft P, Hannaford PC.** Risk factors for acute myocardial infarction in women: evidence from the Royal College of General Practitioners' oral contraception study. BMJ. 1989;298:165-8. [PMID: 2493841]

13. **Sourander L, Rajala T, Räihä I, Mäkinen J, Erkkola R, Helenius H.** Cardiovascular and cancer morbidity and mortality and sudden cardiac death in postmenopausal women on oestrogen replacement therapy (ERT). Lancet. 1998;352:1965-9. [PMID: 9872245]

14. **Sidney S, Petitti DB, Quesenberry CP Jr.** Myocardial infarction and the use of estrogen and estrogen-progestogen in postmenopausal women. Ann Intern Med. 1997;127:501-8. [PMID: 9313017]

15. **Rosenberg L, Palmer JR, Shapiro S.** A case-control study of myocardial infarction in relation to use of estrogen supplements. Am J Epidemiol. 1993;137:54-63. [PMID: 8434573]

16. **Sutton AJ, Abams KR, Jones DR, Sheldon TA, Song F.** Methods for Meta-analysis in Medical Research. Chichester, United Kingdom: J Wiley; 2000.

17. **Talbott E, Kuller LH, Detre K, Perper J.** Biologic and psychosocial risk factors of sudden death from coronary disease in white women. Am J Cardiol. 1977;39:858-64. [PMID: 871112]

18. **Adam S, Williams V, Vessey MP.** Cardiovascular disease and hormone replacement treatment: a pilot case-control study. Br Med J (Clin Res Ed). 1981;282:1277-8. [PMID: 6784816]

19. **Jick H, Dinan B, Rothman KJ.** Noncontraceptive estrogens and nonfatal myocardial infarction. JAMA. 1978;239:1407-9. [PMID: 204804]

20. **La Vecchia C, Franceschi S, Decarli A, Pampallona S, Tognoni G.** Risk factors for myocardial infarction in young women. Am J Epidemiol. 1987;125:832-43. [PMID: 3565357].

21. **Ross RK, Paganini-Hill A, Mack TM, Arthur M, Henderson BE.** Menopausal oestrogen therapy and protection from death from ischaemic heart disease. Lancet. 1981;1:858-60. [PMID: 6112292]

22. **Szklo M, Tonascia J, Gordis L, Bloom I.** Estrogen use and myocardial infarction risk: a case-control study. Prev Med. 1984;13:510-6. [PMID: 6527992]

23. **Psaty BM, Heckbert SR, Atkins D, Lemaitre R, Koepsell TD, Wahl PW, et al.** The risk of myocardial infarction associated with the combined use of estrogens and progestins in postmenopausal women. Arch Intern Med. 1994;154:1333-9. [PMID: 8002685]

24. **Byrd BF Jr, Burch JC, Vaughn WK.** The impact of long term estrogen support after hysterectomy. A report of 1016 cases. Ann Surg. 1977;185:574-80. [PMID: 193450]

25. **McMahon B.** Cardiovascular disease and non-contraceptive oestrogen therapy. In: Oliver MF, ed. Coronary Heart Disease in Young Women. Edinburgh, Scotland: Churchill Livingstone; 1978.

26. **Hammond CB, Jelovsek FR, Lee KL, Creasman WT, Parker RT.** Effects of long-term estrogen replacement therapy. I. Metabolic effects. Am J Obstet Gynecol. 1979;133:525-36. [PMID: 443293]

27. **Henderson BE, Ross RK, Paganini-Hill A, Mack TM.** Estrogen use and cardiovascular disease. Am J Obstet Gynecol. 1986;154:1181-6. [PMID: 3717228]

28. **Hunt K, Vessey M, McPherson K.** Mortality in a cohort of long-term users of hormone replacement therapy: an updated analysis. Br J Obstet Gynaecol.

1990;97:1080-6. [PMID: 2126197]

29. Henderson BE, Paganini-Hill A, Ross RK. Decreased mortality in users of estrogen replacement therapy. Arch Intern Med. 1991;151:75-8. [PMID: 1985611]

30. Falkeborn M, Persson I, Adami HO, Bergström R, Eaker E, Lithell H, et al. The risk of acute myocardial infarction after oestrogen and oestrogen-progestogen replacement. Br J Obstet Gynaecol. 1992;99:821-8. [PMID: 1419993]

31. Lafferty FW, Fiske ME. Postmenopausal estrogen replacement: a long-term cohort study. Am J Med. 1994;97:66-77. [PMID: 8030659]

32. Sturgeon SR, Schairer C, Brinton LA, Pearson T, Hoover RN. Evidence of a healthy estrogen user survivor effect. Epidemiology. 1995;6:227-31. [PMID: 7619927]

33. Ettinger B, Friedman GD, Bush T, Quesenberry CP Jr. Reduced mortality associated with long-term postmenopausal estrogen therapy. Obstet Gynecol. 1996;87:6-12. [PMID: 8532268]

34. Schairer C, Adami HO, Hoover R, Persson I. Cause-specific mortality in women receiving hormone replacement therapy. Epidemiology. 1997;8:59-65. [PMID: 9116097]

35. Grodstein F, Stampfer MJ, Manson JE, Colditz GA, Willett WC, Rosner B, et al. Postmenopausal estrogen and progestin use and the risk of cardiovascular disease. N Engl J Med. 1996;335:453-61. [PMID: 8672166]

36. Stampfer MJ, Willett WC, Colditz GA, Rosner B, Speizer FE, Hennekens CH. A prospective study of postmenopausal estrogen therapy and coronary heart disease. N Engl J Med. 1985;313:1044-9. [PMID: 4047106]

37. Stampfer MJ, Colditz GA, Willett WC, Manson JE, Rosner B, Speizer FE, et al. Postmenopausal estrogen therapy and cardiovascular disease. Ten-year follow-up from the nurses' health study. N Engl J Med. 1991;325:756-62. [PMID: 1870648]

38. Eaker E, Chesebro JH, Sacks FM, Wenger NK, Whisnant JP, Winston M. Special report: cardiovascular disease in women. Special writing group. Heart Dis Stroke. 1994;3:114-9. [PMID: 8199764]

39. Cauley JA, Seeley DG, Browner WS, Ensrud K, Kuller LH, Lipschutz RC, et al. Estrogen replacement therapy and mortality among older women. The study of osteoporotic fractures. Arch Intern Med. 1997;157:2181-7. [PMID: 9342994]

40. Grodstein F, Stampfer MJ, Colditz GA, Willett WC, Manson JE, Joffe M, et al. Postmenopausal hormone therapy and mortality. N Engl J Med. 1997;336:1769-75. [PMID: 9187066]

41. Criqui MH, Suarez L, Barrett-Connor E, McPhillips J, Wingard DL, Garland C. Postmenopausal estrogen use and mortality. Results from a prospective study in a defined, homogeneous community. Am J Epidemiol. 1988;128:606-14. [PMID: 3414664]

42. Bush TL, Barrett-Connor E, Cowan LD, Criqui MH, Wallace RB, Suchindran CM, et al. Cardiovascular mortality and noncontraceptive use of estrogen in women: results from the Lipid Research Clinics Program Follow-up Study. Circulation. 1987;75:1102-9. [PMID: 3568321]

43. Petitti DB, Perlman JA, Sidney S. Noncontraceptive estrogens and mortality: long-term follow-up of women in the Walnut Creek Study. Obstet Gynecol. 1987;70:289-93. [PMID: 3627576]

44. Wolf PH, Madans JH, Finucane FF, Higgins M, Kleinman JC. Reduction of cardiovascular disease-related mortality among postmenopausal women who use hormones: evidence from a national cohort. Am J Obstet Gynecol. 1991;164:489-94. [PMID: 1992690]

45. Folsom AR, Mink PJ, Sellers TA, Hong CP, Zheng W, Potter JD. Hormonal replacement therapy and morbidity and mortality in a prospective study of postmenopausal women. Am J Public Health. 1995;85:1128-32. [PMID: 7625511]

46. Thompson SG, Meade TW, Greenberg G. The use of hormonal replacement therapy and the risk of stroke and myocardial infarction in women. J Epidemiol Community Health. 1989;43:173-8. [PMID: 2592907]

47. Hemminki E, McPherson K. Impact of postmenopausal hormone therapy on cardiovascular events and cancer: pooled data from clinical trials. BMJ. 1997;315:149-53. [PMID: 9251544]

48. Grodstein F, Manson JE, Colditz GA, Willett WC, Speizer FE, Stampfer MJ. A prospective, observational study of postmenopausal hormone therapy and primary prevention of cardiovascular disease. Ann Intern Med. 2000;133:933-41. [PMID: 11119394]

49. Hernandez Avila M, Walker AM, Jick H. Use of replacement estrogens and the risk of myocardial infarction. Epidemiology. 1990;1:128-33. [PMID: 2073499]

50. Varas-Lorenzo C, García-Rodríguez LA, Perez-Gutthann S, Duque-Oliart A. Hormone replacement therapy and incidence of acute myocardial infarction. A population-based nested case-control study. Circulation. 2000;101:2572-8. [PMID: 10840007]

51. Mann RD, Lis Y, Chukwujindu J, Chanter DO. A study of the association between hormone replacement therapy, smoking and the occurrence of myocardial infarction in women. J Clin Epidemiol. 1994;47:307-12. [PMID: 8138842]

52. Heckbert SR, Weiss NS, Koepsell TD, Lemaitre RN, Smith NL, Siscovick DS, et al. Duration of estrogen replacement therapy in relation to the risk of incident myocardial infarction in postmenopausal women. Arch Intern Med. 1997;157:1330-6. [PMID: 9201007]

53. Pfeffer RI, Whipple GH, Kurosaki TT, Chapman JM. Coronary risk and estrogen use in postmenopausal women. Am J Epidemiol. 1978;107:479-97. [PMID: 665662]

54. Beard CM, Kottke TE, Annegers JF, Ballard DJ. The Rochester Coronary Heart Disease Project: effect of cigarette smoking, hypertension, diabetes, and steroidal estrogen use on coronary heart disease among 40- to 59-year-old women, 1960 through 1982. Mayo Clin Proc. 1989;64:1471-80. [PMID: 2557493]

55. Nachtigall LE, Nachtigall RH, Nachtigall RD, Beckman EM. Estrogen replacement therapy II: a prospective study in the relationship to carcinoma and cardiovascular and metabolic problems. Obstet Gynecol. 1979;54:74-9. [PMID: 221871]

56. Stampfer MJ, Colditz GA. Estrogen replacement therapy and coronary heart disease: a quantitative assessment of the epidemiologic evidence. Prev Med. 1991;20:47-63. [PMID: 1826173]

57. Grady D, Rubin SM, Petitti DB, Fox CS, Black D, Ettinger B, et al. Hormone therapy to prevent disease and prolong life in postmenopausal women. Ann Intern Med. 1992;117:1016-37. [PMID: 1443971]

58. Barrett-Connor E, Grady D. Hormone replacement therapy, heart disease, and other considerations. Annu Rev Public Health. 1998;19:55-72. [PMID: 9611612]

59. Rose G, Marmot MG. Social class and coronary heart disease. Br Heart J. 1981;45:13-9. [PMID: 7459161]

60. Barrett-Connor E. Postmenopausal estrogen and prevention bias. Ann Intern Med. 1991;115:455-6. [PMID: 1872493]

61. Persson I, Bergkvist L, Lindgren C, Yuen J. Hormone replacement therapy and major risk factors for reproductive cancers, osteoporosis, and cardiovascular diseases: evidence of confounding by exposure characteristics. J Clin Epidemiol. 1997;50:611-8. [PMID: 9180654]

62. Derby CA, Hume AL, McPhillips JB, Barbour MM, Carleton RA. Prior and current health characteristics of postmenopausal estrogen replacement therapy users compared with nonusers. Am J Obstet Gynecol. 1995;173:544-50. [PMID: 7645633]

63. Bush TL. Evidence for primary and secondary prevention of coronary artery disease in women taking oestrogen replacement therapy. Eur Heart J. 1996;17 Suppl D:9-14. [PMID: 8869876]

64. Humphrey LL, Takano LM, Chan B, Sox H. Postmenopausal Hormone Replacement Therapy and Cardiovascular Disease. Systematic Evidence Review No. 10. Rockville, MD: Agency for Healthcare Research and Quality [In press].

65. Takano L, Chan B, Humphrey LL. Postmenopausal hormone replacement therapy and stroke: a meta-analysis [Abstract]. J Gen Intern Med. 2001;16(Suppl. 1):177.

66. Vandenbroucke JP. How much of the cardioprotective effect of postmenopausal estrogens is real? [Editorial] Epidemiology. 1995;6:207-8. [PMID: 7619923]

67. Redelmeier DA, Tan SH, Booth GL. The treatment of unrelated disorders in patients with chronic medical diseases. N Engl J Med. 1998;338:1516-20. [PMID: 9593791]

68. Hulley S, Grady D, Bush T, Furberg C, Herrington D, Riggs B, et al. Randomized trial of estrogen plus progestin for secondary prevention of coronary heart disease in postmenopausal women. Heart and Estrogen/progestin Replacement Study (HERS) Research Group. JAMA. 1998;280:605-13. [PMID: 9718051]

69. **Petitti DB.** Hormone replacement therapy and heart disease prevention: experimentation trumps observation [Editorial]. JAMA. 1998;280:650-2. [PMID: 9718060]

70. **Horwitz RI, Viscoli CM, Berkman L, Donaldson RM, Horwitz SM, Murray CJ, et al.** Treatment adherence and risk of death after a myocardial infarction. Lancet. 1990;336:542-5. [PMID: 1975045]

71. **Gallagher EJ, Viscoli CM, Horwitz RI.** The relationship of treatment adherence to the risk of death after myocardial infarction in women. JAMA. 1993; 270:742-4. [PMID: 8336377]

72. **Hulley S, Grady D, Bush T, Furberg C, Herrington D, Riggs B, et al.** Randomized trial of estrogen plus progestin for secondary prevention of coronary heart disease in postmenopausal women. Heart and Estrogen/progestin Replacement Study (HERS) Research Group. JAMA. 1998;280:605-13. [PMID: 9718051]

73. HRT Update 2001. National Institutes of Health NH, Lung, and Blood Institute. Women's Health Initiative. Accessed March 2000 at www.nhlbi.nih .gov/whi/hrt.htm.

74. **Price DT, Ridker PM.** Factor V Leiden mutation and the risks for thromboembolic disease: a clinical perspective. Ann Intern Med. 1997;127:895-903. [PMID: 9382368]

75. **Lowe G, Woodward M, Vessey M, Rumley A, Gough P, Daly E.** Thrombotic variables and risk of idiopathic venous thromboembolism in women aged 45-64 years. Relationships to hormone replacement therapy. Thromb Haemost. 2000;83:530-5. [PMID: 10780311]

76. **Psaty BM, Smith NL, Lemaitre RN, Vos HL, Heckbert SR, LaCroix AZ, et al.** Hormone replacement therapy, prothrombotic mutations, and the risk of incident nonfatal myocardial infarction in postmenopausal women. JAMA. 2001; 285:906-13. [PMID: 11180734]

77. **Grodstein F, Manson JE, Stampfer MJ.** Postmenopausal hormone use and secondary prevention of coronary events in the nurses' health study. a prospective, observational study. Ann Intern Med. 2001;135:1-8. [PMID: 11434726]

78. **Alexander KP, Newby LK, Hellkamp AS, Harrington RA, Peterson ED, Kopecky S, et al.** Initiation of hormone replacement therapy after acute myocardial infarction is associated with more cardiac events during follow-up. J Am Coll Cardiol. 2001;38:1-7. [PMID: 11451256]

79. **Heckbert SR, Kaplan RC, Weiss NS, Psaty BM, Lin D, Furberg CD, et al.** Risk of recurrent coronary events in relation to use and recent initiation of postmenopausal hormone therapy. Arch Intern Med. 2001;161:1709-13. [PMID: 11485503]

80. **Wenger NK, Knatterud GL, Canner PL.** Early risks of hormone therapy in patients with coronary heart disease [Letter]. JAMA. 2000;284:41-3. [PMID: 10872009]

81. **Miller J, Chan BK, Nelson HD.** Postmenopausal estrogen replacement and risk for venous thromboembolism: a systematic review and meta-analysis for the U.S. Preventive Services Task Force. Ann Intern Med. 2002;136:680-90. [PMID: 11992304]

82. Risks and benefits of estrogen plus progestin in healthy postmenopausal women: principal results from the Women's Health Initiative randomized trial. JAMA. 2002;288:321-33. [PMID: 12117397]

83. WinBUGS Version 1. 2. User manual program. Cambridge, UK: MRC Biostatistics Unit; 1999.

Aspirin for primary prevention of cardiovascular events

❏ The balance of benefits and harms of the use of aspirin for primary prevention of cardiovascular events is most favorable in patients at high risk for coronary heart disease (5-year risk ≥ 3%).

❏ The optimal dose of aspirin for chemoprevention is not known. Doses of 75 mg/day seem as effective as higher doses. Enteric-coated or buffered preparations do not clearly reduce the adverse gastrointestinal effects of aspirin.

❏ Evidence suggests that diabetic patients benefit equally or even more from aspirin chemoprevention than non-diabetic patients.

❏ The optimal interval for patient discussions related to aspirin therapy is unknown. Reasonable options include every 5 years starting with middle age or when other cardiovascular risk factors are detected.

Aspirin for the Primary Prevention of Cardiovascular Events: A Summary of the Evidence for the U.S. Preventive Services Task Force

Michael Hayden, MD, MPH; Michael Pignone, MD, MPH; Christopher Phillips, MD, MPH; and Cynthia Mulrow, MD, MSc

Background: The use of aspirin to prevent cardiovascular disease events in patients without a history of cardiovascular disease is controversial.

Purpose: To examine the benefits and harms of aspirin chemoprevention.

Data Sources: MEDLINE (1966 to May 2001).

Study Selection: 1) Randomized trials at least 1 year in duration that examined aspirin chemoprevention in patients without previously known cardiovascular disease and 2) systematic reviews, recent trials, and observational studies that examined rates of hemorrhagic strokes and gastrointestinal bleeding secondary to aspirin use.

Data Extraction: One reviewer read and extracted data from each included article and constructed evidence tables. A second reviewer checked the accuracy of the data extraction. Discrepancies were resolved by consensus.

Data Synthesis: Meta-analysis was performed, and the quantitative results of the review were then used to model the consequences of treating patients with different levels of baseline risk for coronary heart disease. Five trials examined the effect of aspirin on cardiovascular events in patients with no previous cardiovascular disease. For patients similar to those enrolled in the trials, aspirin reduces the risk for the combined end point of nonfatal myocardial infarction and fatal coronary heart disease (summary odds ratio, 0.72 [95% CI, 0.60 to 0.87]). Aspirin increased the risk for hemorrhagic strokes (summary odds ratio, 1.4 [CI, 0.9 to 2.0]) and major gastrointestinal bleeding (summary odds ratio, 1.7 [CI, 1.4 to 2.1]). All-cause mortality (summary odds ratio, 0.93 [CI, 0.84 to 1.02]) was not significantly affected.

For 1000 patients with a 5% risk for coronary heart disease events over 5 years, aspirin would prevent 6 to 20 myocardial infarctions but would cause 0 to 2 hemorrhagic strokes and 2 to 4 major gastrointestinal bleeding events. For patients with a risk of 1% over 5 years, aspirin would prevent 1 to 4 myocardial infarctions but would cause 0 to 2 hemorrhagic strokes and 2 to 4 major gastrointestinal bleeding events.

Conclusions: The net benefit of aspirin increases with increasing cardiovascular risk. In the decision to use aspirin chemoprevention, the patient's cardiovascular risk and relative utility for the different clinical outcomes prevented or caused by aspirin use must be considered.

Cardiovascular disease, including ischemic coronary heart disease, stroke, and peripheral vascular disease, is the leading cause of morbidity and death in the United States (1). In 1997, the age-adjusted mortality rate due to coronary heart disease, cerebrovascular disease, and atherosclerotic disease was 194 per 100 000 persons, which is equivalent to more than 500 000 deaths per year (1). The estimated direct and indirect costs of coronary heart disease and stroke were $145 billion for 1999 (2).

Although the benefit of aspirin for patients with known cardiovascular disease is well established (3), the question of whether aspirin reduces the risk for cardiovascular disease in persons without known cardiovascular disease is controversial. Two early randomized trials of aspirin in healthy men, the U.S. Physicians' Health Study (PHS) and the British Male Doctors' Trial (BMD), had conflicting results regarding whether aspirin reduced the risk for myocardial infarction. Neither trial had sufficient power to precisely estimate major harms, such as gastrointestinal bleeding and hemorrhagic stroke (4, 5).

The results of these randomized, controlled trials were available to the members of U.S. Preventive Services Task Force at the time of their 1996 recommendation (4, 5). At that time, the Task Force found insufficient evidence to recommend for or against routine aspirin prophylaxis for the primary prevention of myocardial infarction in asymptomatic persons (6). Two additional large primary prevention trials were published in 1998, and another was reported in January 2001 (7–9). In light of the new evidence, the U.S. Preventive

Table 1. **Summary of Primary Prevention Trials***

Variable	BMD	PHS	TPT	HOT	PPP
Reference	5	4	7	8	9
Year	1988	1989	1998	1998	2001
Location	United Kingdom	United States	United Kingdom	Worldwide	Italy
Duration of therapy, y†	5.8	5	6.8	3.8	3.6
Patients (women), n	5139 (0)	22 071 (0)	2540 (0)	18 790 (8831)	4495 (2583)
Aspirin dosage	500 mg/d	325 mg every other day	75 mg/d (controlled release)	75 mg/d	100 mg/d
Control	No placebo	Placebo	Placebo	Placebo	No placebo
Additional therapies	None	β-Carotene (50% of patients)	Warfarin‡	Felodipine with or without ACE inhibitor or β-blocker	Vitamin E
Included patients	Male physicians	Male physicians	Men at high risk for heart disease	Men and women with a diastolic blood pressure of 100 to 115 mm Hg	>1 major risk factor for CHD
Age	<60 y (46.9%); 60–69 y (39.3%); 70–79 y (13.9%)	Mean, 53 y (range, 40–84 y)	Mean, 57.5 y (range, 45–69 y)	Mean, 61.5 y (range, 50–80 y)	<60 y (29%); 60–69 y (45%); 70–79 y (24%)
Quality	Fair§	Good	Good	Good	Fair§

* ACE = angiotensin-converting enzyme; BMD = British Male Doctors' Trial; CHD = coronary heart disease; HOT = Hypertension Optimal Treatment Trial; PHS = Physicians' Health Study; PPP = Primary Prevention Project; TPT = Thrombosis Prevention Trial.
† Values given are means except for the TPT value, which is the median.
‡ Data from patients who received warfarin are not included in this table.
§ No placebo control or blinding.

Services Task Force sought to reassess the value of aspirin for the primary prevention of cardiovascular events. The Task Force's assessment was performed in partnership with the Agency for Healthcare Research and Quality, Rockville, Maryland, and investigators from the RTI-UNC Evidence-based Practice Center, Research Triangle Park, North Carolina. For this review, we examined three key questions: 1) Does aspirin chemoprevention in patients without known cardiovascular disease reduce the risk for myocardial infarction, stroke, and death? 2) Does aspirin chemoprevention increase major gastrointestinal bleeding, hemorrhagic strokes, or both? 3) What is the balance of benefits and harms for aspirin therapy in patients with different levels of risk for coronary heart disease? The analytic framework of the review can be found in **Appendix Figure 1** (available at www.annals.org).

METHODS
Identification of Relevant Trials

We searched MEDLINE from 1966 to May 2001 to identify studies examining aspirin's ability to prevent cardiovascular events and its likelihood of causing adverse effects. The literature search and data extraction are detailed in the Appendix (available at www.annals.org).

Quality Assessment

We assessed the quality of the trials that examined the benefits of aspirin therapy, considering methods of randomization, blinding, analysis by intention to treat, follow-up rates, and crossover of assigned interventions. To look for differences in estimates of effect, we then performed meta-analyses using only the trials considered to be of good quality.

Modeling

We used our best estimates of the beneficial and harmful effects of aspirin chemoprevention to model its impact on populations of patients with different levels of risk for coronary heart disease. We estimated beneficial effects by using the odds ratios calculated from the meta-analyses; estimates of harmful effects were derived from other systematic reviews, supplemented by studies identified in our literature searches. We based our estimates on 1000 persons receiving aspirin for 5 years and used 95% CIs from the meta-analyses to produce plausible ranges around our point estimates. We also examined how these effects may differ for elderly persons, women, and patients with hypertension or diabetes.

Statistical Analyses

For individual trials, we calculated estimates of unadjusted odds ratios with 95% CIs (10). Because not all of the trials presented their outcomes using the same means of categorization, we contacted the investigators in some cases to determine the actual numbers of certain events and recalculated summary measures to improve comparability. We performed meta-analysis using the DerSimonian and Laird random-effects model in RevMan (Cochrane Collaboration, Oxford, United Kingdom) (11). Heterogeneity was assessed by using graphs of the outcomes and the Mantel–Haenszel chi-square test.

DATA SYNTHESIS

Literature Searches

The results of our search strategy are shown in the Appendix (available at www.annals.org). We identified 5 randomized, controlled trials that had been designed to assess the efficacy of aspirin in the primary prevention of cardiovascular disease: the British Male Doctors' Trial (BMD), the Physicians' Health Study (PHS), the Thrombosis Prevention Trial (TPT), the Hypertension Optimal Treatment Trial (HOT), and the Primary Prevention Project (PPP) (4, 5, 7–9). We excluded 2 large trials that examined the effect of aspirin in patients with diabetes or with stable angina because more than 10% of the participants had definite or suspected vascular disease (12, 13). From our search for articles on adverse effects, we identified 9 articles that examined the effect of aspirin on gastrointestinal bleeding and hemorrhagic stroke (3, 14–21).

Trial Characteristics

The characteristics of the 5 randomized trials, which included a total of more than 50 000 patients, are shown in **Table 1**. The duration of the trials ranged from 3 to 7 years. Only 2 trials (HOT and PPP) included women. Aspirin dosage was 500 mg daily in BMD and 162 mg or less per day in the other 4 trials. Most participants were middle-aged, although 4 of the 5

trials included substantial numbers of patients who were 70 to 80 years of age.

Assessment of Study Quality

Overall, the quality of the trials examining the effectiveness of aspirin was high. All 5 trials concealed allocation of randomization. Researchers and participants were blinded in 3 trials (PHS, HOT, and TPT). In BMD and PPP, participants were not blinded and were not given placebo pills. Analyses in all trials were by intention to treat. Fewer than 1% of participants were lost to follow-up in BMD, PHS, and TPT, and 2.6% were lost to follow-up in HOT. In PPP, 7.7% of patients were lost to clinical follow-up, but data on vital status were obtained from census offices for 99.3% of the total sample.

During BMD, 39% of participants in the aspirin group discontinued therapy, primarily because of dyspepsia; 11% of participants assigned to no therapy began taking aspirin during the course of the trial. In contrast, in PHS, 14% of participants crossed over to the opposing treatment groups but rates of gastrointestinal discomfort did not differ significantly in each group. In PPP, 19% of patients assigned to aspirin discontinued taking it (8% due to side effects) and 7% of patients assigned to "no aspirin" were taking aspirin at the trial's conclusion. Crossover rates were not explicitly reported in TPT and HOT, although approximately 50% of patients participating in TPT withdrew for unreported reasons. However, the rate of withdrawal in TPT did not differ between the treatment and control groups. On the basis of these features, we rated the quality of

Table 2. **Effect of Aspirin on Risk for Coronary Heart Disease in Primary Prevention Trials***

Trial (Reference)	Aspirin Events/Patients	Control Events/Patients	Odds Ratio (95% CI)	Duration of Therapy†	Annual Risk for a CHD Event among Control Patients	Approximate Vascular Events Avoided per 1000 Patients Treated per Year
	n/n (%)			*y*	*%*	*n*
BMD (5)	169/3429 (4.93)	88/1710 (5.15)	0.96 (0.73–1.24)	5.8	0.89	0.4
PHS (4)	163/11 037 (1.48)	266/11 034 (2.41)	0.61 (0.50–0.74)	5	0.48	1.9
TPT (7)	83/1268 (6.55)	107/1272 (8.41)	0.76 (0.57–1.03)	6.8	1.24	2.7
HOT (8)	82/9399 (0.87)	127/9391 (1.35)	0.64 (0.49–0.85)	3.8	0.36	1.3
PPP (9)	26/2226 (1.17)	35/2269 (1.54)	0.75 (0.45–1.26)	3.6	0.43	1.0

* BMD = British Male Doctors' Trial; CHD = coronary heart disease; HOT = Hypertension Optimal Treatment Trial; PHS = Physicians' Health Study; PPP = Primary Prevention Project; TPT = Thrombosis Prevention Trial.
† Values given are means except for the TPT value, which is the median.

Figure 1. **Meta-analysis of total coronary heart disease events.**

Study (Reference)	Aspirin, *n/n*	Control, *n/n*	OR (95% CI Random)	Weight, %	OR (95% CI Random)
BMD (5)	169 / 3429	88 / 1710		22.0	0.96 (0.73–1.24)
PHS (4)	163 / 11 037	266 / 11 034		27.8	0.61 (0.50–0.74)
TPT (7)	83 / 1268	107 / 1272		19.6	0.76 (0.57–1.03)
HOT (8)	82 / 9399	127 / 9391		20.9	0.64 (0.49–0.85)
PPP (9)	26 / 2226	35 / 2269		9.7	0.75 (0.45–1.26)
Total (95% CI)	523 / 27 359	623 / 25 676		100.0	0.72 (0.60–0.87)

0.20   0.50   1.0   2.0   5.0
Favors Aspirin   Favors Control

BMD = British Male Doctors' Trial; HOT = Hypertension Optimal Treatment Trial; OR = odds ratio; PHS = Physicians' Health Study; PPP = Primary Prevention Project; TPT = Thrombosis Prevention Trial. The result of the chi-square test for heterogeneity was 8.07 ($P = 0.089$).

PHS, TPT, and HOT as "good" and the quality of BMD and PPP as "fair."

Effect of Aspirin on Coronary Heart Disease

All trials had point estimates suggesting that aspirin prevented total coronary heart disease events, defined as nonfatal myocardial infarction or death due to coronary heart disease (fatal myocardial infarction or sudden death) (**Table 2**). In PHS and TPT, aspirin use was associated with increases in sudden death that did not reach statistical significance: 22 events with aspirin versus 12 events with placebo in PHS (odds ratio, 1.83 [95% CI, 0.91 to 3.71]) (4), and 18 events with aspirin versus 11 with placebo in TPT (odds ratio, 1.65 [CI, 0.78 to 3.51]) (22).

Meta-analysis of the 5 trials for the combined outcome of confirmed nonfatal myocardial infarction or death from coronary heart disease produced a summary odds ratio of 0.72 (CI, 0.60 to 0.87) (**Figure 1**). The Mantel–Haenszel test suggested possible heterogeneity ($P = 0.089$), reflecting the anomalous result of BMD. In that study, no difference was found in the rate of myocardial infarction between the intervention and control groups.

Mortality data for coronary heart disease (fatal myocardial infarctions and sudden death) from HOT and PPP were not reported separately in the main papers but were obtained from the authors (Hannson L. Personal communication, 2000; Roncaglioni C. Personal communication, 2001). Of the 5 trials, only PHS reported a statistically significant decrease in risk with aspirin (odds ratio, 0.64 [CI, 0.42 to 0.99]). Cumulative mortality rates for coronary heart disease in the placebo group were low, ranging from 0.15% in HOT to 2.7% in BMD and TPT. Meta-analysis of the 5 trials found a summary odds ratio of 0.87 (CI, 0.70 to 1.09) (**Figure 2**, *top*). There was no significant heterogeneity in trial results ($P > 0.2$).

Effect of Aspirin on Stroke

It is difficult to interpret the overall effect of aspirin on stroke because the effect differs according to stroke subtype (**Table 3**). Data from secondary prevention trials suggest that aspirin prevents ischemic strokes but show that aspirin can also cause hemorrhagic stroke. The effect of aspirin on the total incidence of stroke depends on the patient's underlying risk for each stroke subtype (23). Overall stroke rates were lower than expected (based on age and risk factors) in all 5 primary prevention trials (**Table 4**). In each trial, control participants who had not been given aspirin had a less than 2% incidence of total strokes over 5 years. Because of the lower-than-expected stroke rates, the individual trials had limited statistical power to reliably detect the true effect of aspirin on stroke. Point estimates in PPP and TPT suggested modest decreases in total strokes, but CIs were wide (7, 23). In HOT, no effect of aspirin on overall rates of stroke was seen. In BMD and PHS, trends toward increased risk for stroke in aspirin-treated patients were observed but did not reach statistical significance (4, 5). The summary estimate (**Figure 2**, *middle*) showed no difference in total stroke overall (odds ratio, 1.02 [CI, 0.85 to 1.23]), and the results displayed no significant heterogeneity ($P > 0.2$).

The low number of strokes and the imperfect classification of stroke subtypes limited our ability to estimate the independent effect of aspirin on ischemic stroke in primary prevention settings. Rates of ischemic stroke were not specifically reported in HOT (8), and BMD did not use neuroimaging to differentiate ischemic from hemorrhagic strokes (5). In PHS, 91 ischemic strokes were seen with aspirin and 82 were seen with placebo (odds ratio, 1.11 [CI, 0.83 to 1.50]) (5). In TPT, 10 ischemic strokes occurred in the aspirin group and 18 occurred in the placebo group (odds ratio, 0.55 [CI, 0.25 to 1.20]) (7). Fourteen ischemic strokes in the intervention group and 21 in the "no aspirin" group were reported in PPP (9).

Despite the uncertainty of stroke classification, Hart and colleagues (19) combined data from the first 4 primary prevention trials (4, 5, 7, 8) and concluded that aspirin appeared to have no effect on ischemic strokes in

Figure 2. Meta-analysis of the effect of aspirin on coronary heart disease mortality (*top*), fatal and nonfatal stroke events (*middle*), and all-cause mortality (*bottom*).

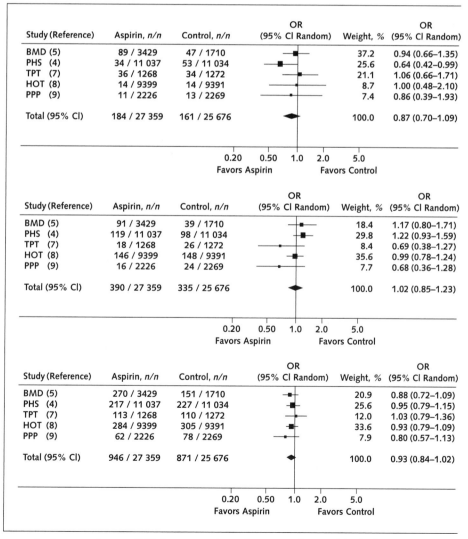

Results of the chi-square test for heterogeneity were 2.96 for coronary heart disease mortality, 5.36 for fatal and nonfatal stroke events, and 1.58 for all-cause mortality ($P > 0.2$ in all cases). BMD = British Male Doctors' Trial; HOT = Hypertension Optimal Treatment Trial; OR = odds ratio; PHS = Physicians' Health Study; PPP = Primary Prevention Project; TPT = Thrombosis Prevention Trial.

Table 3. **Estimates of the Role of Aspirin in Primary Prevention of Total Fatal and Nonfatal Stroke***

Trial (Reference)	Aspirin Events/Patients	Control Events/Patients	Odds Ratio (95% CI)	Duration of Therapy†	Annual Risk for Stroke among Control Patients	Vascular Events Avoided per 1000 Patients Treated per Year	Vascular Events Caused per 1000 Patients Treated per Year
	n/n (%)			*y*	*%*	*n*	
BMD (5)	91/3429 (2.65)	39/1710 (2.28)	1.17 (0.80–1.71)	5.8	0.39	–	0.6
PHS (4)	119/11 037 (1.08)	98/11 034 (0.89)	1.22 (0.93–1.59)	5	0.18	–	0.4
TPT (7)	18/1268 (1.42)	26/1272 (2.04)	0.69 (0.38–1.27)	6.8	0.30	0.9	–
HOT (8)	146/9399 (1.55)	148/9391 (1.58)	0.99 (0.78–1.24)	3.8	0.41	0.1	–
PPP (9)	16/2226 (0.72)	24/2269 (1.06)	0.68 (0.36–1.28)	3.6	0.29	0.9	–

* BMD = British Male Doctors' Trial; HOT = Hypertension Optimal Treatment Trial; PHS = Physicians' Health Study; PPP = Primary Prevention Project; TPT = Thrombosis Prevention Trial.
† Values given are means except for the TPT value, which is the median.

the middle-aged, relatively low-risk patients (relative risk, 1.03 [CI, 0.87 to 1.21]) (19).

Effect of Aspirin on All-Cause Mortality

None of the 5 trials found significant differences between aspirin-treated and control groups for all-cause mortality rates. Five-year mortality rates in the control groups of the individual trials ranged from 2% to 10%. The summary odds ratio for the effect of aspirin on all-cause mortality was 0.93 (CI, 0.84 to 1.02), consistent with a small or no reduction in all-cause mortality over 3 to 7 years (**Figure 2**, *bottom*).

Effectiveness of Aspirin Chemoprevention in Patient Subgroups

Most of the participants in the 5 randomized trials were middle-aged men. Limited data are available to examine whether the effect of aspirin differs in other demographic groups, including elderly persons, women, and persons with diabetes or hypertension. The following data come primarily from subgroup analyses and should be interpreted with caution.

Age

In PHS, aspirin reduced the relative risk for myocardial infarction for patients 70 to 84 years of age (relative risk, 0.49) as much as or more than it did for patients 60 to 69 years of age (relative risk, 0.46) and patients 50 to 59 years of age (relative risk, 0.58). In HOT, aspirin's effectiveness in patients older than 65 years of age (30% of the study sample) did not differ from its effect in those 50 to 64 years of age (24). In TPT, however, patients 65 to 69 years of age did not

benefit from aspirin (relative risk, 1.12) but younger patients did. Relative risks were 0.75 for patients 50 to 59 years of age and 0.61 for patients 60 to 64 years of age.

Sex

Only 2 of the 5 primary prevention trials included women (HOT and PPP). Kjeldsen and coworkers (24) performed a subgroup analysis of HOT to examine the influence of patient sex on the effectiveness of aspirin chemoprevention. Aspirin reduced the incidence of myocardial infarction in men (2.9/1000 patient-years in the aspirin group vs. 5/1000 patient-years in controls; relative risk, 0.58 [CI, 0.41 to 0.81]). However, its effect in women was smaller and not statistically significant (1.7/1000 person-years in the aspirin group vs. 2.1/1000 patient-years in controls; relative risk, 0.81 [CI, 0.49 to 1.31]). Sex differences in the effect of aspirin were not seen for stroke or all-cause mortality. In PPP, the investigators noted that women seemed to derive the same level of benefit from reduction of coronary heart disease as men, but specific data were not presented.

The question of whether sex modifies the effect of aspirin remains unclear. The Women's Health Study, a primary prevention trial that will test low-dose aspirin in approximately 40 000 patients, is expected to clarify risks and benefits among women (10).

Patients with Diabetes Mellitus

The proportion of patients with diabetes mellitus was small in each trial (PPP, 17%; HOT, 8%; PHS, 2%; BMD, 2%; TPT, 2%). In PHS, patients with diabetes derived greater benefit from aspirin than those without diabetes (relative risk, 0.39 vs. 0.60). Pooled data from aspirin trials in secondary prevention settings (23) and a single trial in diabetic patients with and without coronary heart disease (12) also suggested that diabetic patients benefit as much or more from aspirin as nondiabetic patients.

Patients with Hypertension

The influence of hypertension on the effectiveness of aspirin chemoprevention has been examined in subgroup analyses. In TPT, Meade and Brennan (22) found that aspirin reduced total cardiovascular events in patients whose systolic blood pressure was less than 130 mm Hg (relative risk, 0.59) but not in patients whose systolic blood pressure was greater than 145 mm Hg (relative risk, 1.08). Patients with systolic blood pressure between 130 and 145 mm Hg also had reduced risk (relative risk, 0.68). In PHS, patients who were taking aspirin and had systolic blood pressure greater than 150 mm Hg had a relative risk of 0.65 for myocardial infarction, compared with relative risks of 0.55 for those with systolic blood pressure between 130 and 149 mm Hg and 0.52 for those with systolic blood pressure between 110 and 129 mm Hg (4). Significant reductions in coronary heart disease events were seen in HOT among patients with treated hypertension, but HOT did not have a comparison group of patients without hypertension (8).

On the basis of these data, aspirin seems to reduce risk for coronary heart disease in patients with treated hypertension, but its effects may be attenuated in patients with poorly controlled blood pressure.

Effect of Study Quality on Effectiveness of Aspirin

We performed an additional set of meta-analyses using only the 3 trials we rated as good (PHS, TPT,

HOT). The reduction in total coronary heart disease events was slightly larger (summary odds ratio, 0.65 [CI, 0.56 to 0.75]), but other outcomes were similar to our main analysis.

Adverse Effects of Aspirin Therapy
Hemorrhagic Stroke

The event rates for hemorrhagic strokes, including intracranial hemorrhage, were higher among aspirin-exposed participants than controls in BMD, PHS, and TPT, although these differences did not reach statistical significance in any single trial (**Table 4**) (4, 5, 7). In BMD, most strokes (>60%) were of unknown cause because computed tomography was not performed in most cases (5). In HOT and PPP, hemorrhagic strokes were almost equally common in the intervention and control groups (8, 9).

Two systematic reviews and meta-analyses have examined the effect of aspirin on the incidence of hemorrhagic stroke in the primary prevention trials. Hart and colleagues (19) pooled the results of the first 4 primary prevention studies and estimated that the relative risk for hemorrhagic stroke due to long-term aspirin use was 1.36 (CI, 0.88 to 2.1). Sudlow (25) recently performed a similar analysis using all 5 trials and reached a similar effect estimate (odds ratio, 1.4 [CI, 0.9 to 2.0]). In this analysis, the estimated annual excess risk with aspirin was 0.1 event per 1000 users.

He and coworkers (3) performed a meta-analysis of 16 trials (14 secondary prevention trials and the 2 older primary prevention trials [BMD and PHS]) that reported stroke subtype. Taken together, the trials involved more than 55 000 participants. Participants had a mean age of 59 years, and 86% were men. The mean

Table 4. Estimates of the Role of Aspirin in Hemorrhagic Stroke and Intracranial Hemorrhage*

Trial (Reference)	Aspirin Events/Patients	Control Events/Patients	Odds Ratio (95% CI)	Duration of Therapy	Annual Approximate Control Group Risk	Approximate Excess Bleeding Events per 1000 Patients Treated per Year	Approximate Bleeding Events Avoided per 1000 Patients Treated per Year
	n/n (%)			*y*	*%*		*n*
BMD (5)	13/3429 (0.38)	6/1710 (0.35)	1.08 (0.41–2.85)	5.8	0.06	0.05	–
PHS (4)	23/11 037 (0.21)	12/11 034 (0.11)	1.92 (0.95–3.86)	5	0.02	0.2	–
TPT (7)	3/1268 (0.24)	2/1272 (0.16)	1.51 (0.25–9.03)	6.8	0.02	0.12	–
HOT (8)	14/9399 (0.15)	15/9391 (0.16)	0.93 (0.45–1.93)	3.8	0.04	–	0.03
PPP (9)	2/2226 (0.08)	3/2269 (0.13)	0.67 (NR)	3.6	0.04	–	0.12

* BMD = British Male Doctors' Trial; HOT = Hypertension Optimal Treatment Trial; NR = not reported; PHS = Physicians' Health Study; PPP = Primary Prevention Project; TPT = Thrombosis Prevention Trial.

Table 5. **Estimates of the Role of Aspirin in Gastrointestinal Bleeding***

Trial (Reference)	Type of Gastrointestinal Bleeding	Cumulative Incidence		P Value	Excess Bleeding Events per 1000 Patients Treated per Year	Fatal Gastrointestinal Bleeding Events	
		Aspirin Group	Control Group			Aspirin Group	Control Group
		%			← n →		
BMD (5)	Self-reported peptic ulcer disease	2.6	1.6	<0.05	1.7	3	3
PHS (4)	Upper gastrointestinal ulcers	1.5	1.3	0.08	0.4	1	0
TPT (7)	Major or intermediate bleeding†	1.7	0.8	NR	1.3	0	1
HOT (8)	Fatal and nonfatal major gastrointestinal bleeding events‡	0.8	0.4	NR	1.1	5	3
PPP (9)	Gastrointestinal bleeding§	0.8	0.2	NR	1.5	0	0

* BMD = British Male Doctors' Trial; HOT = Hypertension Optimal Treatment Trial; NR = not reported; PHS = Physicians' Health Study; PPP = Primary Prevention Project; TPT = Thrombosis Prevention Trial.
† Major bleeding included fatal and life-threatening hemorrhages that required transfusion, surgery, or both. Intermediate episodes were bleeding events that prompted patients to notify research coordinators separately from routine questionnaires.
‡ Major bleeding was not defined.
§ Described as severe but nonfatal.

dosage of aspirin was 273 mg/d, and the mean duration of treatment was 37 months. The summary relative risk for hemorrhagic stroke with aspirin use was 1.84 (CI, 1.24 to 2.74). He and coworkers estimated that aspirin increased the absolute risk for hemorrhagic stroke by 12 events (CI, 5 to 20 events) per 10 000 persons over approximately 3 years, or about 0.4 excess event per 1000 users annually. This estimate is higher than that in Sudlow's meta-analysis, which included only primary prevention trials. He and coworkers also concluded that the absolute risk for hemorrhagic stroke did not vary significantly according to preexisting cardiovascular disease, mean age, sample size, dosage of aspirin, or study duration, although the statistical power to detect such differences was low because of the small number of total events.

The small number of primary prevention trials makes it difficult to examine the influence of other factors on the relationship between aspirin and hemorrhagic stroke. He and coworkers' systematic review did not find that age was an independent predictor of risk for hemorrhagic stroke, but the power of the review to detect such differences was low. In the large Stroke Prevention in Atrial Fibrillation II trial (26), advanced age was associated with an increased incidence of bleeding during aspirin therapy in patients with atrial fibrillation. The rate of intracranial hemorrhage with aspirin use was 0.2% per year in patients 75 years of age or younger and 0.8% per year in patients older than 75 years of age.

The question of whether there is a "safe" dose of aspirin with respect to hemorrhagic stroke has been ad-

dressed only in observational studies. A case–control study from Australia (27) examined the relationship between the use of aspirin or other nonsteroidal anti-inflammatory medications and the risk for hemorrhagic stroke. Reported use of low-dosage aspirin (<1225 mg/wk) was not associated with an increased risk for hemorrhagic stroke (odds ratio, 1.00 [CI, 0.60 to 1.66]) in multivariate risk-adjusted analyses. Larger amounts of aspirin were associated with hemorrhagic stroke (odds ratio, 3.05 [CI, 1.02 to 9.14]).

Gastrointestinal Bleeding

Aspirin increased the rates of gastrointestinal bleeding in all 5 primary prevention trials. Detection of events, definition of a "significant" bleeding event, and reporting of location of upper gastrointestinal bleeding varied across trials (**Table 5**).

Pooling the data on major extracranial bleeding from the 5 primary prevention trials, Sudlow estimated that aspirin increased the risk for major extracranial bleeding (odds ratio, 1.7 [CI, 1.4 to 2.1]). This translates to an excess risk for major, mostly gastrointestinal bleeding events of 0.7 (CI, 0.4 to 0.9) per 1000 patients treated with aspirin per year (25).

Several other systematic reviews have examined the risk for gastrointestinal bleeding with aspirin use (14–16, 28). Roderick and associates (15) performed a systematic review of 21 trials from the Antiplatelet Trialists' Collaboration (1990), all but 1 of which were secondary prevention studies. They estimated pooled odds ratios of 1.5 to 2.0 for gastrointestinal bleeding due to aspirin. The risk for bleeding was greater in trials that used dosages exceeding 300 mg/d than in trials using lower dosages, but the difference was not statistically significant. Dickinson and Prentice (14) updated the Roderick review using data from trials that lasted more than 1 month. They determined that ongoing use of aspirin would produce an excess of two major gastrointestinal bleeding events per 1000 patient-years of exposure.

Recently, Derry and Loke (28) performed a systematic review and meta-analysis of trials published through 1999 that examined the risk for gastrointestinal hemorrhage with long-term (>1 year) aspirin use. They identified 24 randomized trials with a total of 66 000 participants and an average duration of 28 months. Aspirin use increased the odds of gastrointestinal hemorrhage (summary odds ratio, 1.68 [CI, 1.51 to 1.88]). The absolute risk difference was 1.05%. The authors estimated that treating 106 patients with aspirin for 28 months would lead to one excess episode of hemorrhage. Stalnikowicz-Darvasi performed a meta-analysis of 9 trials of low-dose aspirin prevention that had lasted at least 3 months (16); the pooled odds ratio for all gastrointestinal bleeding was 1.5 (CI, 1.3 to 1.7).

Derry and Loke (28) used meta-regression to examine the effect of aspirin dosage on the incidence of gastrointestinal hemorrhage and did not detect a statistically significant relationship (odds ratio, 1.015 [CI, 0.984 to 1.047] per 100-mg change in dose; $P > 0.2$). Cappelleri and colleagues (17) performed a meta-analysis and meta-regression to determine the effect of dosage on the risk for gastrointestinal bleeding with aspirin use among persons at high risk for vascular disease. They did not find a relationship between aspirin dose and risk for gastrointestinal bleeding but concluded that the likelihood of other gastrointestinal symptoms (for example, dyspepsia) increased with higher aspirin doses.

In a case–control study in Great Britain, Weil and coworkers (20) found that the risk for gastrointestinal bleeding was greater with all doses of aspirin compared with no usage but was higher with larger doses (odds ratios, 2.3 for 75 mg/d vs. 3.9 for 300 mg/d). Kelly and associates (18), in another case–control study, found an estimated relative odds of 2.6 for dosages less than 325 mg/d and 5.8 for larger doses. Enteric-coated or buffered preparations did not seem to reduce risk. Concomitant use of other nonsteroidal anti-inflammatory agents or anticoagulants further increased risk.

Table 6. **Summary Estimates of the Effect of Aspirin***

Outcome	Odds Ratio (95% CI)
Benefits	
Myocardial infarction	0.72 (0.60–0.87)
CHD death	0.87 (0.70–1.09)
Total stroke	1.02 (0.85–1.23)
All-cause mortality	0.93 (0.84–1.02)
Harms	
Hemorrhagic stroke	1.4 (0.9–2.0)
Major gastrointestinal bleeding event	1.7 (1.4–2.1)

* CHD = coronary heart disease.

Silagy and colleagues (21) examined the adverse effects of low-dosage aspirin (100 mg/d) in a randomized, double-blind, placebo-controlled trial of 400 patients older than 70 years of age who did not have preexisting vascular disease. The reported absolute rate of any gastrointestinal bleeding in the aspirin group was 3% after 1 year. One case of bleeding duodenal ulcer required hospitalization for transfusion and emergency surgery. No gastrointestinal bleeding was reported for patients in the control group. Existing meta-analyses have not determined (3) or have not examined (28) whether age modifies the effect of aspirin on gastrointestinal hemorrhage, although cohort data suggest that the absolute risk for bleeding is higher in elderly persons (26).

Gastrointestinal Bleeding: Summary

Aspirin chemoprevention, even at low doses, seems to increase the risk for gastrointestinal bleeding by a factor of 1.5 to 2. The absolute excess risk for major bleeding events appears to be approximately 3 per 1000 middle-aged men receiving low-dose aspirin for more than 5 years. Higher rates (up to 2/1000 persons per year) are likely in elderly patients and perhaps among those using higher doses of aspirin.

Modeling a Risk Threshold for Aspirin Chemoprevention

Table 6 presents a summary of the effect estimates for the most important outcomes related to aspirin use. The estimates are based on the results of meta-analyses of data from the 5 primary prevention trials and therefore are most valid for middle-aged men (50 to 65 years of age) taking low-dosage aspirin ($\leq$162 mg/d).

We used our best estimates of the beneficial and harmful effects of aspirin chemoprevention to model its impact on populations of patients with different levels of

Table 7. **Estimated Benefits and Harms of Aspirin Therapy for Patients at Different Levels of Risk for Coronary Heart Disease Events***

Outcome	Estimated 5-Year Risk for CHD Events at Baseline		
	1%	3%	5%
Effect on all-cause mortality	No change	No change	No change
CHD events avoided, n	3 (1–4)	8 (4–12)	14 (6–20)
Ischemic strokes avoided, n	0	0	0
Hemorrhagic strokes precipitated, n	1 (0–2)	1 (0–2)	1 (0–2)
Major gastrointestinal bleeding events precipitated, n	3 (2–4)	3 (2–4)	3 (2–4)

* Estimates based on 1000 patients receiving aspirin for 5 years and a relative risk reduction of 28% for coronary heart disease (CHD) events in those who received aspirin. CHD events = nonfatal acute myocardial infarction, fatal CHD. Values in parentheses are 95% CIs. The following caveats apply to these estimates. 1) Reduction in CHD risk may be smaller in women, but data are limited. 2) For elderly persons, absolute risk for hemorrhagic stroke and major gastrointestinal bleeding may be two to three times higher in patients receiving aspirin; however, aspirin may provide benefit in elderly persons by reducing ischemic stroke, the incidence of which increases with age. Aspirin does not appear to improve incidence of ischemic stroke in middle-aged patients. 3) Risk for hemorrhagic stroke may be greater with larger doses of aspirin. 4) Aspirin may not prevent myocardial infarction in patients with uncontrolled hypertension (systolic blood pressure > 150 mm Hg). 5) Long-term outcomes (>5–7 years) are unknown. 6) Patients at high risk (≥10% 5-year risk) may derive greater benefit from aspirin, including a 15% to 20% reduction in ischemic stroke and all-cause mortality, because their risk is similar to that of patients with known CHD.

risk for coronary heart disease over 5 years. **Table 7** shows the net impact of low-dose aspirin chemoprevention on patients with different levels of risk. Treating patients with a moderately high risk (a 5-year risk of 5%) would prevent 14 events (range, 6 to 20). In low-risk patients, such as those with a 5-year risk of 1%, aspirin would prevent 3 events (range, 1 to 4). Low-dose aspirin is estimated to result in an excess of 1 hemorrhagic stroke (range, 0 to 2) and 3 major gastrointestinal bleeding events (range, 2 to 4) among 1000 persons treated in each group, independent of risk for coronary heart disease.

DISCUSSION

For patients without known cardiovascular disease who are similar to those enrolled in the 5 large primary prevention trials, our systematic review suggests that aspirin chemoprevention reduces myocardial infarction but has no effect on ischemic stroke or all-cause mortality over 5 years. Aspirin therapy also increases the risk for gastrointestinal bleeding and hemorrhagic stroke. Aspirin chemoprevention is probably beneficial for patients who have no previous diagnosis of cardiovascular

disease but are at high risk for developing coronary heart disease in the next 5 years. Conversely, patients at low risk for coronary heart disease probably do not benefit from and may even be harmed by aspirin because the risk for adverse events may exceed the benefits of chemoprevention (6, 29).

To aid in applying these general results to individual patients, we have attempted to define quantitatively the benefits and harms of aspirin at various levels of risk for coronary heart disease. The advantage of such an approach is that it allows a more specific and accurate discussion and consideration of the potential consequences of using or not using aspirin for each individual patient.

Utilization of our results in shared decision making with patients requires an estimation of a given patient's absolute risk for coronary heart disease as well as his or her willingness to accept the risks of low-dose aspirin to avoid coronary heart disease. Risk for future coronary heart disease events can be predicted from coronary risk algorithms (30). Factors used to estimate risk include sex, age, blood pressure, serum total cholesterol level (or low-density lipoprotein cholesterol level), high-density lipoprotein cholesterol level, diabetes mellitus, cigarette smoking, and left ventricular hypertrophy. Several easy-to-use risk assessment tools, most based on risk equations derived from the Framingham Heart Study, are available on the Internet (for example, at www.intmed .mcw.edu/clincalc/heartrisk.html) or in printed form (30). Some tools calculate only 10-year risk estimates; in these cases, half of the 10-year estimate is a reasonable approximation of the 5-year risk for which we project our potential outcomes. Framingham data have recently been shown to generalize adequately to other populations (31). We have also provided a risk calculator at www.med-decisions.com to facilitate risk calculation.

Estimates of benefits and harms should be interpreted and compared cautiously. The principal beneficial effect of aspirin, a reduction in nonfatal myocardial infarction, cannot be directly equated to an adverse event, such as a stroke or gastrointestinal bleeding. We modeled outcomes over a period of 5 years because the trials included in our review ranged from 3 to 7 years in duration. However, outcomes from the use of aspirin chemoprevention will affect not only patients' current health status but also their future risk for coronary heart disease. For example, a nonfatal myocardial infarction may produce a relatively small decrement in the patient's current health status but may also increase the future risk for a more disabling condition, such as recurrent myocardial infarction or congestive heart failure, and may lead to premature death.

The value that individual patients place on the outcomes affected by aspirin will vary. Decision analysts have measured mean values in representative populations. Augustovski and associates (32) used existing studies to estimate utility values as follows: nonfatal myocardial infarction, 0.88; disabling stroke, 0.50; nondisabling stroke, 0.75; and gastrointestinal bleeding, 0.97. Our estimates of expected event rates and these mean utility values can provide an initial framework for discussion with individual patients, who may weigh or value outcomes differently.

Others have attempted to quantitate the benefits and harms of aspirin therapy (19, 33). Sanmuganathan and colleagues (34) performed a meta-analysis of the first four primary prevention trials and reached similar estimates of the beneficial effects of aspirin. In their analysis, they combined data on harms into a single category of "major bleeding events" induced, and they calculated that the number of bleeding events induced equaled the number of cardiovascular events averted when the cardiovascular event rate was 0.22% per year. They further estimated that the upper end of the 95% confidence interval for this point estimate occurred at an event rate of 0.8% per year for cardiovascular disease; this is equivalent to an event rate of 0.6% per year for coronary heart disease. Sanmuganathan and colleagues concluded that aspirin was "safe and worthwhile" for persons whose risk for coronary heart disease events exceeded 1.5% per year and was "unsafe" for persons whose risk was less than 0.5% per year. However, their analysis treated the beneficial and harmful outcomes as equal in magnitude, an assumption that oversimplifies the clinical dilemma.

Augustovski and associates (32) used a Markov decision analysis model to consider the effect of low-dose aspirin for primary prevention in patients with different risk factor profiles. Effect estimates were based on the evidence available at the time of the analysis, which was before publication of the three most recent trials. Outcomes were measured as changes in quality-adjusted life-days. For 55-year-old patients, those at low risk (0 risk factors in men; 0 or 1 risk factor in women) were

harmed by aspirin therapy, whereas those at moderate to high risk ($\geq$2 risk factors) seemed to benefit. However, because outcomes were presented in mean life-days gained or lost, it is difficult to translate their findings for use in counseling of individual patients.

On the basis of our review, we conclude that aspirin appears to reduce myocardial infarction but increases gastrointestinal and intracranial bleeding. The net effect of aspirin improves with increasing risk for coronary heart disease. Consideration of underlying risk for coronary heart disease, as well as the relative values patients attach to the main outcomes, can help patients and providers decide whether aspirin chemoprevention is warranted.

From University of North Carolina at Chapel Hill, Chapel Hill, North Carolina; and Air Force Medical Operations Agency and University of Texas Health Science Center at San Antonio, San Antonio, Texas.

Disclaimers: The authors of this article are responsible for its contents, including any clinical or treatment recommendations. No statement in this article should be construed as an official position of the Agency for Healthcare Research and Quality, the U.S. Department of Defense, or the U.S. Department of Health and Human Services.

Acknowledgments: The authors thank Kathleen Lohr, PhD; Sonya Sutton, BSPH; and Sheila White of Research Triangle Institute and Carol Krasnov of the University of North Carolina at Chapel Hill.

Grant Support: This study was developed by the RTI-UNC Evidence-based Practice Center under contract to the Agency for Healthcare Research and Quality (290-97-0011).

Requests for Single Reprints: Reprints are available from the Agency for Healthcare Research and Quality Web site (www.ahrq.gov/clinic/prevenix .htm) and in print through the Agency for Healthcare Research and Quality Publications Clearinghouse (800-358-9295).

Current Author Addresses: Dr. Hayden: Division of General Medicine, Department of Medicine, 11C Ambulatory Care, Veterans Administration Medical Center.
Dr. Pignone: University of North Carolina Division of General Internal Medicine, CB 7110, 5039 Old Clinic Building, University of North Carolina Hospitals, Chapel Hill, NC 27599-7110.
Dr. Phillips: AFMOA/SGZZ, Population Health Support Division, 2606 Doolittle Road, Building 804, Brooks Air Force Base, TX 78235-5249.
Dr. Mulrow: Department of Medicine, University of Texas Health Science Center at San Antonio, 7400 Merton Minter Boulevard (11C6), San Antonio, TX 78284.

References

1. **Hoyert D, Kochanek K, Murphy SL.** Deaths: Final Data for 1997. National Vital Statistics Reports. Hyattsville, MD: National Center for Health Statistics; 1999.

2. 1999 Heart and Stroke Statistical Update. American Heart Association. Dallas, TX: American Heart Association; 1998.

3. **He J, Whelton PK, Vu B, Klag MJ.** Aspirin and risk of hemorrhagic stroke: a meta-analysis of randomized controlled trials. JAMA. 1998;280:1930-5. [PMID: 9851479]

4. Final report on the aspirin component of the ongoing Physicians' Health Study. Steering Committee of the Physicians' Health Study Research Group. N Engl J Med. 1989;321:129-35. [PMID: 2664509]

5. **Peto R, Gray R, Collins R, Wheatley K, Hennekens C, Jamrozik K, et al.** Randomised trial of prophylactic daily aspirin in British male doctors. Br Med J (Clin Res Ed). 1988;296:313-6. [PMID: 3125882]

6. Guide to Clinical Preventive Services. Report of the U.S. Preventive Services Task Force. 2nd ed. Baltimore: Williams & Wilkins; 1996.

7. Thrombosis prevention trial: randomised trial of low-intensity oral anticoagulation with warfarin and low-dose aspirin in the primary prevention of ischaemic heart disease in men at increased risk. The Medical Research Council's General Practice Research Framework. Lancet. 1998;351:233-41. [PMID: 9457092]

8. **Hansson L, Zanchetti A, Carruthers SG, Dahlöf B, Elmfeldt D, Julius S, et al.** Effects of intensive blood-pressure lowering and low-dose aspirin in patients with hypertension: principal results of the Hypertension Optimal Treatment (HOT) randomised trial. HOT Study Group. Lancet. 1998;351:1755-62. [PMID: 9635947]

9. Low-dose aspirin and vitamin E in people at cardiovascular risk: a randomised trial in general practice. Collaborative Group of the Primary Prevention Project. Lancet. 2001;357:89-95. [PMID: 11197445]

10. **Rexrode KM, Lee IM, Cook NR, Hennekens CH, Buring JE.** Baseline characteristics of participants in the Women's Health Study. J Womens Health Gend Based Med. 2000;9:19-27. [PMID: 10718501]

11. Reviewer Manager (RevMan). The Cochrane Collaboration. Oxford, England: The Cochrane Collaboration; 1999.

12. Aspirin effects on mortality and morbidity in patients with diabetes mellitus. Early Treatment Diabetic Retinopathy Study report 14. ETDRS Investigators. JAMA. 1992;268:1292-300. [PMID: 1507375]

13. **Juul-Möller S, Edvardsson N, Jahnmatz B, Rosén A, Sørensen S, Omblus R.** Double-blind trial of aspirin in primary prevention of myocardial infarction in patients with stable chronic angina pectoris. The Swedish Angina Pectoris Aspirin Trial (SAPAT) Group. Lancet. 1992;340:1421-5. [PMID: 1360557]

14. **Dickinson JP, Prentice CR.** Aspirin: benefit and risk in thromboprophylaxis. QJM. 1998;91:523-38. [PMID: 9893756]

15. **Roderick PJ, Wilkes HC, Meade TW.** The gastrointestinal toxicity of aspirin: an overview of randomised controlled trials. Br J Clin Pharmacol. 1993;35:219-26. [PMID: 8471398]

16. **Stalnikowicz-Darvasi R.** Gastrointestinal bleeding during low-dose aspirin administration for prevention of arterial occlusive events. A critical analysis. J Clin Gastroenterol. 1995;21:13-6. [PMID: 7560825]

17. **Cappelleri JC, Lau J, Kupelnick B, Chalmers TC.** Efficacy and safety of different aspirin dosages on vascular diseases in high-risk patients. A metaregression analysis. Online J Curr Clin Trials. 1995;174. [PMID: 7889238]

18. **Kelly JP, Kaufman DW, Jurgelon JM, Sheehan J, Koff RS, Shapiro S.** Risk of aspirin-associated major upper-gastrointestinal bleeding with enteric-coated or buffered product. Lancet. 1996;348:1413-6. [PMID: 8937281]

19. **Hart RG, Halperin JL, McBride R, Benavente O, Man-Son-Hing M, Kronmal RA.** Aspirin for the primary prevention of stroke and other major vascular events: meta-analysis and hypotheses. Arch Neurol. 2000;57:326-32. [PMID: 10714657]

20. **Weil J, Colin-Jones D, Langman M, Lawson D, Logan R, Murphy M, et al.** Prophylactic aspirin and risk of peptic ulcer bleeding. BMJ. 1995;310:827-30. [PMID: 7711618]

21. **Silagy CA, McNeil JJ, Donnan GA, Tonkin AM, Worsam B, Campion K.** Adverse effects of low-dose aspirin in a healthy elderly population. Clin Pharmacol Ther. 1993;54:84-9. [PMID: 8330469]

22. **Meade TW, Brennan PJ.** Determination of who may derive most benefit from aspirin in primary prevention: subgroup results from a randomised controlled trial. BMJ. 2000;321:13-7. [PMID: 10875825]

23. Collaborative overview of randomised trials of antiplatelet therapy—I: Prevention of death, myocardial infarction, and stroke by prolonged antiplatelet therapy in various categories of patients. Antiplatelet Trialists' Collaboration. BMJ. 1994;308:81-106. [PMID: 8298418]

24. **Kjeldsen SE, Kolloch RE, Leonetti G, Mallion JM, Zanchetti A, Elmfeldt D, et al.** Influence of gender and age on preventing cardiovascular disease by antihypertensive treatment and acetylsalicylic acid. The HOT study. Hypertension Optimal Treatment. J Hypertens. 2000;18:629-42. [PMID: 10826567]

25. **Sudlow C.** Antithrombotic treatment. In: Clinical Evidence. American College of Physicians–American Society of Internal Medicine. 5th ed. London: BMJ Publishing Group; 2001.

26. Warfarin versus aspirin for prevention of thromboembolism in atrial fibrillation: Stroke Prevention in Atrial Fibrillation II Study. Lancet. 1994;343:687-91. [PMID: 7907677]

27. **Thrift AG, McNeil JJ, Forbes A, Donnan GA.** Risk of primary intracerebral haemorrhage associated with aspirin and non-steroidal anti-inflammatory drugs: case-control study. BMJ. 1999;318:759-64. [PMID: 10082697]

28. **Derry S, Loke YK.** Risk of gastrointestinal haemorrhage with long term use of aspirin: meta-analysis. BMJ. 2000;321:1183-7. [PMID: 11073508]

29. **Hennekens CH, Dyken ML, Fuster V.** Aspirin as a therapeutic agent in cardiovascular disease: a statement for healthcare professionals from the American Heart Association. Circulation. 1997;96:2751-3. [PMID: 9355934]

30. **Wilson PW, D'Agostino RB, Levy D, Belanger AM, Silbershatz H, Kannel WB.** Prediction of coronary heart disease using risk factor categories. Circulation. 1998;97:1837-47. [PMID: 9603539]

31. **D'Agostino RB Sr, Grundy S, Sullivan LM, Wilson P.** Validation of the Framingham coronary heart disease prediction scores: results of a multiple ethnic groups investigation. JAMA. 2001;286:180-7. [PMID: 11448281]

32. **Augustovski FA, Cantor SB, Thach CT, Spann SJ.** Aspirin for primary prevention of cardiovascular events. J Gen Intern Med. 1998;13:824-35. [PMID: 9844080]

33. **Hebert PR, Hennekens CH.** An overview of the 4 randomized trials of aspirin therapy in the primary prevention of vascular disease. Arch Intern Med. 2000;160:3123-7. [PMID: 11074741]

34. **Sanmuganathan PS, Ghahramani P, Jackson PR, Wallis EJ, Ramsay LE.** Aspirin for primary prevention of coronary heart disease: safety and absolute benefit related to coronary risk derived from meta-analysis of randomised trials. Heart. 2001;85:265-71. [PMID: 11179262] 17

APPENDIX: DETAILED DESCRIPTION OF SEARCH STRATEGY AND DATA EXTRACTION

Search Strategy

We used the following MeSH headings for the beneficial effects of aspirin: aspirin AND cardiovascular disease AND (randomized controlled trial or controlled clinical trial or randomized controlled trials or random allocation or double blind method or single blind method). The MeSH headings aspirin AND (gastrointestinal bleeding or cerebral hemorrhage) were used for the adverse effects of aspirin. We supplemented our basic search strategies by examining bibliographies from other relevant articles and systematic reviews and by seeking the advice of content experts. Our search strategy is detailed in **Appendix Figures 2 and 3.**

Inclusion Criteria

For studies examining the benefits of aspirin chemoprevention, we included randomized trials of at least 1 year in duration that met the following criteria: 1) compared aspirin with placebo or no aspirin; 2) included patients with no previous history of cardiovascular disease, including myocardial infarction, stroke, angina, transient ischemic attack, or peripheral vascular disease (trials in which >10% of participants had known vascular disease were excluded); and 3) measured the outcomes of myocardial infarction, stroke, and mortality (**Figure 1**).

For harms data, we examined case–control studies, randomized trials, and systematic reviews or meta-analyses of randomized trials that examined rates of hemorrhagic stroke or gastrointestinal bleeding from aspirin use.

Appendix Figure 2. **Search strategy: beneficial effects.**

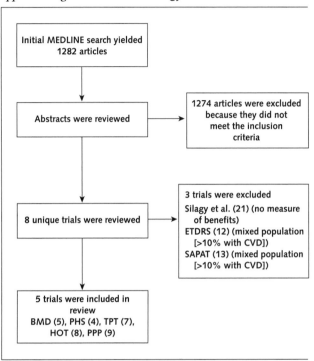

BMD = British Male Doctors' Trial; CVD = coronary vascular disease; ETDRS = Early Treatment Diabetic Retinopathy Study; HOT = Hypertension Optimal Treatment Trial; PHS = Physicians' Health Study; PPP = Primary Prevention Project; SAPAT = Swedish Angina Pectoris Aspirin Trial; TPT = Thrombosis Prevention Trial.

Appendix Figure 1. **Analytic framework: aspirin to prevent cardiovascular events.**

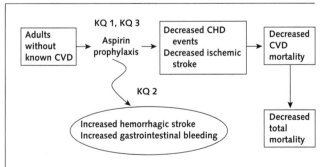

CHD = coronary heart disease; CVD = cardiovascular disease; KQ = key question. KQ 1: Does aspirin chemoprevention in patients without known cardiovascular disease reduce the risk for myocardial infarction, stroke, and death? KQ 2: Does aspirin chemoprevention increase major gastrointestinal bleeding, hemorrhagic strokes, or both? KQ 3: What is the balance of benefits and harms for aspirin therapy in patients with different levels of cardiovascular risk?

Data Extraction and Definition of Outcomes

Two reviewers examined all abstracts and excluded those that they agreed were clearly outside the scope of the review. The same reviewers then examined the full articles for the remaining studies and determined final eligibility by consensus. Two independent reviewers abstracted the included studies. Disagreements were resolved by consensus. Potentially beneficial outcomes examined were the efficacy of aspirin versus placebo in reducing the following events: 1) nonfatal acute myocardial infarction or death due to coronary heart disease, including fatal acute myocardial infarction or death from other ischemic heart disease; 2) fatal or nonfatal stroke; 3) total cardiovascular events (nonfatal acute myocardial infarction, death from coronary heart disease, and fatal or nonfatal stroke); and 4) all-cause mortality. Major harms examined were hemorrhagic stroke and major gastrointestinal bleeding.

Appendix Figure 3. **Search strategy: harmful effects.**

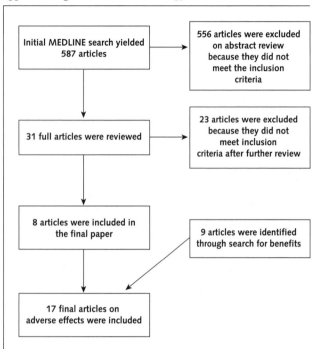

Key Points

Breast cancer

❏ There is strong evidence that screening mammography every 12 to 33 months decreases mortality in women aged 50 to 69.

❏ The evidence that screening mammography decreases mortality in women aged 40 to 49 is not as strong, and the evidence is not clear as to an optimal screening interval in this age group.

❏ The evidence is unclear as to the benefits/harms of clinical breast examination and self-breast examination.

❏ The precise age at which to discontinue screening mammography is uncertain; very few trials enrolled women over age 69. However, women with significant co-morbidities are unlikely to benefit from continued screening.

Breast Cancer Screening: A Summary of the Evidence for the U.S. Preventive Services Task Force

Linda L. Humphrey, MD, MPH; Mark Helfand, MD, MS; Benjamin K.S. Chan, MS; and Steven H. Woolf, MD, MPH

Purpose: To synthesize new data on breast cancer screening for the U.S. Preventive Services Task Force.

Data Sources: MEDLINE; the Cochrane Controlled Trials Registry; and reference lists of reviews, editorials, and original studies.

Study Selection: Eight randomized, controlled trials of mammography and 2 trials evaluating breast self-examination were included. One hundred fifty-four publications of the results of these trials, as well as selected articles about the test characteristics and harms associated with screening, were examined.

Data Extraction: Predefined criteria were used to assess the quality of each study. Meta-analyses using a Bayesian random-effects model were conducted to provide summary relative risk estimates and credible intervals (CrIs) for the effectiveness of screening with mammography in reducing death from breast cancer.

Data Synthesis: For studies of fair quality or better, the summary relative risk was 0.84 (95% CrI, 0.77 to 0.91) and the number needed to screen to prevent one death from breast cancer

after approximately 14 years of observation was 1224 (CrI, 665 to 2564). Among women younger than 50 years of age, the summary relative risk associated with mammography was 0.85 (CrI, 0.73 to 0.99) and the number needed to screen to prevent one death from breast cancer after 14 years of observation was 1792 (CrI, 764 to 10 540). For clinical breast examination and breast self-examination, evidence from randomized trials is inconclusive.

Conclusions: In the randomized, controlled trials, mammography reduced breast cancer mortality rates among women 40 to 74 years of age. Greater absolute risk reduction was seen among older women. Because these results incorporate several rounds of screening, the actual number of mammograms needed to prevent one death from breast cancer is higher. In addition, each screening has associated risks and costs.

B reast cancer is the second leading cause of cancer death among North American women. Approximately 1 in 8.2 women will receive a diagnosis of breast cancer during her lifetime, and 1 in 30 will die of the disease (1). Breast cancer incidence increases with age (1), and although significant progress has been made in identifying risk factors and genetic markers, more than 50% of cases occur in women without known major predictors (2–5).

This review was commissioned to assist the current U.S. Preventive Services Task Force (USPSTF) in updating its recommendations on breast cancer screening. We focus on information that was not available in 1996, when the second USPSTF examined the issue (6). Our goal was to critically appraise and synthesize evidence about the overall effectiveness of breast cancer screening, as well as its effectiveness among women younger than 50 years of age.

METHODS

The analytic framework, literature search, and data extraction are described in detail in the Appendix (available at www.annals.org). Briefly, we searched the Cochrane Controlled Trials Registry, MEDLINE, PREMEDLINE, and reference lists (6–8) for randomized, controlled trials of screening with death from breast cancer as an outcome. In all, we reviewed 154 publications from eight eligible randomized trials of screening mammography and two trials of breast self-examination (BSE). We abstracted details about patient population, design, quality, data analysis, and published results at each reported length of follow-up. We also evaluated previous meta-analyses of these trials

and of screening test characteristics and studies evaluating the harms associated with false-positive test results.

We used predefined criteria developed by the current USPSTF to assess the internal validity of the trials (9). Two authors rated the internal validity of each study as "good," "fair," or "poor." Disagreements were resolved by further review and discussion. In the USPSTF system, a study that meets all the criteria for internal validity is rated as good quality (9). The rating reflects a judgment that the results of the study are very likely to be correct. The fair-quality rating is used for studies that have important but not major flaws and implies that the findings are probably valid. A study that has a major flaw in design or execution—one that is serious enough to invalidate the results of the study—is rated as poor quality. We based our quality ratings on the entire set of publications from a trial rather than on individual articles.

The USPSTF criteria for internal validity are listed in **Appendix Table 1**, available at www.annals.org. All of the mammography trials met the first three criteria: They clearly defined interventions, measured important outcomes, and used intention-to-treat analysis. Therefore, our quality ratings reflect differences among the studies on the remaining criteria: 1) initial assembly of comparable groups; 2) maintenance of comparable groups and minimization of differential loss to follow-up or overall loss to follow-up; and 3) use of outcome measurements that were equal, reliable, and valid. The Appendix (available at www.annals.org) describes our approach to applying these criteria in more detail.

We conducted new meta-analyses to incorporate new information about the quality of the trials and longer follow-up results. Breast cancer is known for its biological heterogeneity (10) as well as for late recurrences (10). Thus, longer follow-up is relevant in evaluating mortality rates, particularly in younger women. In addition, for several of the trials, the most recent analyses correct flaws in earlier reports.

Six of the eight mammography trials were designed to assess the effectiveness of mammography over a broad age range, rather than its comparative effectiveness in various age subgroups. One trial specifically examined women 40 to 49 years of age because the earliest trial seemed to show no benefit in this subgroup. The USPSTF posed these questions for the meta-analysis: 1) Does mammography reduce breast cancer mortality rates among women over a broad range of ages when compared with usual care? and 2) If so, does mammography reduce breast cancer mortality rates among women 40 to 49 years of age when compared with usual care?

We answered each question in two parts. First, using WinBUGS software (MRC Biostatistics Unit, Cambridge, United Kingdom), we constructed a two-level Bayesian random-effects model to estimate the effect size from multiple data points for each study and to derive a pooled estimate of relative risk reduction and credible intervals (CrIs) for a given length of follow-up (11). Second, we pooled the most recent results of each trial to calculate the absolute and relative risk reduction, using the results of the first analysis to estimate the mean length of follow-up.

To avoid bias that could result from excluding any data from valid studies, we included the results of all trials of fair quality or better in the base-case analysis. The disadvantage of this approach is that it combines results from two distinct types of studies.

The six population-based trials randomly assigned women to an invitation-to-screening group or to a control group that received "usual care" and was followed passively. In these trials, women who were invited to screening but chose not to be screened were included in the analysis of the "screened" group. Two trials from Canada, the Canadian National Breast Cancer Screening Study-1 (CNBSS-1) and the Canadian National Breast Cancer Screening Study-2 (CNBSS-2), differed from the other six trials. First, the Canadian trials used mass media to recruit a sample of volunteers, and all women randomly assigned to mammography had mammography at least once (12, 13). Second, in CNBSS-2, the control group was screened periodically with clinical breast examination (CBE). To estimate the relative risk reduction and the number needed to *invite* to screening to prevent one breast cancer death compared with usual care, we reanalyzed the data excluding the results of the Canadian studies.

This study was funded by the U.S. Agency for Healthcare Research and Quality. Agency staff and members of the USPSTF reviewed and made substantive recommenda-

tions about the analyses and final manuscript. Agency approval was required before the manuscript could be submitted for publication.

RESULTS
Description of Trials

The eight randomized trials of mammography identified in our review (12–23) varied in recruitment of participants, mammography protocol, control groups, and size (Table 1). Six trials examined the effectiveness of screening among women between 40 and 74 years of age; one trial enrolled women in their 40s, and one enrolled only women in their 50s. Four trials from Sweden tested mammography only (14–17, 23–26), and the other four, from Canada, New York, and Edinburgh, Scotland, tested mammography and CBE (12, 13, 18–22, 27).

Study Quality

We found important methodologic limitations in all of the trials and rated all but one as fair, using USPSTF criteria. Table 1 lists the flaws of each trial and indicates how they influenced the overall ratings. The two reviewers rated the Swedish and Canadian trials as fair. Their initial ratings for the Edinburgh study and for the Health Insurance Plan of Greater New York (HIP) study differed. After extensive peer review, and detailed review of these trials' associated publications, the reviewers reached a consensus that the HIP study should be rated as fair and the Edinburgh study should be rated as poor.

The HIP trial (conducted from 1963 to 1966) was the first trial of breast cancer screening. It is difficult to critically appraise because publications that describe it differ in detail from more recent publications. We found several limitations of this trial, including inadequate description of allocation concealment and poor reporting of intervention and control group numbers. In addition, we found better ascertainment of clinical variables (including previous mastectomy) among the invitation-to-screening cohort than among the passively followed control group. However, we viewed this as an expected consequence of a study design in which a control group receives usual care and is not contacted. The screening and control groups differed from each other slightly in education, menopausal status, and previous breast lumps; however, the differences were not systematic and did not favor one group over the other. The strengths of the trial included intention-to-treat analysis, little contamination, and blind review of deaths. We did not find the faults severe enough to rate the study as poor quality and rated it as fair, which signifies that the results were probably valid at the time the study was conducted.

The Canadian trials met all of the USPSTF criteria for a rating of good quality, except for adequacy of allocation concealment. They differed from the other trials because all participants had a history and physical examination before randomization. This design permitted exclusion of pa-

Table 1. Controlled Trials of Mammography and Clinical Breast Examination*

Variable	Trial (Reference)							
	HIP (19)	CNBSS-1 (13)	CNBSS-2 (13, 20)	Edinburgh (18)	Gothenburg (14, 23)	Stockholm (17)	Malmö (15)	Swedish Two-County Trial (16)
Description								
Year study began	1963	1980	1980	1978	1982	1981	1976–1978	1977
Setting or population	New York health plan members	15 centers in Canada, self-selected participants	15 centers in Canada, self-selected participants	All women aged 45–64 y from 87 general practices in Edinburgh	Entire female population, born between 1923–1944, of one Swedish town	Residents of southeast greater Stockholm, Sweden	All women born between 1927–1945 living in Malmö, Sweden	From Ostergotland (E-County) and Kopparberg (W-County)
Age at enrollment, y	40–64	40–49	50–59	45–64	39–59	40–64	45–70	40–74
Interventions								
Method of randomization	Age- and family size–stratified pairs of women randomly assigned individually by drawing from a list	Blocks (stratified by center and 5-year age group) after CBE		Cluster, based on general practitioner practices	Cluster, based on day of birth for 1923–1935 cohort (18%), by individual for 1936–1944 cohort (82%)	Individual, by day of month; ratio of screening to control group, 2:1	Individual, within birth year	Cluster, based on geographic units; blocks designed to be demographically homogeneous
Study groups	Mammography + CBE vs. usual care	Mammography + CBE vs. usual care (all women prescreened and instructed in BSE)	Mammography + CBE vs. CBE (all women pre-screened and instructed in BSE)	Mammography + CBE vs. usual care	Mammography vs. usual care; controls offered screening after year 5, completed screening at approximately year 7	Mammography vs. usual care; controls offered screening after year 5	Mammography vs. usual care; controls offered screening after year 14	Mammography vs. usual care; controls offered screening after year 7
Screening protocol								
Interval, mo	12	12	12	24	18	24–28	18–24	24–33
Rounds, n	4	4–5	4–5	4	5	2	9	3
Views, n	2	2	2	2 (1)	2 (1)	1	2 (1)	1
Participants, n								
Study group	30 239	25 214	19 711	28 628	20 724	40 318	21 088	77 080
Control group	30 256	25 216	19 694	26 015	28 809	19 943	21 195	55 985
Longest follow-up by 2002, y	18	13	13	14	12†	11.4†	11–13	20
							15.5†	15.5†
Trial quality								
Assembly of comparable groups								
Allocation concealment and baseline groups	*Use of lists and pairs made subversion possible. More menopausal women and women with previous breast lumps in a sample of controls; more education in the screened group*	*Use of lists and blocks made subversion possible.* 17 in women in mammography group vs. 5 in control group had tumors with 4 nodes on initial screening	*Use of lists and blocks made subversion possible*	Allocation concealment not described; *significantly lower SES and higher all-cause mortality in control group suggest inadequate randomization*	Allocation concealment not described	*Allocation concealment not described*	*Allocation concealment not described*	Allocation concealment not described; intervention women slightly older than controls

Continued on following page

Table 1—**Continued**

Variable	Trial (Reference)							
	HIP (19)	CNBSS-1 (13)	CNBSS-2 (13, 20)	Edinburgh (18)	Gothenburg (14, 23)	Stockholm (17)	Malmö (15, 25)	Swedish Two-County Trial (16)
Relative risk for all-cause mortality (screened vs. control group)	0.98	1.02	1.06	*0.8 (statistically significant)*	0.98	NR	0.99	1
Maintenance of comparable groups								
Screening attendance	Round 1, 67%; round 2, 54%; round 3, 50%; round 4, 46%	Round 1, 100%; rounds 2 and 4, 85%–89%	Round 1, 100%; round 2, 90.4%, round 5, 86.5%	Round 1, 61%; round 7, 44%	Round 1, 85%; rounds 2–5, 75%–78%; control group, 66%	Round 1, 81%; round 2, 81%; control group, 77%	Round 1, 74%; rounds 2–5, 70%; control group, ???	Round 1, 89%; round 2, 83%; round 3, 84%; control group, ???
Contamination, %	Unknown, probably small	25	16	Not reported	20	Not reported	25	13
Post-randomization exclusions	Yes	No	No	Yes	One fewer death in screening group included in 1997 results	Yes	Yes	Yes
Validity of outcome assessment								
Deaths included in analysis (follow-up vs. evaluation method)	*Breast cancer deaths diagnosed within 7 years of follow-up*	Follow-up method	Follow-up method	Follow-up method and evaluation method	Initially, all four trials used the evaluation method of analysis (breast cancer cases diagnosed after screening period were excluded from count of breast cancer deaths), but this was corrected in reanalyses of the data in 1993 and in 2002. *Control screening was delayed relative to the last screen in the mammography groups, resulting in bias because more cases of cancer were included in the control groups than in the intervention groups.*			
Method for verifying breast cancer deaths	Blinded review of the death certificate and medical records; *unclear how deaths were selected for review*	Blinded review of all deaths of women known to have breast cancer whose death certificates mentioned liver, lung, or colon cancer or unknown primary, or whose medical records raised a question of breast cancer		All deaths, with breast cancer deaths diagnosed within 14 years of follow-up; *not masked*	In the 1993 analysis, an independent panel used an explicit protocol to perform blinded assessment of cause of death			
Analysis method								
Intention-to-treat analysis; completeness of reporting‡	*Did not provide relative risk, confidence intervals, or P values in recent report; estimated the number of participants*	Appropriate	Appropriate	–	Sample sizes differed for different publications because different methods were used to estimate the size of the underlying population.			
External validity	Poor mammography technique; only a third of cancer cases found by mammography alone	Many women with screening abnormalities (especially on CBE) were "deemed not to require a diagnostic procedure," potentially reducing the sensitivity of screening		–	19% of controls and 13% of study women had mammography in the 2 years before the study	25% of all women entering the study had had mammography	–	In the age group of 40–49 y, 3 women died after being invited to screening and 1 died before invitation but after randomization
Grade								
USPSTF internal validity	Fair	Fair or better	Fair or better	Poor	Fair	Fair	Fair	Fair

* Italic type indicates aspects of the design or conduct of the trials that influenced the quality rating. BSE = breast self-examination; CBE = clinical breast examination; CNBSS = Canadian National Breast Screening Study; HIP = Health Insurance Plan of Greater New York; NR = not reported; USPSTF = U.S. Preventive Services Task Force.
† Most recent results for age 40 to 49 years, if different.
‡ All studies were analyzed by using intention-to-treat methods.

tients who had a history of breast cancer and extensive examination of the baseline differences between groups.

The Swedish trials all had limitations that resulted in a rating of fair rather than good. The Stockholm and Malmö trials, which were individually randomized, did not report whether allocation was concealed. The Gothenburg trial and Swedish Two-County Study, which were cluster randomized trials, had small differences in mean age between the invited and control groups. Such differences are expected to occur in a cluster-randomized trial, do not indicate failure of randomization or a problem in the trial execution, and can be adjusted for in statistical analyses (28). Both the Gothenburg trial and the Swedish Two-County Trial provided insufficient data to determine whether randomization distributed other important confounders equally among the groups, but comparison of overall mortality rates in the invited and control groups do not suggest that a major imbalance occurred (29).

As originally conducted, the Swedish trials had important flaws related to measurement of the primary outcome measure, death from breast cancer. In the Swedish Two-County Trial and the Gothenburg and Stockholm trials, review of deaths was unblinded and criteria for the assignment of cause of death were unclear. Another concern about the Swedish trials as a group related to screening of the control groups. Originally, the Swedish trials used the "evaluation" method of analysis, in which mortality rates in the screened population were calculated only for cancer diagnosed between the time of randomization and the last mammographic examination. When the evaluation method of analysis is used, control group screening can introduce bias unless it is performed concurrently with the final instance of mammography in the screened group (30, 31). This method is inferior to the "follow-up" method of analysis, in which all deaths that occur after randomization are included in the analysis. The follow-up method of analysis dilutes relative benefit over time, particularly in studies that offered screening to the control group and in areas where widespread screening is adopted.

We considered these flaws to be adequately corrected in subsequent analyses by the trialists. In a 1993 overview of the trials, an independent end point committee used an explicit protocol to perform blind assessment of cause of death (32). Participants were linked to an external cancer registry and were excluded from the analysis if breast cancer had been diagnosed before the trial began. For the Swedish trials as a whole, death from every cause except breast cancer was similar in the compared groups (33). In the Swedish Two-County Trial, the reduction in rates of advanced breast cancer (34), which are not related to judgments about the causes of death, was similar to the reduction in breast cancer mortality rates (35). The overview also reanalyzed the data by using the follow-up method of analysis and found very little difference between the recalculated and original relative risk values. A recent review (8) critical of the Swedish studies raised concern about bias in

postrandomization exclusions, as evidenced by variation in the reported number of participants. This concern was effectively addressed in a recent update of these trials, which explained that this variation was due to the use of different methods for estimating the number of women in each birth cohort rather than to manipulation after randomization (23). The update also reported more recent results of the Swedish trials by using both the follow-up and evaluation methods of analysis.

We rated the Edinburgh study as poor quality because of a serious imbalance between the control and screened groups. General practitioners' practices were randomized in clusters without matching for socioeconomic factors. As a result, socioeconomic status, a predictor of stage at diagnosis as well as death from breast cancer, was significantly lower in the control group than in the mammography group. All-cause mortality was dramatically higher in the control group than in the screened group (20.1 more deaths per 10 000 person-years [95% CI, 13.3 to 26.9]) (29). This difference is close to 25 times larger than the difference in breast cancer deaths between the groups and confirms our assessment that the trial was severely flawed.

Sensitivity of Mammography

Since no gold standard can be applied to the entire screened population, the denominator used for estimating sensitivity is the total number of breast cancer cases diagnosed in a given interval. The results of recent, good-quality systematic reviews of the accuracy of mammography in the screening trials are summarized in **Table 2** (36, 37). The overall sensitivity for all rounds of screening was lowest in the HIP trial. Otherwise, one study was not clearly better or worse than another. For a 1-year screening interval, the sensitivity of first mammography ranged from 71% to 96%. Sensitivity was substantially lower for women in their 40s than for older women.

The data in **Table 2** cannot be applied to individual patients because they are not adjusted for several factors that are known to affect sensitivity. These include patient factors (use of hormone replacement therapy, mammographic breast density), technical factors (the quality of mammography, the number of mammographic views), and provider factors (the experience of radiologists and their propensity to label the results of an examination abnormal, the choice of follow-up evaluation for abnormal mammograms) (36, 38–42).

Specificity and Positive Predictive Value

In the randomized trials, the specificity of a single mammographic examination was 94% to 97% (36, 43–44). This indicates that 3% to 6% of women who did not have cancer underwent further diagnostic evaluation, typically a clinical examination, more mammographic views, or ultrasonography. The positive predictive value of one-time mammography ranged from 2% to 22% for abnormal results requiring further evaluation and from 12% to 78% for abnormal results requiring biopsy (36, 45, 46) (**Table**

Table 2. **Sensitivity of Mammography***

Study	All Rounds			First Round Only	
	Cases of Cancer Detected by Screening	Total Cases of Cancer	Estimated Sensitivity of Mammography (Rounds)†	Sensitivity of Screening at 1-Year Intervals	Sensitivity of Screening at 2-Year Intervals
	n	*n (%)*	*% (n)*	%	
HIP					
40–64 y	73	173 (0.42)	39 (4)		
Malmö					
45–49 y				73	
50–59 y				71	
60–69 y				85	
70–74 y				81	
45–69 y	176	227 (0.78)	61 (2)	92	
Swedish Two-County Trial					
40–49 y	39	82 (0.48)		81	
50–59 y	102	137 (0.74)		96	
60–69 y	184	220 (0.84)		95	
70–74 y	101	112 (0.90)		98	
40–74 y				95	86
Stockholm					
40–49 y	24	45 (0.53)	64		53
50–59 y	71	95 (0.75)	89		75
60–64 y	33	48 (0.69)			69
40–64 y				86	68
CNBSS-1					
40–49 y	162	286 (0.57)	61 (4)	77	56
CNBSS-2					
50–59 y	243	347 (0.70)	66 (4)	88	56

* The Gothenburg trial is not listed because of insufficient data; the Edinburgh trial is excluded. Empty cells indicate lack of sufficient data. All data are taken from reference 36, using the "detection" method, unless otherwise noted. CNBSS = Canadian National Breast Screening Study; HIP = Health Insurance Plan of Greater New York.
† Data taken from reference 37.

3). Estimates from community settings suggest a graded, continuous increase in predictive value with age. For example, among 31 814 average-risk women screened in California from 1985 to 1992, the positive predictive value for further evaluation was 1% to 4% among those 40 to 49 years of age, 4% to 9% among those 50 to 59 years of age, 10% to 19% among those 60 to 69 years of age, and 18% to 20% among those 70 years of age and older (47).

Effectiveness of Mammography in Reducing Breast Cancer Mortality

Table 4 summarizes the most recent results from trials that included at least some participants older than 50 years of age. The four Swedish trials that compared two to six rounds of mammography with usual care (23, 26) reported 9% to 32% reductions in the risk for death from breast cancer. The results of the trials have changed little over time (Figure). The reduction was statistically significant in only one of these trials (the Swedish Two-County Trial) (relative risk, 0.68 [CI, 0.59 to 0.80]) (26). The number of times mammography was performed and the frequency of screening did not seem to explain the variation among the Swedish studies. A previous meta-analysis found little change when the individual trial results were adjusted for type of randomization and degree of adherence (48).

Of the four studies that evaluated the combination of mammography and CBE (Table 4), three were of at least fair quality (12, 13, 18, 27, 49). The HIP trial reported a relative risk reduction that began 5 years after randomization and remained below 1 after 16 or more years of follow-up (relative risk, 0.79). The CNBSS-2, which compared annual mammography and CBE with annual CBE among women 50 to 59 years of age, showed no benefit 13

Table 3. **Specificity and Positive Predictive Value***

Study	Specificity of the Work-up Method	Positive Predictive Value	
		Work-up Method	Biopsy Method
		%	
HIP	NR	12	20
Malmö	97.4	10–22	33–61
Swedish Two-County Trial	95.6	12	50–75
Stockholm	95.1	8–10	62–78
CNBSS-1	93.5	2	12
CNBSS-2		4–6	20
Gothenburg		3–7 (complete mammography)	
		12–18 (CBE and FNA biopsy)	

* Adapted from references 36 and 45. Work-up method = mammogram requiring further evaluation; biopsy method = mammogram resulting in biopsy. CBE = clinical breast examination; CNBSS = Canadian National Breast Screening Study; FNA = fine-needle aspiration; HIP = Health Insurance Plan of Greater New York; NR = not reported.

years after the study began (12, 20). The CNBSS-1, which compared annual mammography and CBE with usual care in women 40 to 49 years of age, also showed no benefit.

In our meta-analysis of results from all age groups combined, we excluded the Edinburgh trial (which we rated as poor) and used the results from both Canadian trials. The summary relative risk was 0.84 (95% CrI, 0.77 to 0.91), equivalent to a number needed to screen of 1224 (CrI, 665 to 2564) an average of 14 years after study entry. To estimate the effectiveness of an invitation to screen compared with usual care, we also excluded the Canadian trials, which recruited volunteers. The relative risk reduction was 0.81 (CrI, 0.73 to 0.89), and the number needed to invite to screening was 1008 (CrI, 531 to 2128). The relative risks by year of observation (including trial plus follow-up time) are shown in the Figure, which suggests a gradual decrease in benefit with longer observation time.

Effectiveness of Mammography among Women 40 to 49 Years of Age

Since 1963, seven randomized, controlled trials have included women 40 to 49 years of age, approximately 200 000 participants. With the exception of one of the Canadian studies, none of the trials was planned to evaluate breast cancer screening in this age group and none had sufficient power. Two trials, the Stockholm trial and CNBSS-1, showed no benefit for this age group even with longer follow-up (Table 5). The other five trials suggest a benefit (risk reduction, 13% to 42%), and one (the Gothenburg trial) observed a statistically significant risk reduction since 1996. These findings reflect results after 11 to 19 years of observation; the median period of active screening was 6 years (range, 4 to 15 years).

In our meta-analysis, excluding the Edinburgh trial, the summary relative risk was 0.85 (CrI, 0.73 to 0.99) after 14 years of observation, with a number needed to screen of 1792 (CrI, 764 to 10 540) to prevent one death from

breast cancer. Some might argue that the Canadian study should be excluded in calculating the number needed to invite to screening because its participants were pre-screened volunteers who may have differed from the general population. When the Canadian study was excluded, the summary relative risk was 0.80 (CrI, 0.67 to 0.96) and the number needed to invite to screening was 1385 (CrI, 659 to 6060). The Figure shows an increasing screening benefit among this age group with a longer period of observation.

Among women 50 years of age or older, the summary relative risk was 0.78 (CrI, 0.70 to 0.87) after 14 years of observation, with a number needed to screen of 838 (CrI, 494 to 1676) to prevent one death from breast cancer. As shown in the Figure, the benefit has decreased with longer duration of follow-up.

We found seven meta-analyses of the effectiveness of mammography in women 40 to 49 years of age (Table 6) (8, 30, 32, 48, 50–58). Our results, which reflect exclusion of one flawed trial, longer follow-up in six of the trials, and corrected results for the Swedish trials, were consistent with those of most previous meta-analyses. Two meta-analyses (8, 51), including one from the Cochrane Collaboration, produced results that differed substantially from ours. The Cochrane review reported a summary relative risk of 1.03 (CI, 0.77 to 1.38) but based this on only two trials.

Effectiveness of Mammography in Older Women

Direct evidence of effectiveness among older women is limited to two trials that included women older than 65 years of age. Both of these trials reported relative risk reductions among women 65 to 74 years of age (relative risk, 0.68 [CI, 0.51 to 0.89] [25] and 0.79 [59] among women 70 to 74 years of age). In the recent Swedish overview, the summary relative risk among women 65 to 74 years of age was 0.78 (CI, 0.62 to 0.99) (23, 60).

Table 4. **Results of Randomized, Controlled Trials of Mammography among Women 39 to 74 Years of Age***

Study (Reference)	Age	Median Follow-up	Breast Cancer Deaths/Total Women		Breast Cancer Death Rate per 1000 Women		Relative Risk for Death from Breast Cancer (95% CI)	Absolute Risk Reduction per 1000 Women	Number Needed To Invite to Screening†
			Screened Group	Control Group	Screened Group	Control Group			
		y	*n/n*						
Mammography alone									
Stockholm (23)	40–64	13.8	82/39 139	50/20 978	2.10	2.38	0.91 (0.65–1.27)	0.288	3468
Gothenburg (23)	39–59	12.8	62/20 724	113/29 200	2.99	3.87	0.76 (0.56–1.04)	0.878	1139
Malmö (23)	45–70	17.1	161/21 088	198/21 195	7.63	9.35	0.82 (0.67–1.00)	1.712	584
Swedish Two-County Trial (26)	40–74	17	319/77 080	333/55 985	4.14	5.95	0.68 (0.59–0.80)	1.809	553
Mammography plus CBE									
CNBSS-1 (22)	40–49	13	105/25 214	108/25 216	4.16	4.28	0.97 (0.74–1.27)	0.12	–
CNBSS-2 (20)	50–59	13	107/19 711	105/19 694	5.43	5.33	1.02 (0.78–1.33)	−0.097	–
HIP (19)	40–64	16	232/30 239	281/30 256	5.46	6.89	0.79	1.438	883
Edinburgh (18)	45–64	13	156/22 926	167/21 342	6.80	7.82	0.79 (0.60–1.02)	1.020	980

* CBE = clinical breast examination; CNBSS = Canadian National Breast Screening Study; HIP = Health Insurance Plan of Greater New York.
† Number needed to invite to screening to prevent one death from breast cancer 13–20 years after randomization.

Figure. **Relative risk compared with average years of follow-up for women 40 to 49 years of age, women 50 to 74 years of age, and all women.**

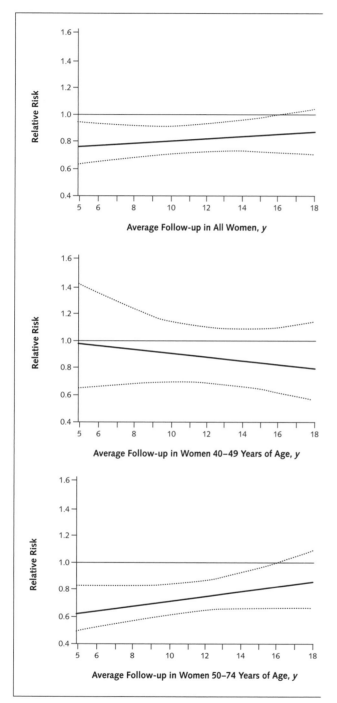

Estimated curves are from a hierarchical meta-regression model. Dotted curves represent 95% credible intervals.

Clinical Breast Examination

The test characteristics of CBE, based on data from trials designed specifically for breast cancer screening, were recently reviewed (61). Sensitivity ranged from 40% to 69%, specificity from 88% to 99%, and positive predictive value from 4% to 50% when mammography and interval

cancer were used as the criterion standard. One community study showed that over 10 years of biennial screening, 13.4% of women had false-positive results on CBE at least once; risk for such results was higher among women younger than 50 years of age (62).

No trial has compared CBE alone with no screening. However, two randomized, controlled trials involving the use of mammography and CBE had mortality reductions of 29% and 14% (18, 27, 63). A controlled, nonrandomized United Kingdom trial of CBE and mammography showed a nonsignificant mortality reduction of 14% (relative risk, 0.86 [CI, 0.73 to 1.01]) (64).

What is the contribution of CBE to these reductions in mortality rate? Among studies showing a benefit of screening, mortality reductions in trials of CBE with mammography are similar to those in trials including mammography only. In the CNBSS-2, in which women 50 to 59 years of age were randomly assigned to annual CBE and mammography or to annual CBE (65), the relative risk for death was 0.97 (CI, 0.62 to 1.52) (13). This suggests that mammography has little additive benefit in the setting of a careful, detailed CBE.

Breast Self-Examination

Because neither CBE nor mammography is 100% sensitive, BSE has been advised as an important screening method among women older than 20 years of age. However, its effectiveness in decreasing death from breast cancer has been controversial because evidence from clinical trials is limited. Observational studies evaluating BSE and breast cancer stage at diagnosis or death have had mixed results (45, 66).

In two randomized, controlled trials with 5 to 10 years of follow-up, both conducted outside the United States, breast cancer mortality rates were similar in women instructed in BSE and in noninstructed controls (67–69). Both studies involved large numbers of women who were meticulously trained with proper technique and had numerous reinforcement sessions; mammography was not part of routine screening in the countries involved. In both trials, physician visits and biopsy for benign breast lesions increased among those educated in BSE. To date, no studies have evaluated other potential adverse outcomes of BSE, such as anxiety and subsequent screening behavior.

Adverse Effects

The most frequently discussed adverse effects of mammography are the anxiety, discomfort, and cost associated with positive test results, many of which are false positive, and the diagnostic procedures they generate. For a woman undergoing regular mammography, cumulative specificity may be more relevant than the specificity of a single examination. In one community setting involving 2400 women 40 to 69 years of age, 6.5% of mammography results requiring further evaluation were false positive (specificity, 93.5%). When evaluated on an individual basis, however, approximately 23% of women had at least one false-positive result on mammography requiring further work-up during 10 years of biennial screening (average of 4 mammograms per woman), indicating a 10-year cumulative specificity of 76.2%. For every $100 spent on screening, $33 was spent on the evaluation of false-positive results (62).

Anxiety over an abnormal mammogram is documented in some (70–74) but not all (71, 75) studies. These studies generally suggest that anxiety dissipates after cancer is ruled out, but some studies suggest that some women worry persistently (72, 74–76). The anxiety associated with an abnormal mammogram does not seem to dissuade women from undergoing further screening (77) and may even be associated with improved adherence to recommended screening intervals (70, 78, 79). Many women are willing to accept the risk for false-positive results. In one survey, 99% of women understood that false-positive examination results occur with screening, although they underestimated the likelihood. Of importance, 63% stated that they would accept 500 instances of false-positive examination results to save one life (80).

Some view diagnosis and treatment of ductal carcinoma in situ (DCIS) as potential adverse consequences of mammography. There is incomplete evidence regarding the natural history of DCIS, the need for treatment, and treatment efficacy, and some women may receive treatment of DCIS that poses little threat to their health. In a 1992 study, 44% of women with DCIS were treated with mastectomy and 23% to 30% were treated with lumpectomy or radiation (81, 82). In one survey, only 6% of women were aware that mammography might detect nonprogressive breast cancer (80).

Radiation exposure is also a potential risk associated with mammography (83). Using risk estimates provided by the Biological Effects of Ionizing Radiation report of the U.S. National Academy of Sciences, and assuming a 4-mGy mean glandular dose from each two-views-per-breast bilateral mammography, Feig and Hendrick estimated that annual mammography of 100 000 women for 10 years beginning at 40 years of age would induce no more than eight deaths from breast cancer (84). Women with an inherited susceptibility to ionizing radiation damage have higher risk for radiogenic breast cancer (10, 85), although this has not been documented in association with mammography.

DISCUSSION

Fair-quality, relatively consistent evidence suggests that mammography screening reduces breast cancer death among women 40 to 74 years of age. We found no evidence that inclusion of CBE conferred greater benefit than mammography alone. We also found no evidence supporting the role of BSE in reducing breast cancer mortality.

Over the three decades in which mammography trial data have been available, critical reviewers and the investigators themselves have discussed limitations and irregularities in data reporting. One highly publicized review by the Cochrane Collaboration criticized the trials in regard to randomization, postrandomization exclusions, and determination of deaths from breast cancer (8). It found all but two of the trials, the Malmö trial and the Canadian trials, severely flawed or of poor quality and prompted some official bodies to question their support for screening mammography.

We identified many of the same design problems highlighted in the Cochrane review but reached different conclusions about their bearing on the validity of the findings. With the exception of the Edinburgh trial, we found inadequate evidence to conclude that the specific flaws identified introduced biases of sufficient magnitude or direction to invalidate the findings or to cause us to reject the inference that screening mammography reduces breast cancer mortality rates.

The effectiveness of screening in women 40 to 49 years of age is a longstanding controversy. In early years, it

Table 5. **Results of Mammography Trials among Women Younger Than 50 Years of Age***

Study (Reference)	Age	Median Follow-up	Breast Cancer Deaths/Total Women		Breast Cancer Death Rate per 1000 Women		Relative Risk for Death from Breast Cancer (95% Credible Interval)	Absolute Risk Reduction per 1000 Women	Number Needed To Invite to Screening†	Follow-up Year or Years in Which Controls Were Screened
			Screened Group	Control Group	Screened Group	Control Group				
		y	*n/n*							
Mammography alone										
Stockholm (23)	40–49	14.3	34/14 842	13/7103	2.29	1.83	1.52 (0.8–2.88)	No reduction	–	5
Gothenburg (23)	39–49	12.7	22/11 724	46/14 217	1.88	3.24	0.58 (0.35–0.96)	1.36	736	7
Malmö (23)	45–50	13.3	53/13 568	66/12 279	3.91	5.38	0.73 (0.51–1.04)	1.47	681	4
Swedish Two-County Trial (16)	40–49	13	45/19 844	39/15 604	2.27	2.50	0.87 (0.54–1.41)	0.23	4316	7–8
Mammography plus CBE										
CNBSS-1 (22)	40–49	13	105/25 214	108/25 216	4.16	4.28	0.97 (0.74–1.27)	0.12	–	–
HIP (19, 27)	40–49	14	64/13 740	82/13 740	4.66	5.97	0.78 (0.56–1.08)	1.31	763	–
Edinburgh (18)	45–49	13	49/11 749	53/10 267	4.17	5.16	0.75 (0.48–1.18)	0.99	1008	6–10

* CBE = clinical breast examination; CNBSS = Canadian National Breast Screening Study; HIP = Health Insurance Plan of Greater New York.
† Number needed to invite to screening to prevent one death from breast cancer 11 to 16 years after randomization.

Table 6. Meta-Analyses of Randomized Trials of Screening Mammography among Women 40 to 49 Years of Age*

Study (Reference), Year	Assessed Quality?	Included Trials	Methods	Follow-up, y	Relative Risk (95% CI)	Number Needed To Screen
Larsson et al. (50), 1997 Nyström et al. (32), 1993	No	5 Swedish trials	Weighted relative risks	12.8	0.77 (0.59–1.01)	
Cox (51), 1997 Elwood et al. (52), 1993	No	All 8 trials	Fixed effects	10	0.93 (0.77–1.11)	
Glasziou and Irwig (53), 1997 Glasziou (54), 1992	Yes. Rated all studies as "good." Rated Malmö and CNBSS highest and the Swedish Two-County Trial and Gothenburg lowest	All 8 trials	Variance weighted	13.13	0.85 (0.71–1.01)	
Hendrick et al. (55), 1997 Smart et al. (56), 1995	No	All 8 trials†	Fixed effects	12.7	0.82 (0.71–0.95)	1540
Kerlikowske et al. (57), 1995 Kerlikowske (58), 1997	No	All 8 trials	Fixed effects	Approximately 12	0.84 (0.71–0.99)	2500
Berry (30), 1998	No	All 8 trials	Random effects‡	12–15	0.82 (0.49–1.17)	
Olsen and Gøtzsche (8), 2001	Yes. Excluded 6 trials rated "flawed" or "poor"	Canadian, Malmö	Fixed effects	13	1.03 (0.77–1.38)	
Current study, 2002	Yes. Rated Edinburgh "poor" and others fair or better	7 trials, excluding Edinburgh	Random effects	Approximately 14	0.85 (0.73–0.99)	1698

* For multiple publications, data from the most recent update are recorded. CNBSS = Canadian National Breast Screening Study.
† Included an additional 17 000 patients from the Malmö II trial.
‡ Hierarchical Bayes model; estimates are for the "next trial" analysis.

centered on the lack of evidence that observed risk reductions were statistically significant (6, 52, 86). That argument has dissipated over time as more evidence has shown a significant separation in survival curves with longer follow-up. The delay in the separation of those curves, however, has prompted some to question whether the observed benefits are due to the detection of cancer after 50 years of age, suggesting little incremental benefit from initiating screening at 40 years of age and exposing women to the harms of screening for an extra decade (87, 88). We found little evidence to convincingly address this concern and some evidence that some benefit from screening women 40 to 49 years of age would be sacrificed if screening began at age 50 years (27, 89).

The use of 50 years of age as a threshold is somewhat arbitrary (except that it approximates the age of menopause). The risks for developing and dying of breast cancer are continuous variables that increase with age, and the greatest increase in incidence actually occurs before menopause (90, 91). We found that the relative risk reduction achieved with mammography screening does not differ substantially by age, although the time required to obtain the benefit is longer for younger women. On the other hand, younger women have more potential years of life to gain by screening. Thus, the variable most affected by age

is absolute risk reduction, which increases as a continuum with age while the number needed to screen decreases. The age of 50 years has no special bearing on this pattern, and some question the scientific rationale for treating women 40 to 49 years of age as a special entity (92).

What emerges as a more important concern, across all age groups, is whether the magnitude of benefit is sufficient to outweigh the harms. The risk for false-positive results and their consequences decreases with age. Thus, although mammography at any age poses a tradeoff of benefits and harms, the balance between increasing absolute risk reduction and decreasing harms grows more favorable over time. The age at which this tradeoff becomes acceptable is a subjective judgment that cannot be answered on scientific grounds, since early evidence suggests that women will tolerate a high risk for false-positive results. As noted earlier, 63% of women in one study stated that they would accept 500 instances of false-positive results to save one life (80). On the basis of the results of our meta-analysis, we calculated that over 10 years of biennial screening among 40-year-old women invited to be screened, approximately 400 women would have false-positive results on mammography and 100 women would undergo biopsy or fine-needle aspiration for each death from breast cancer prevented.

A limitation of our meta-analysis is that we combined

studies that used different methods of analysis. In the most recent report from the Swedish trials (23), Nyström and colleagues did not report individual study–level data using the follow-up method. The pooled follow-up analysis reported by Nyström and colleagues in 2002 suggest that the use of the follow-up method would have resulted in a smaller estimate of relative risk reduction.

Women older than 70 years of age have the highest incidence of breast cancer, and test performance in these women is likely to be similar to that in women 50 to 70 years of age. Therefore, theoretically, mammography should be at least as effective for women older than 65 years of age as it is for younger women. Offsetting this potential benefit, however, is the greater comorbidity observed in elderly persons. The potential benefit of early detection is unlikely to be realized in women who have other diseases that diminish life expectancy, in those who would not tolerate evaluation or treatment, and in those with impaired quality of life (for example, dementia) (93). In addition, no data from randomized, controlled trials provide information about the morbidity associated with screening, follow-up, and treatment among women older than 74 years of age. Finally, a major concern in elderly women is the diagnosis and treatment of DCIS, since mortality rates from DCIS are low (1% to 2% at 10 years) and 99% of DCIS is treated surgically (94).

The interval at which mammography was performed in the screening trials varied between 12 and 33 months, but annual mammography was no more effective than biennial mammography. Data from the Swedish Two-County Trial indicate that the period in which breast cancer can be detected before it presents clinically is shorter for women 40 to 49 years of age (95–97). Annual screening may be more important in this age group than in older women, but we found no direct proof for this hypothesis in the controlled trials that have been completed so far.

We found no evidence that CBE or BSE reduces breast cancer mortality. Whether the BSE trials are generalizable to the United States, where the use of CBE and mammography and the incidence of breast cancer are higher, is uncertain. It is also uncertain whether BSE might be beneficial to women who are not in the age ranges at which mammography is recommended or do not avail themselves of mammography. In the setting of CBE and mammography, the probability of finding a significant decrease in mortality rates is likely to be small.

In summary, when judged as population-based trials of cancer screening, most mammography trials are of fair quality. Their flaws reflect tradeoffs in planning that make the trial results widely generalizable but decrease internal validity. In absolute terms, the mortality benefit of mammography screening is small enough that biases in the trials could erase or create it. However, we found that although these trials were flawed in design or execution, there is insufficient evidence to conclude that most were seriously biased and consequently invalid.

Future research should be directed toward developing new screening methods as well as methods of improving the sensitivity and specificity of mammography. Methods of reducing surgical biopsy rates and complications of treatment should also be studied, as should communication of the risks and benefits associated with screening to patients. Finally, efforts to identify breast cancer risk factors with high attributable risk, as well as appropriate prevention strategies, should continue. Even in the best screening settings, most deaths from breast cancer are not currently prevented.

APPENDIX
Analytic Framework

Because of the availability of population-based, randomized trials, mammography has the most direct type of evidence of any cancer screening program (98). Nevertheless, mammography has been controversial since it was first proposed in the 1960s. To understand why, it is helpful to consider the assumptions underlying the steps in the causal chain from screening test to health outcomes. In the analytic framework (**Appendix Figure 1**), this evidence is shown by the overarching arc connecting screening with the outcomes, reduced morbidity and mortality. Mammography is aimed at early detection of invasive cancer, which is treated by major surgery (mastectomy or tumorectomy). This differs from screening for colorectal cancer and cervical cancer, which is aimed at detecting and removing precancerous lesions to prevent invasive cancer and to preserve the involved organ (colon or uterine cervix). This is one reason why, although it may be reasonable to endorse one cancer screening test (Papanicolaou smear) based on observational, indirect evidence, it may also be reasonable to require experimental evidence before endorsing another (mammography or prostate cancer screening).

It is important to note that the mammography trials do not necessarily provide the highest level of evidence about the efficacy of early treatment. While there is no doubt that screening results in earlier diagnosis of invasive breast cancer, the efficacy of earlier treatment of invasive cancer has not been established independently of the trials (99). That is, there is no direct evidence from trials of surgical therapy (versus watchful waiting) that earlier treatment of invasive cancer reduces mortality. The mammography trials do not attempt to link specific treatments, such as radical mastectomy or adjuvant radiation, to improved outcomes.

The reliance on a theory of treatment rather than on evidence about the efficacy of treatment increases the burden of proof placed on the trials of mammography. It also distinguishes cancer screening from other screening services considered by the USPSTF, such as chlamydia, depression, or osteoporosis screening, for which randomized, placebo-controlled trials of treatment have been done.

The threshold for sufficient evidence about efficacy

also depends on the balance of benefits and harms. Because mammography technology, the timing and type of information provided to patients, and treatment approaches have changed over time, the adverse consequences of screening in current practice might be very different from those in the trials. Other sources of data must be used to estimate these consequences.

Identification and Selection of Articles

We identified controlled trials and meta-analyses by searching the Cochrane Controlled Trials Registry (all dates), as well as searching for recent publications in MEDLINE (January 1994 to December 2001). Other sources were a PREMEDLINE search (December 2001 through February 2002); the reference lists of previous reviews, commentaries, and meta-analyses (5, 8, 27, 32, 50, 53, 56, 55, 60, 87, 100–103); the results of a broader search conducted for the systematic evidence review on which this article is based (46); and suggestions from experts.

In the electronic searches, the terms *breast neoplasms* and *breast cancer* were combined with the terms *mammography* and *mass screening* and with terms for controlled or randomized trials to yield 954 citations. Titles and abstracts were reviewed to identify publications that were randomized, controlled trials of breast cancer screening and had a relevant clinical outcome (advanced breast cancer, breast cancer mortality, or all-cause mortality). In all, the searches identified 146 controlled trials, of which 132 were excluded at the title and abstract phase because they concerned promoting screening rather than the efficacy of mammography (**Appendix Figure 2**). Four of the remaining 12 trials were excluded. Two were randomized trials of screening with mammography that have not yet presented outcomes of mortality or advanced breast cancer (104, 105). The third was a controlled trial that reported a reduction in breast cancer mortality but was not randomized (106, 107). The fourth, the Malmö Prevention Study, was apparently a randomized trial of a variety of preventive interventions, including mammography (108). It reported significantly fewer deaths from cancer among women younger than 40 years of age at study entry but provided no information about the mammography protocol, referring reader to another randomized trial, the Malmö Mammographic Screening Program, for further information. We believe that the two trials were in fact separate and that the results of the Malmö Mammographic Screening Program probably do not include results for the 8000 women who participated in the Malmö Prevention Study.

The remaining eight randomized trials of mammography were conducted between 1963 and 1994. Four of these were Swedish studies: the Malmö, Kopparberg, Ostergotland, Stockholm, and Gothenburg studies. (Kopparberg and Ostergotland together are known as the Swedish Two-County Trial.) The remaining studies were the Edinburgh study, the HIP study, and the two Canadian National Breast Screening Studies (CNBSS-1 and CNBSS-2).

Using the electronic searches and other sources, we retrieved the full text of 157 publications about these trials (these are listed in the bibliography accompanying the full systematic evidence review [46]). We also identified 10 previous systematic reviews of the trials. Seven of these concerned breast cancer mortality, and three addressed test performance (36, 37, 45). The searches identified three nonrandomized, controlled trials (109–111) that are not included in the meta-analysis but are discussed in the larger report (46). Two randomized trials of BSE were identified and reviewed.

Two of the authors abstracted information about each randomized, controlled trial. We compiled an appendix consisting of detailed information about the patient population, design, potential flaws, missing information, and analysis conducted in each trial. For the primary end point of breast cancer mortality, we abstracted results for each reported length of follow-up. Whenever possible, we abstracted data separately for participants by decade of age.

The randomized trials of screening provide little information about morbidity or the adverse effects of screening or treatment. A systematic review of adverse effects was beyond the scope of our review. In examining titles and abstracts, we obtained the full text of and reviewed recent articles reporting the frequency of false-positive results on screening mammography in the community and surveys of women's reactions to positive results on screening tests.

Assessment of Study Quality: General Approach

We used predefined criteria developed by the third USPSTF to assess the internal validity of each study (**Appendix Table 1**) (9). Two authors rated each study as "good," "fair," or "poor," resolving disagreements by discussion among the authors after review of the data and of comments by 12 peer reviewers of earlier drafts of the report. We tried to apply the same standards to the mammography trials as we have applied to other prevention topics. We based our quality ratings on the entire set of publications from a trial rather than on individual articles.

The USPSTF criteria were designed to be adaptable to the circumstances of different clinical questions. Like other current systems to assess the quality of trials, the criteria are based as much as possible on empirical evidence of bias in relation to study characteristics. However, although the body of such evidence is growing, it does not permit a high degree of certainty about the importance of specific quality criteria in judging the mammography trials. This is because nearly all empirical evidence of the impact of bias on effect size examined drug treatment or other therapies, rather than screening (112, 113). Generalization of these findings to large, population-based trials of screening is not straightforward. In recognition of this fact, cancer screening literature from the 1970s emphasizes that design standards for conventional trials of treatment should not always be applied to cancer screening trials (114).

The quality of reporting of trials limits precision in

critical appraisal (115). This is a particular issue in the mammography screening trials, many of which were conducted in the 1960s and 1970s. Their methods were poorly described, which limits precision in critical appraisal. Although some reviewers have promoted extensive query of trial authors to fill in gaps in published articles, the reliability of such data, as well as the appropriate interpretation of query data that contradicts what has been published in multiauthored, peer-reviewed papers, is uncertain. Moreover, authors are often unable to provide clarifying information (116).

Assessment of Study Quality: Application of Specific Criteria

All of the trials clearly defined interventions and co-interventions (CBE and BSE), all considered mortality outcomes, and all used intention-to-screen analysis. For this reason, the following received particular emphasis in judging the quality of the mammography trials: 1) initial assembly of comparable groups, 2) maintenance of comparable groups and minimization of differential or overall loss to follow-up, 3) and use of outcome measurements that were equal, reliable, and valid. As described below, we used a systematic approach to assess the flaws of the trials in each of these areas.

Initial Assembly of Comparable Groups

In the mammography trials, randomization was done individually or by clusters. Randomization of individuals is preferable because it is less likely to result in baseline differences among compared groups. In individually randomized trials, we classified *allocation concealment* as adequate, inadequate, or poorly described, according to the criteria used by Schulz and colleagues (115). In a cluster-randomized trial, it is impossible to conceal the assignment of individual patients, and the importance of concealing the allocation of clusters is unclear. Accordingly, we placed more importance on concealment in individually randomized trials.

We rated the way in which each trial compared participants in the screened and control groups. To obtain the highest rating in this category, a trial had to obtain baseline data on possible covariates before randomization, and the distribution of these covariates had to be similar in screening and control groups. In a large, individually randomized trial, baseline differences in sociodemographic variables would suggest that randomization failed, especially if there were opportunities for subversion (that is, if allocation was not concealed).

This standard applies only if baseline data can be reliably collected in all patients in both groups. In several of the mammography screening trials, participants in the usual care group were followed passively, and there was no opportunity to collect baseline data from all of them. The decision not to contact each individual in the control group has logistic advantages and probably reduced contamination, but it limits comparison between the screened and control groups. Moreover, when clusters are used, some baseline differences in the compared groups are almost inevitable.

We evaluated whether the method of identifying clusters (for example, geographic areas, month or year of birth) was likely to result in bias and whether measures such as matching were used to reduce it. If bias in assigning clusters to intervention or control groups seemed likely, we considered this a major flaw that was enough to invalidate the findings and rated the study as "poor." However, in contrast to individually randomized trials, we did not take small differences in the mean age of compared groups as an indicator that randomization failed to distribute more important confounders equally among the groups.

Several of the trials measured mortality rates from causes other than breast cancer to establish the comparability of the mammography and control groups. We recorded this information when it was available. Although comparable total mortality supports balanced randomization, it does not assure it. However, if there were dramatic differences in death from other causes, we considered it to be evidence that randomization failed.

Maintenance of Comparable Groups and Minimization of Differential or Overall Loss to Follow-up

Exclusions after randomization are considered to be a serious flaw in the execution of randomized trials, although empirical evidence of this bias is inconsistent (112, 113). Postrandomization exclusions were poorly described in several of the mammography trials and could have resulted in bias if the exclusions resulted in different levels of risk for death from breast cancer between the groups. In most of the mammography trials, however, exclusion of participants after randomization was an expected consequence of the protocol; some exclusion criteria, such as previous mastectomy, could not be applied to all participants before randomization because participants were not individually contacted. We examined the number of, reasons for, and methods for exclusion of participants after randomization. We based our rating on whether the methods used to ascertain patients were objective and consistent, not on the numbers of exclusions in the compared groups. Since ascertainment of clinical variables that might result in exclusion of a participant will be greater among intervention participants and is an expected consequence of the study design, we did not consider unequal numbers of excluded participants in the treatment and control groups after randomization to be definitive evidence of bias.

Use of Outcome Measurements That Were Equal, Reliable, and Valid (Including Masking of Outcome Assessment)

Over the duration of most of the trials, death from breast cancer (the primary end point) occurred in 2 to 9 per 1000 participants. The relatively low numbers of events means that misclassification or biased exclusion of a few deaths could change the direction and statistical significance of the trial results. For this reason, selection of cases for review of cause of death on broad criteria, use of reliable sources of information to ascertain vital status (death certificates, medical records, autopsies, registries), and use of independent blinded review of the cause of death are important measures to prevent bias. We considered blinded review of deaths a requirement for a quality rating of fair or better.

Approach to Multiple Analyses

The mammography trials have been criticized for decades (99, 117–119), and the trialists have responded by conducting additional analyses intended to address these criticisms. In our assessment of quality, we took into account the results of these supplemental analyses. For example, the cluster-randomized trials have been criticized because they analyzed results using statistical methods appropriate only to individually randomized trials. However, an independent reanalysis using the correct statistical method found that the results were unchanged (48). The Canadian trialists addressed criticisms that women who had palpable nodes might have been enrolled preferentially in the mammography group (120) by reanalyzing their data and showing that the exclusion of these participants did not affect the results (22).

Data Synthesis

Four of the trials compared mammography alone with usual care, and four compared mammography plus CBE with usual care. Because of lack of certainty that CBE is effective, and in consultation with USPSTF members, we decided that these trials were qualitatively homogeneous. The homogeneity of the trials was also assessed by using the standard chi-square test. The P value was greater than 0.1, indicating the effect sizes estimated by the studies are homogeneous.

We conducted two meta-analyses to address two key questions posed by the USPSTF: 1) Does mammography reduce breast cancer mortality rates among women over a broad range of ages when compared with usual care? and 2) If so, does mammography reduce breast cancer mortality rates among women 40 to 49 years of age when compared with usual care? In the first analysis, we included all data from the seven fair-quality trials, treating the two Canadian studies as one trial in participants 40 to 59 years of age. In the second analysis, we included the six fair-quality trials that reported results for women younger than 50 years of age.

We conducted each meta-analysis in two parts. First, using WinBUGS software, we constructed a two-level Bayesian random-effects model to estimate the effect size from multiple data points for each study and to derive a pooled estimate of relative risk reduction and credible interval for a given length of follow-up (11). The purpose of this analysis was to use repeated measures of the effect over time to estimate the relationship between length of follow-up and effect size. **Appendix Table 2** shows the data we used in this analysis. Second, we pooled the most recent

results of each trial to calculate the absolute and relative risk reduction, using the results of the first analysis to estimate the mean length of observation. Risks were modeled on the logit scale.

To model the relationship between length of follow-up and relative risk, a two-level hierarchical model was used. The first level was the result of a trial at a given average or median follow-up time, x_{ij}, where i indexes the trial and j indexes the data point within a trial. The second level was the trial itself. The model allows for within-trial and between-trial variability. Specifically, the model was:

$$\alpha^* \sim \text{Normal}(\cdot,\cdot)$$
$$\beta^* \sim \text{Normal}(\cdot,\cdot)$$
$$\alpha_i \cdot \sim \text{Normal}(\alpha^*, \sigma^2_\alpha$$
$$\beta_i \cdot \sim \text{Normal}(\beta^*, \sigma^2_\beta \cdot$$
$$\mu_{ij} = \alpha_i + \beta_i x_{ij} + \tau \cdot z_{ij}$$
$$\tau \cdot \sim \Gamma(\cdot,\cdot)$$
$$z_{ij} \sim \text{Normal}(0,1)$$
$$\log RR_{ij} \sim \text{Normal}(\mu_{ij}, s^2).$$

A global regression curve was estimated as $\log RR = \alpha^* + \beta^* x$. The random effect was $\tau \cdot z_{ij}$. The model to estimate summary risk was

$$\# \text{deaths}_{\text{control}, i} \sim \text{Binomial}(\pi_{\text{control},i}, n_{\text{control},i})$$
$$\# \text{deaths}_{\text{intervention},i} \sim \text{Binomial}(\pi_{\text{intervention},i}, n_{\text{intervention}, i})$$

$$\text{logit}(\pi_{\text{control},i}) = \alpha + \tau \cdot z_i$$
$$\text{logit}(\pi_{\text{intervention},i}) = \alpha + \beta + \tau \cdot z_i$$
$$\alpha \sim \text{Normal}(\cdot,\cdot)$$
$$\beta^* \sim \text{Normal}(\cdot,\cdot)$$
$$\tau \cdot \sim \Gamma(\cdot,\cdot)$$

Absolute risk difference was calculated as $\pi_{\text{control},i} - \pi_{\text{intervention},i}$. Relative risk was calculated as $\exp(\beta)$.

The models were estimated by using a Bayesian data analytic framework (121). The data were analyzed by using WinBUGS (11), which uses Gibbs sampling to simulate posterior probability distributions. Noninformative (proper) prior probability distributions were used: $\text{Normal}(0, 10^6)$ and $\Gamma(0.001, 0.001)$. Five separate Markov chains with overdispersed initial values were used to generate draws from posterior distributions. Point estimates (mean) and 95% credible intervals (2.5 and 97.5 percentiles) were derived from the subsequent $5 \times 10\,000$ draws after reasonable convergence of the five chains was attained. The code to model the data in WinBUGS is available from the authors on request.

Peer Review and Revisions

Our review was begun early in 2000. A first draft was presented to the USPSTF in December 2000. Throughout 2001, the manuscript underwent extensive critical review by a broad range of experts. Subsequent versions were reviewed by the USPSTF in September 2001 and in January 2002.

Appendix Figure 1. **Analytic framework.**

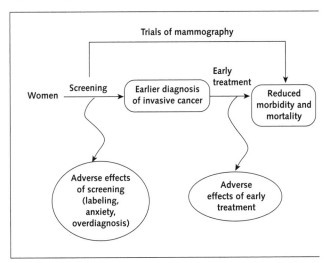

Trials of mammography link screening to health outcomes, but do not address the intermediate steps (screening and early treatment) or harms (adverse effects of screening and early treatment). Arrows indicating screening and early treatment represent the intermediate steps in the causal chain linking screening with improved mortality and morbidity.

Appendix Figure 2. **Selection of randomized trials for the systematic review and meta-analysis.**

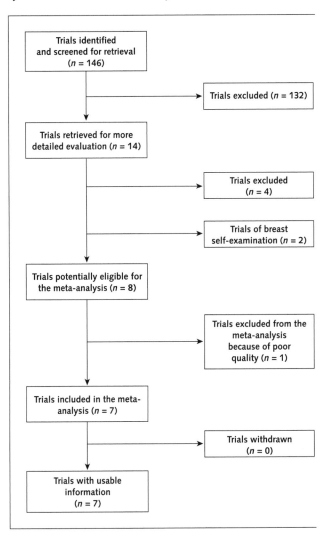

Appendix Table 1. **Criteria for Grading the Internal Validity of Individual Studies**

Randomized, controlled trials
  Clear definition of interventions
  All important outcomes considered
  Intention-to-treat analysis
  Initial assembly of comparable groups
    Adequate randomization, including first concealment and whether potential confounders were distributed equally among groups
    Similar all-cause mortality among groups
  Maintenance of comparable groups (includes attrition, crossovers, adherence, contamination)
  Important differential loss to follow-up or overall high loss to follow-up
  Equal, reliable, and valid measurements (includes masking of outcome assessment)
Systematic reviews
  Comprehensiveness of sources considered and search strategy used
  Standard appraisal of included studies
  Validity of conclusions
  Recency and relevance (especially important)

Appendix Table 2. **Data Used in the Analysis***

Study, Year (Reference)	Age	Mean Follow-up	Intervention Group				Control Group				RR (95% CI)
			Deaths	Partici-pants	Life-Years	Rate/10 000 Women	Deaths	Partici-pants	Life-Years	Rate/10 000 Women	
	y		*n*				*n*				
CNBSS											
Miller, unpublished manuscript	40–49	13.0	105	25 214	282 606	3.7	108	25 216	282 575	3.8	0.97 (0.74–1.27)
Miller et al., 1997 (21)†	40–49	10.5	82	25 214	264 747	3.1	72	25 216	264 768	2.7	1.14 (0.83–1.56)
Miller et al., 1992 (12)	40–49	8.5	38	25 214	214 319	1.8	28	25 216	214 336	1.3	1.36 (0.84–2.21)
	40–59	13.0	212	44 925	584 025	3.6	213	44 910	583 830	3.6	1.00 (0.82–1.20)
	40–59	8.5	76	44 925	381 863	2.0	67	44 910	381 735	1.8	1.13 (0.82–1.57)
Miller et al., 2000 (20)	50–59	13.0	107	19 711	216 133	5.0	105	19 694	216 042	4.9	1.02 (0.78–1.33)
Miller et al., 1992 (13)	50–59	8.3	38	19 711	163 601	2.3	39	19 694	163 460	2.4	0.97 (0.62–1.52)
HIP											
Shapiro, 1997 (27)†	40–49	18.0	49	13 740	247 320	2.0	65	13 740	247 320	2.6	0.75 (0.52–1.09)
Habbema et al., 1986 (122)	40–49	14.0	64	13 740	192 360	3.3	82	13 740	192 360	4.3	0.78 (0.56–1.08)
Shapiro et al., 1988 (19)	40–49	10.0	39	13 740	137 400	2.8	51	13 740	137 400	3.7	0.76 (0.50–1.16)
Shapiro et al., 1988 (19)	40–49	5.0	19	13 740	68 700	2.8	20	13 740	68 700	2.9	0.95 (0.51–1.78)
Shapiro et al., 1988 (19)	40–64	18.0	126	30 245	544 410	2.3	163	30 245	544 410	3.0	0.77 (0.61–0.98)
Shapiro et al., 1985 (123)	40–64	16.0	236	30 239	483 824	4.9	281	30 756	492 096	5.7	0.85 (0.72–1.02)
Habbema et al., 1986 (122)	40–64	14.0	165	30 245	423 430	3.9	212	30 245	423 430	5.0	0.78 (0.64–0.95)
Shapiro et al., 1988 (19)	40–64	10.0	95	30 245	302 450	3.1	133	30 245	302 450	4.4	0.71 (0.55–0.93)
Shapiro et al., 1988 (19)	40–64	5.0	39	30 245	151 225	2.6	63	30 245	151 225	4.2	0.62 (0.42–0.92)
Shapiro et al., 1988 (19)	50–64	18.0	77	16 505	297 090	2.6	98	16 505	297 090	3.3	0.79 (0.58–1.06)
Habbema et al., 1986 (122)	50–64	14.0	101	16 505	231 070	4.4	130	16 505	231 070	5.6	0.78 (0.60–1.01)
Shapiro et al., 1988 (19)	50–64	10.0	56	16 505	165 050	3.4	82	16 505	165 050	5.0	0.68 (0.49–0.96)
Shapiro et al., 1988 (19)	50–64	5.0	20	16 505	82 525	2.4	43	16 505	82 525	5.2	0.47 (0.27–0.79)
Gothenburg											
Bjurstam et al., 1997 (24)†	39–49	11.8	18	11 724	138 402	1.3	40	14 217	168 025	2.4	0.55 (0.31–0.96)
Nyström et al., 2002 (23)	40–49	12.7	22	10 888	138 000	1.6	46	13 203	167 000	2.8	0.58 (0.35–0.96)
Larsson et al., 1997 (50)	40–49	9.8	16	10 821	106 000	1.5	33	13 101	129 000	2.6	0.59 (0.33–1.06)
Nyström et al., 2002 (23)	40–59	12.8	62	21 000	268 000	2.3	113	29 200	373 000	3.0	0.76 (0.56–1.04)
Nyström et al., 1993 (32)	40–59	6.3	27	20 724	129 000	2.1	47	28 809	181 000	2.6	0.86 (0.54–1.37)
Nyström et al., 2002 (23)	50–59	12.9	40	10 112	130 000	3.1	67	15 997	206 000	3.3	0.94 (0.62–1.43)
Stockholm											
Nyström et al., 2002 (23)	40–49	14.3	34	14 303	203 000	1.7	13	8021	117 000	1.1	1.52 (0.80–2.88)
Frisell and Lidbrink, 1997b (124)†	40–49	11.9	24	14 842	173 866	1.4	12	7103	87 826	1.4	1.08 (0.54–2.17)
Larsson et al., 1997 (50)	40–49	11.5	23	14 185	162 000	1.4	10	7985	94 000	1.1	1.34 (0.64–2.80)
Frisell et al., 1991 (125)	40–49	7.2	16	14 375	99 155	1.6	8	7103	54 446	1.5	1.09 (0.40–3.00)
Frisell et al., 1997a (17)	40–64	11.8	66	40 318	473 153	1.4	45	19 943	239 460	1.9	0.74 (0.50–1.10)
Frisell et al., 1991 (125)	40–64	7.1	39	39 164	270 247	1.4	30	19 943	147 373	2.0	0.71 (0.40–1.20)
Nyström et al., 2002 (23)	40–65	13.8	82	39 139	535 000	1.5	50	20 978	296 000	1.7	0.91 (0.65–1.27)
Nyström et al., 1993 (32)	40–65	7.6	53	38 525	287 000	1.8	40	20 651	164 000	2.4	0.80 (0.53–1.22)
Nyström et al., 2002 (23)	50–59	13.7	25	15 946	217 000	1.2	24	8421	118 000	2.0	0.56 (0.32–0.97)
Frisell et al., 1997a (17)	50–64	11.8	42	25 476	299 287	1.4	33	12 840	151 634	2.2	0.62 (0.38–1.00)
Frisell et al., 1991 (125)	50–64	7.0	23	24 789	171 092	1.3	22	12 840	92 927	2.4	0.57 (0.30–1.10)
Malmö I + II											
Nyström et al., 2002 (23)	43–49	13.3	53	13 568	184 000	2.9	66	12 279	160 000	4.1	0.73 (0.51–1.04)
Andersson and Janzon, 1997 (15)†	43–49	12.0	57	13 528	165 596	3.4	78	12 242	144 036	5.4	0.64 (0.45–0.89)
Nyström et al., 2002 (23)	43–70	15.3	190	30 669	473 000	4.0	231	29 407	448 000	5.2	0.79 (0.65–0.96)
Nyström et al., 2002 (23)	45–49	18.0	24	3987	71 000	3.4	33	4067	74 000	4.5	0.74 (0.44–1.25)
Larsson et al., 1997 (50)	45–49	15.4	15	3945	61 000	2.5	23	4017	62 000	3.7	0.67 (0.35–1.27)
Nyström et al., 2002 (23)	45–54	18.2	71	8673	158 000	4.5	78	8311	151 000	5.2	0.87 (0.63–1.20)
Andersson et al., 1988 (25)	45–54	9.0	28	7981	71 775	3.9	22	8082	72 635	3.0	1.29 (0.74–2.25)
Andersson et al., 1988 (25)	45–69	8.8	63	21 088	186 297	3.4	66	21 195	187 016	3.5	0.96 (0.68–1.35)
Nyström et al., 2002 (23)	45–70	17.1	161	21 088	360 000	4.5	198	21 195	362 000	5.5	0.82 (0.67–1.00)
Nyström et al., 1993 (32)	45–70	11.5	87	20 695	239 000	3.6	108	20 783	240 000	4.5	0.81 (0.62–1.07)
Nyström et al., 2002 (23)	50–70	16.9	137	17 101	289 000	4.7	165	17 128	288 000	5.7	0.83 (0.66–1.04)
Nyström et al., 2002 (23)	55–64	17.2	63	8194	141 000	4.5	83	8679	149 000	5.6	0.80 (0.57–1.12)
Andersson et al., 1988 (25)	55–69	8.7	35	13 107	114 522	3.1	44	13 113	114 381	3.8	0.79 (0.51–1.24)
Nyström et al., 2002 (23)	55–70	16.3	90	12 415	202 000	4.5	120	12 884	211 000	5.7	0.78 (0.59–1.02)
Swedish Two-County Trial, Kopparberg											
Tabár et al., 2000 (26)	40–49	17.3	NR	NR	NR	**NR**	NR	NR	NR	**NR**	0.76 (0.42–1.40)
Tabár et al., 1995 (16)	40–49	13.0	22	9582	124 566	1.8	16	5031	65 403	2.4	0.73 (0.37–1.41)

Continued on following page

Appendix Table 2—**Continued**

Study, Year (Reference)	Age	Mean Follow-up	Intervention Group				Control Group				RR (95% CI)
			Deaths	Partici-pants	Life-Years	Rate/ 10 000 Women	Deaths	Partici-pants	Life-Years	Rate/ 10 000 Women	
	y		*n*				*n*				
Tabár et al., 1989 (28)	40–49	7.9	13	9582	**75 698**	1.7	9	5031	**39 745**	2.3	**0.76 (0.32–1.77)**
Tabár et al., 1985 (35)	40–49	6.0	8	9625	**57 750**	1.4	3	5053	**30 318**	1.0	**1.40 (0.37–5.28)**
Tabár et al., 2000 (26)	40–74	17.3	152	NR	672 482	2.3	121	NR	326 091	3.7	0.61 (NR–NR)
Tabár et al., 1995 (16)	40–74	13.0	126	38 589	**501 657**	2.5	104	18 582	241 566	4.3	**0.60 (0.46–0.79)**
Tabár et al., 1989 (28)	40–74	7.9	77	38 589	**304 853**	2.5	58	18 582	**146 798**	4.0	**0.64 (0.46–0.90)**
Tabár et al., 1985 (35)	40–74	6.0	51	39 051	**234 306**	2.2	39	18 846	**113 076**	3.4	**0.63 (0.42–0.96)**
Tabár et al., 2000 (26)	50–59	17.3	NR	NR	NR	**NR**	NR	NR	NR	**NR**	0.46 (0.30–0.71)
Tabár et al., 1995 (16)	50–59	13.0	34	11 728	**152 464**	2.2	34	5557	**72 241**	4.7	**0.48 (0.29–0.77)**
Tabár et al., 1989 (28)	50–59	7.9	20	9582	**75 698**	2.6	20	5031	**39 745**	5.0	**0.53 (0.28–0.98)**
Tabár et al., 1995 (16)	50–74	13.0	104	29 007	**377 091**	2.8	88	13 551	**176 163**	5.0	**0.58 (0.43–0.78)**
Tabár et al., 1989 (28)	50–74	7.9	64	29 007	**229 155**	2.8	49	13 551	**107 053**	4.6	**0.61 (0.42–0.89)**
Tabár et al., 1985 (35)	50–74	6.0	43	29 426	**176 556**	2.4	36	13 793	**82 758**	4.4	**0.56 (0.36–0.87)**
Swedish Two-County Trial, Ostergötland											
Tabár et al., 2000 (26)	40–49	**17.3**	NR	NR	NR	**NR**	NR	NR	**NR**	NR	1.06 (0.65–1.76)
Nyström et al., 2002 (23)	40–49	**16.8**	31	10 285	172 000	**1.8**	30	10 459	176 000	**1.7**	1.05 (0.64–1.71)
Tabár et al., 1995 (16)	40–49	13.0	23	10 262	**133 406**	1.7	23	10 573	**137 449**	1.7	1.02 (0.52–1.99)
Tabár et al., 1989 (28)	40–49	7.9	15	10 262	**81 070**	1.9	15	10 573	**83 527**	1.8	**1.03 (0.50–2.11)**
Tabár et al., 1985 (35)	40–49	6.0	8	10 312	**61 872**	1.3	7	10 625	**63 750**	1.1	**1.18 (0.43–3.25)**
Tabár et al., 2000 (26)	40–74	17.3	167	NR	660 242	2.5	213	NR	643 696	3.3	**0.76 (NR–NR)**
Nyström et al., 2002 (23)	40–74	15.2	177	38 942	589 000	3.0	190	37 675	572 000	3.3	**0.90 (0.73–1.11)**
Tabár et al., 1995 (16)	40–74	13.0	135	38 491	**500 383**	2.7	173	37 403	**486 239**	3.6	0.78 (0.60–1.01)
Tabár et al., 1989 (28)	40–74	7.9	83	38 491	**304 079**	2.7	109	37 403	**295 484**	3.7	**0.74 (0.56–0.98)**
Tabár et al., 1985 (35)	40–74	6.0	36	39 034	**234 204**	1.5	47	37 936	**227 616**	2.1	**0.74 (0.48–1.15)**
Tabár et al., 2000 (26)	50–59	17.3	NR	NR	NR	**NR**	NR	NR	NR	**NR**	0.76 (0.53–1.10)
Nyström et al., 2002 (23)	50–59	16.1	53	12 011	194 000	2.7	54	11 495	185 000	2.9	**0.94 (0.66–1.35)**
Tabár et al., 1995 (16)	50–59	13.0	44	11 757	**152 841**	2.9	51	11 248	**146 224**	3.5	**0.85 (0.52–1.38)**
Tabár et al., 1989 (28)	50–59	7.9	25	11 757	**92 880**	2.7	34	11 248	**88 859**	3.8	**0.70 (0.42–1.18)**
Nyström et al., 2002 (23)	50–74	14.9	146	28 657	**417 000**	3.5	160	25 920	396 000	4.0	**0.83 (0.66–1.03)**
Tabár et al., 1995 (16)	50–74	13.0	112	28 229	**366 977**	3.1	150	26 830	**348 790**	4.3	**0.73 (0.56–0.97)**
Tabár et al., 1989 (28)	50–74	7.9	68	28 229	**223 009**	3.0	94	26 830	**211 957**	4.4	**0.69 (0.50–0.94)**
Tabár et al., 1985 (35)	50–74	6.0	28	28 722	**172 332**	1.6	40	27 311	**163 866**	2.4	**0.67 (0.41–1.08)**
Swedish Two-County Trial, Kopparberg + Ostergötland											
Tabár et al., 1995 (16)	40–49	13.0	45	19 844	**257 972**	1.7	39	15 604	**202 852**	1.9	0.87 (0.54–1.41)
Tabár et al., 1989 (28)	40–49	7.9	28	19 844	**156 768**	1.8	24	15 604	**123 272**	1.9	0.92 (0.52–1.60)
Tabár et al., 1989 (28)	40–49	7.9	28	19 844	**156 768**	1.8	24	15 604	**123 272**	1.9	**0.92 (0.53–1.58)**
Tabár et al., 1985 (35)	40–49	6.0	16	19 937	**119 622**	1.3	10	15 678	**94 068**	1.1	**1.26 (0.56–2.84)**
Tabár et al., 2000 (26)	40–74	17.3	319	77 080	1 332 724	2.4	334	55 985	969 787	3.4	**0.68 (0.59–0.80)**
Tabár et al., 1995 (16)	40–74	12.5	269	77 080	965 405	2.8	277	55 985	701 207	4.0	**0.69 (0.57–0.84)**
Tabár et al., 1989 (28)	40–74	7.9	160	77 080	**608 932**	2.6	167	55 985	**442 282**	3.8	**0.70 (0.56–0.86)**
Tabár et al., 1985 (35)	40–74	6.0	87	78 085	**468 510**	1.9	86	56 782	**340 692**	2.5	**0.69 (0.51–0.92)**
Tabár et al., 1995 (16)	50–59	13.0	78	23 485	**305 305**	2.6	85	16 805	**218 465**	3.9	**0.66 (0.46–0.93)**
Tabár et al., 1989 (28)	50–59	7.9	45	23 485	**185 532**	2.4	54	16 805	**132 760**	4.1	**0.60 (0.40–0.89)**
Tabár et al., 1995 (16)	50–74	13.0	224	57 236	**744 068**	3.0	238	55 985	**727 805**	3.3	**0.66 (0.54–0.81)**
Tabár et al., 1989 (28)	50–74	7.9	132	57 236	**452 164**	2.9	143	40 381	**319 010**	4.5	**0.65 (0.51–0.83)**
Tabár et al., 1985 (35)	50–74	6.0	71	58 148	**348 888**	2.0	76	41 104	**246 624**	3.1	**0.61 (0.44–0.84)**
Edinburgh											
Alexander et al., 1999 (18)	45–49	12.2	47	11 479	139 868	3.4	53	10 267	126 413	4.2	**0.75 (0.48–1.18)**
Alexander, 1997 (126)†	45–49	12.2	46	NR	139 871	3.3	52	NR	126 417	4.1	**0.88 (0.55–1.41)**
Alexander et al., 1994 (127)	45–49	8.5	25	11 505	97 206	2.6	31	10 269	88 766	3.5	**0.78 (0.46–1.31)**
Roberts et al., 1990 (128)	45–49	6.9	13	5913	40 851	3.2	13	5810	40 009	3.2	**0.98 (NR–NR)**
Alexander et al., 1999 (18)	45–64	13.0	156	22 926	301 155	5.2	167	21 342	276 363	6.0	0.79 (0.60–1.02)
Alexander et al., 1994 (127)	45–64	9.5	96	22 944	219 215	4.4	106	21 344	201 821	5.3	**0.82 (0.61–1.11)**
Roberts et al., 1990 (128)	45–64	6.8	68	23 226	157 946	4.3	76	21 904	147 854	5.1	**0.83 (0.58–1.18)**
Alexander et al., 1999 (18)	50–64	12.9	129	17 149	222 393	5.8	134	15 748	200 637	6.7	**0.87 (NR–NR)**
Alexander et al., 1994 (127)	50–64	9.4	79	17 149	162 465	4.9	85	15 748	147 233	5.8	**0.85 (0.62–1.15)**
Roberts et al., 1990 (128)	50–64	6.7	55	17 313	117 095	4.7	63	16 094	107 845	5.8	**0.80 (0.54–1.17)**

* Numbers in boldface type were calculated from data in the spreadsheet; all other numbers were taken from publications. CNBSS = Canadian National Breast Screening Study; HIP = Health Insurance Plan of Greater New York; NR = not reported; RR = relative risk.
† Used in reference 30.

From Oregon Health & Science University and Portland Veterans Affairs Medical Center, Portland, Oregon; and Medical College of Virginia, Virginia Commonwealth University, Fairfax, Virginia.

Note: This manuscript is based on a longer systematic evidence review that was reviewed by outside experts and representatives of professional societies. A complete list of peer reviewers is available online at www.ahrq.gov/clinic/usstfix.htm.

Disclaimer: The authors of this article are responsible for its contents, including any clinical or treatment recommendations. No statement in this article should be construed as an official position of the Agency for Healthcare Research and Quality or the U.S. Department of Health and Human Services.

Acknowledgments: The authors thank Stephanie Detlefsen, MD, for her contribution to this evidence review and David Atkins, MD, MPH, from the Agency for Healthcare Research and Quality and members of the U.S. Preventive Services Task Force for their comments on earlier versions of this review. They also thank Kathryn Pyle Krages, AMLS, MA, Susan Carson, MPH, Patty Davies, MS, Susan Wingenfeld, and Jim Wallace for their help with preparation of the manuscript and the full systematic evidence review.

Grant Support: This study was conducted by the Oregon Health & Science University Evidence-based Practice Center under contract to the Agency for Healthcare Research and Quality (contract no. 290-97-0018, task order no. 2), Rockville, Maryland.

Requests for Single Reprints: Reprints are available from the Agency for Healthcare Research and Quality Web site (www.preventiveservices.ahrq.gov) or the Agency for Healthcare Research and Quality Publications Clearinghouse (800-358-9295).

Current author addresses, the Appendix, Appendix Figures, and Appendix Tables are available at www.annals.org.

Current Author Addresses: Drs. Humphrey and Helfand and Mr. Chan: Oregon Health & Science University, Mailcode BICC, 3181 SW Sam Jackson Park Road, Portland, OR 97201-3098.
Dr. Woolf: Virginia Commonwealth University, 3712 Charles Stewart Drive, Fairfax, VA 22033.

References

1. Cancer Facts and Figures 2001. American Cancer Society. Accessed at www.cancer.org/downloads/STT/F&F2001.pdf on 16 July 2002.

2. Gail MH, Brinton LA, Byar DP, Corle DK, Green SB, Schairer C, et al. Projecting individualized probabilities of developing breast cancer for white females who are being examined annually. J Natl Cancer Inst. 1989;81:1879-86. [PMID: 2593165]

3. Colditz GA, Willett WC, Hunter DJ, Stampfer MJ, Manson JE, Hennekens CH, et al. Family history, age, and risk of breast cancer. Prospective data from the Nurses' Health Study. JAMA. 1993;270:338-43. [PMID: 8123079]

4. Seidman H, Stellman SD, Mushinski MH. A different perspective on breast cancer risk factors: some implications of the nonattributable risk. CA Cancer J Clin. 1982;32:301-13. [PMID: 6811109]

5. Strax P. Mass screening of asymptomatic women. In: Ariel IM, Cleary J, eds. Breast Cancer: Diagnosis and Treatment. New York: McGraw-Hill; 1987:145-51.

6. Guide to Clinical Preventive Services. 2nd ed. US Preventive Services Task Force. Baltimore, MD: Williams & Wilkins; 1996.

7. Sirovich BE, Sox HC Jr. Breast cancer screening. Surg Clin North Am. 1999;79:961-90. [PMID: 10572546]

8. Olsen O, Gøtzsche PC. Cochrane review on screening for breast cancer with mammography [Letter]. Lancet. 2001;358:1340-2. [PMID: 11684218]

9. Harris RP, Helfand M, Woolf SH, Lohr KN, Mulrow CD, Teutsch SM, et al. Current methods of the US Preventive Services Task Force: a review of the process. Am J Prev Med. 2001;20:21-35. [PMID: 11306229]

10. Harrison TR. Breast cancer. In: Fauci AS, ed. Principles of Internal Medicine. 14th ed. New York: McGraw Hill; 1998:564-7.

11. WinBUGS Version 1.2 User Manual. Cambridge, United Kingdom: MRC Biostatistics Unit; 1999.

12. Miller AB, Baines CJ, To T, Wall C. Canadian National Breast Screening Study: 1. Breast cancer detection and death rates among women aged 40 to 49 years. CMAJ. 1992;147:1459-76. [PMID: 1423087]

13. Miller AB, Baines CJ, To T, Wall C. Canadian National Breast Screening Study: 2. Breast cancer detection and death rates among women aged 50 to 59 years. CMAJ. 1992;147:1477-88. [PMID: 1423088]

14. Bjurstam N, Björneld L, Duffy SW, Smith TC, Cahlin E, Erikson O, et al. The Gothenburg Breast Cancer Screening Trial: preliminary results on breast cancer mortality for women aged 39-49. J Natl Cancer Inst Monogr. 1997:53-5. [PMID: 9709276]

15. Andersson I, Janzon L. Reduced breast cancer mortality in women under age 50: updated results from the Malmö Mammographic Screening Program. J Natl Cancer Inst Monogr. 1997:63-7. [PMID: 9709278]

16. Tabar L, Fagerberg G, Chen HH, Duffy SW, Smart CR, Gad A, et al. Efficacy of breast cancer screening by age. New results from the Swedish Two-County Trial. Cancer. 1995;75:2507-17. [PMID: 7736395]

17. Frisell J, Lidbrink E, Hellström L, Rutqvist LE. Followup after 11 years–update of mortality results in the Stockholm mammographic screening trial. Breast Cancer Res Treat. 1997;45:263-70. [PMID: 9386870]

18. Alexander FE, Anderson TJ, Brown HK, Forrest AP, Hepburn W, Kirkpatrick AE, et al. 14 years of follow-up from the Edinburgh randomised trial of breast-cancer screening. Lancet. 1999;353:1903-8. [PMID: 10371567]

19. Shapiro S, Venet W, Strax P, Venet L. Current results of the breast cancer screening randomized trial: the health insurance plan (HIP) of greater New York study. In: Day NE, Miller AB, eds. Screening for Breast Cancer. Toronto: Hans Huber; 1988:3-15.

20. Miller AB, To T, Baines CJ, Wall C. Canadian National Breast Screening Study-2: 13-year results of a randomized trial in women aged 50-59 years. J Natl Cancer Inst. 2000;92:1490-9. [PMID: 10995804]

21. Miller AB, To T, Baines CJ, Wall C. The Canadian National Breast Screening Study: update on breast cancer mortality. J Natl Cancer Inst Monogr. 1997:37-41. [PMID: 9709273]

22. Miller AB, To T, Baines CJ, Wall C. The Canadian National Breast Cancer Screening Study-1: breast cancer mortality after 11 to 16 years of follow-up. A randomized screening trial of mammography in women age 40 to 49 years. Ann Intern Med. 2002;137:305-12.

23. Nyström L, Andersson I, Bjurstam N, Frisell J, Nordenskjöld B, Rutqvist LE. Long-term effects of mammography screening: updated overview of the Swedish randomised trials. Lancet. 2002;359:909-19. [PMID: 11918907]

24. Bjurstam N, Björneld L, Duffy SW, Smith TC, Cahlin E, Eriksson O, et al. The Gothenburg breast screening trial: first results on mortality, incidence, and mode of detection for women ages 39-49 years at randomization. Cancer. 1997;80:2091-9. [PMID: 9392331]

25. Andersson I, Aspegren K, Janzon L, Landberg T, Lindholm K, Linell F, et al. Mammographic screening and mortality from breast cancer: the Malmö mammographic screening trial. BMJ. 1988;297:943-8. [PMID: 3142562]

26. Tabár L, Vitak B, Chen HH, Duffy SW, Yen MF, Chiang CF, et al. The Swedish Two-County Trial twenty years later. Updated mortality results and new insights from long-term follow-up. Radiol Clin North Am. 2000;38:625-51. [PMID: 10943268]

27. Shapiro S. Periodic screening for breast cancer: the HIP Randomized Controlled Trial. Health Insurance Plan. J Natl Cancer Inst Monogr. 1997:27-30. [PMID: 9709271]

28. Tabar L, Fagerberg G, Duffy SW, Day NE. The Swedish two county trial of mammographic screening for breast cancer: recent results and calculation of benefit. J Epidemiol Community Health. 1989;43:107-14. [PMID: 2512366]

29. Black WC, Haggstrom DA, Welch HG. All-cause mortality in randomized trials of cancer screening. J Natl Cancer Inst. 2002;94:167-73. [PMID:

11830606]

30. Berry DA. Benefits and risks of screening mammography for women in their forties: a statistical appraisal. J Natl Cancer Inst. 1998;90:1431-9. [PMID: 9776408]

31. Sjönell G, Ståhle L. [Mammographic screening does not reduce breast cancer mortality]. Lakartidningen. 1999;96:904-5, 908-13. [PMID: 10089737]

32. Nyström L, Rutqvist LE, Wall S, Lindgren A, Lindqvist M, Rydén S, et al. Breast cancer screening with mammography: overview of Swedish randomised trials. Lancet. 1993;341:973-8. [PMID: 8096941]

33. Nystrom L, Larsson LG, Wall S, Rutqvist LE, Andersson I, Bjurstam N, et al. An overview of the Swedish randomised mammography trials: total mortality pattern and the representivity of the study cohorts. J Med Screen. 1996;3:85-7. [PMID: 8849766]

34. Tabár L, Gad A, Holmberg L, Ljungquist U. Significant reduction in advanced breast cancer. Results of the first seven years of mammography screening in Kopparberg, Sweden. Diagn Imaging Clin Med. 1985;54:158-64. [PMID: 3896614]

35. Tabár L, Fagerberg CJ, Gad A, Baldetorp L, Holmberg LH, Gröntoft O, et al. Reduction in mortality from breast cancer after mass screening with mammography. Randomised trial from the Breast Cancer Screening Working Group of the Swedish National Board of Health and Welfare. Lancet. 1985;1:829-32. [PMID: 2858707]

36. Mushlin AI, Kouides RW, Shapiro DE. Estimating the accuracy of screening mammography: a meta-analysis. Am J Prev Med. 1998;14:143-53. [PMID: 9631167]

37. Shen Y, Zelen M. Screening sensitivity and sojourn time from breast cancer early detection clinical trials: mammograms and physical examinations. J Clin Oncol. 2001;19:3490-9. [PMID: 11481355]

38. Laya MB, Larson EB, Taplin SH, White E. Effect of estrogen replacement therapy on the specificity and sensitivity of screening mammography. J Natl Cancer Inst. 1996;88:643-9. [PMID: 8627640]

39. Greendale GA, Reboussin BA, Sie A, Singh HR, Olson LK, Gatewood O, et al. Effects of estrogen and estrogen-progestin on mammographic parenchymal density. Postmenopausal Estrogen/Progestin Interventions (PEPI) Investigators. Ann Intern Med. 1999;130:262-9. [PMID: 10068383]

40. Marugg RC, van der Mooren MJ, Hendriks JH, Rolland R, Ruijs SH. Mammographic changes in postmenopausal women on hormonal replacement therapy. Eur Radiol. 1997;7:749-55. [PMID: 9166577]

41. Kerlikowske K, Grady D, Barclay J, Sickles EA, Ernster V. Effect of age, breast density, and family history on the sensitivity of first screening mammography. JAMA. 1996;276:33-8. [PMID: 8667536]

42. Kerlikowske K, Grady D, Barclay J, Sickles EA, Ernster V. Likelihood ratios for modern screening mammography. Risk of breast cancer based on age and mammographic interpretation. JAMA. 1996;276:39-43. [PMID: 8667537]

43. Eddy DM. Screening for breast cancer. Ann Intern Med. 1989;111:389-99. [PMID: 2504094]

44. Lidbrink E, Elfving J, Frisell J, Jonsson E. Neglected aspects of false positive findings of mammography in breast cancer screening: analysis of false positive cases from the Stockholm trial. BMJ. 1996;312:273-6. [PMID: 8611781]

45. Fletcher SW, Black W, Harris R, Rimer BK, Shapiro S. Report of the International Workshop on Screening for Breast Cancer. J Natl Cancer Inst. 1993;85:1644-56. [PMID: 8105098]

46. Humphrey L, Helfand M. Screening for Breast Cancer. Rockville, MD: Agency for Healthcare Research and Quality; 2002.

47. Kerlikowske K, Grady D, Barclay J, Sickles EA, Eaton A, Ernster V. Positive predictive value of screening mammography by age and family history of breast cancer. JAMA. 1993;270:2444-50. [PMID: 8230621]

48. Glasziou PP, Woodward AJ, Mahon CM. Mammographic screening trials for women aged under 50. A quality assessment and meta-analysis. Med J Aust. 1995;162:625-9. [PMID: 7603372]

49. Miller AB, Baines CJ, To T, Wall C. Screening mammography re-evaluated [Letter]. Lancet. 2000;355:747; discussion 752. [PMID: 10703818]

50. Larsson LG, Andersson I, Bjurstam N, Fagerberg G, Frisell J, Tabár L, et al. Updated overview of the Swedish Randomized Trials on Breast Cancer Screening with Mammography: age group 40-49 at randomization. J Natl Cancer Inst Monogr. 1997;57-61. [PMID: 9709277]

51. Cox B. Variation in the effectiveness of breast screening by year of follow-up.

J Natl Cancer Inst Monogr. 1997;69-72. [PMID: 9709279]

52. Elwood JM, Cox B, Richardson AK. The effectiveness of breast cancer screening by mammography in younger women. Online J Curr Clin Trials. 1993;Doc No 32:[23,227 words; 195 paragraphs]. [PMID: 8305999]

53. Glasziou P, Irwig L. The quality and interpretation of mammographic screening trials for women ages 40-49. J Natl Cancer Inst Monogr. 1997:73-7. [PMID: 9709280]

54. Glasziou PP. Meta-analysis adjusting for compliance: the example of screening for breast cancer. J Clin Epidemiol. 1992;45:1251-6. [PMID: 1432006]

55. Hendrick RE, Smith RA, Rutledge JH 3rd, Smart CR. Benefit of screening mammography in women aged 40-49: a new meta-analysis of randomized controlled trials. J Natl Cancer Inst Monogr. 1997;87-92. [PMID: 9709282]

56. Smart CR, Hendrick RE, Rutledge JH 3rd, Smith RA. Benefit of mammography screening in women ages 40 to 49 years. Current evidence from randomized controlled trials. Cancer. 1995;75:1619-26. [PMID: 8826919]

57. Kerlikowske K, Grady D, Ernster V. Benefit of mammography screening in women ages 40-49 years: current evidence from randomized controlled trials [Letter]. Cancer. 1995;76:1679-81. [PMID: 8635076]

58. Kerlikowske K. Efficacy of screening mammography among women aged 40 to 49 years and 50 to 69 years: comparison of relative and absolute benefit. J Natl Cancer Inst Monogr. 1997:79-86. [PMID: 9709281]

59. Tabar L, Fagerberg G, Chen HH, Duffy SW, Gad A. Screening for breast cancer in women aged under 50: mode of detection, incidence, fatality, and histology. J Med Screen. 1995;2:94-8. [PMID: 7497163]

60. Larsson LG, Nyström L, Wall S, Rutqvist L, Andersson I, Bjurstam N, et al. The Swedish randomised mammography screening trials: analysis of their effect on the breast cancer related excess mortality. J Med Screen. 1996;3:129-32. [PMID: 8946307]

61. Barton MB, Harris R, Fletcher SW. The rational clinical examination. Does this patient have breast cancer? The screening clinical breast examination: should it be done? How? JAMA. 1999;282:1270-80. [PMID: 10517431]

62. Elmore JG, Barton MB, Moceri VM, Polk S, Arena PJ, Fletcher SW. Ten-year risk of false positive screening mammograms and clinical breast examinations. N Engl J Med. 1998;338:1089-96. [PMID: 9545356]

63. Shapiro S. Evidence on screening for breast cancer from a randomized trial. Cancer (Philadelphia). 1977;39:2772-82.

64. 16-year mortality from breast cancer in the UK Trial of Early Detection of Breast Cancer. Lancet. 1999;353:1909-14. [PMID: 10371568]

65. Baines CJ. The Canadian National Breast Screening Study: responses to controversy. Womens Health Issues. 1992;2:206-11. [PMID: 1486284]

66. Richert-Boe KE, Humphrey LL. Screening for cancers of the cervix and breast. Arch Intern Med. 1992;152:2405-11. [PMID: 1456849]

67. Semiglazov VF, Moiseyenko VM, Bavli JL, Migmanova NSh, Seleznyov NK, Popova RT, et al. The role of breast self-examination in early breast cancer detection (results of the 5-years USSR/WHO randomized study in Leningrad). Eur J Epidemiol. 1992;8:498-502. [PMID: 1397215]

68. Semiglazov VF, Moiseenko VM, Manikhas AG, Protsenko SA, Kharikova RS, Popova RT, et al. [Interim results of a prospective randomized study of self-examination for early detection of breast cancer (Russia/St.Petersburg/WHO)]. Vopr Onkol. 1999;45:265-71. [PMID: 10443229]

69. Thomas DB, Gao DL, Self SG, Allison CJ, Tao Y, Mahloch J, et al. Randomized trial of breast self-examination in Shanghai: methodology and preliminary results. J Natl Cancer Inst. 1997;89:355-65. [PMID: 9060957]

70. Pisano ED, Earp J, Schell M, Vokaty K, Denham A. Screening behavior of women after a false-positive mammogram. Radiology. 1998;208:245-9. [PMID: 9646820]

71. Ekeberg O, Skjauff H, Karesen R. Screening for breast cancer is associated with a low degree of psychological distress. The Breast. 2001;10:20-4.

72. Lampic C, Thurfjell E, Bergh J, Sjödén PO. Short- and long-term anxiety and depression in women recalled after breast cancer screening. Eur J Cancer. 2001;37:463-9. [PMID: 11267855]

73. Meystre-Agustoni G, Paccaud F, Jeannin A, Dubois-Arber F. Anxiety in a cohort of Swiss women participating in a mammographic screening programme. J Med Screen. 2001;8:213-9. [PMID: 11743038]

74. Lerman C, Trock B, Rimer BK, Boyce A, Jepson C, Engstrom PF. Psychological and behavioral implications of abnormal mammograms. Ann Intern Med. 1991;114:657-61. [PMID: 2003712]

75. **Rimer BK, Bluman LG.** The psychosocial consequences of mammography. J Natl Cancer Inst Monogr. 1997:131-8. [PMID: 9709289]

76. **Olsson P, Armelius K, Nordahl G, Lenner P, Westman G.** Women with false positive screening mammograms: how do they cope? J Med Screen. 1999; 6:89-93. [PMID: 10444727]

77. **O'Sullivan I, Sutton S, Dixon S, Perry N.** False positive results do not have a negative effect on reattendance for subsequent breast screening. J Med Screen. 2001;8:145-8. [PMID: 11678554]

78. **Lipkus IM, Kuchibhatla M, McBride CM, Bosworth HB, Pollak KI, Siegler IC, et al.** Relationships among breast cancer perceived absolute risk, comparative risk, and worries. Cancer Epidemiol Biomarkers Prev. 2000;9:973-5. [PMID: 11008917]

79. **Burman ML, Taplin SH, Herta DF, Elmore JG.** Effect of false-positive mammograms on interval breast cancer screening in a health maintenance organization. Ann Intern Med. 1999;131:1-6. [PMID: 10391809]

80. **Schwartz LM, Woloshin S, Sox HC, Fischhoff B, Welch HG.** US women's attitudes to false positive mammography results and detection of ductal carcinoma in situ: cross sectional survey. BMJ. 2000;320:1635-40. [PMID: 10856064]

81. **Harstall C.** Mammography Screening: Mortality Rate Reduction and Screening Interval. Edmonton, Canada: Alberta Heritage Foundation for Medical Research; 2000.

82. **Ernster VL, Barclay J.** Increases in ductal carcinoma in situ (DCIS) of the breast in relation to mammography: a dilemma. J Natl Cancer Inst Monogr. 1997:151-6. [PMID: 9709292]

83. **Mattsson A, Leitz W, Rutqvist LE.** Radiation risk and mammographic screening of women from 40 to 49 years of age: effect on breast cancer rates and years of life. Br J Cancer. 2000;82:220-6. [PMID: 10638993]

84. **Feig SA, Hendrick RE.** Radiation risk from screening mammography of women aged 40-49 years. J Natl Cancer Inst Monogr. 1997:119-24. [PMID: 9709287]

85. **Swift M, Morrell D, Massey RB, Chase CL.** Incidence of cancer in 161 families affected by ataxia-telangiectasia. N Engl J Med. 1991;325:1831-6. [PMID: 1961222]

86. Guide to Clinical Preventive Services. U.S. Preventive Services Task Force. Baltimore: Williams and Wilkins; 1989.

87. **Kerlikowske K, Grady D, Rubin SM, Sandrock C, Ernster VL.** Efficacy of screening mammography. A meta-analysis. JAMA. 1995;273:149-54. [PMID: 7799496]

88. **Fletcher SW.** Why question screening mammography for women in their forties? Radiol Clin North Am. 1995;33:1259-71. [PMID: 7480669]

89. **Tabár L, Duffy SW, Chen HH.** Re: Quantitative interpretation of age-specific mortality reductions from the Swedish Breast Cancer-Screening Trials [Letter]. J Natl Cancer Inst. 1996;88:52-5. [PMID: 8847728]

90. **McPherson K, Steel CM, Dixon JM.** ABC of breast diseases. Breast cancer-epidemiology, risk factors, and genetics. BMJ. 2000;321:624-8. [PMID: 10977847]

91. **Ries LA, Eisner MP, Kosary CL, et al.** SEER Cancer Statistics Review, 1973-1997, NIH pub. no. 00-2789. Bethesda, MD: National Cancer Institute ;2000.

92. **Kopans DB.** An overview of the breast cancer screening controversy. J Natl Cancer Inst Monogr. 1997:1-3. [PMID: 9709266]

93. **Satariano WA, Ragland DR.** The effect of comorbidity on 3-year survival of women with primary breast cancer. Ann Intern Med. 1994;120:104-10. [PMID: 8256968]

94. **Kerlikowske K, Salzmann P, Phillips KA, Cauley JA, Cummings SR.** Continuing screening mammography in women aged 70 to 79 years: impact on life expectancy and cost-effectiveness. JAMA. 1999;282:2156-63. [PMID: 10591338]

95. **Tabár L, Faberberg G, Day NE, Holmberg L.** What is the optimum interval between mammographic screening examinations? An analysis based on the latest results of the Swedish two-county breast cancer screening trial. Br J Cancer. 1987;55:547-51. [PMID: 3606947]

96. **Duffy SW, Day NE, Tabár L, Chen HH, Smith TC.** Markov models of breast tumor progression: some age-specific results. J Natl Cancer Inst Monogr. 1997:93-7. [PMID: 9709283]

97. **Duffy SW, Chen HH, Tabar L, Fagerberg G, Paci E.** Sojourn time, sensitivity and positive predictive value of mammography screening for breast cancer in women aged 40-49. Int J Epidemiol. 1996;25:1139-45. [PMID: 9027517]

98. **Kramer BS, Brawley OW.** Cancer screening. Hematol Oncol Clin North Am. 2000;14:831-48. [PMID: 10949776]

99. **Skrabanek P.** False premises and false promises of breast cancer screening. Lancet. 1985;2:316-20. [PMID: 2862479]

100. **Ringash J.** Preventive health care, 2001 update: screening mammography among women aged 40-49 years at average risk of breast cancer. CMAJ. 2001; 164:469-76. [PMID: 11233866]

101. **Tabár L, Vitak B, Chen HH, Yen MF, Duffy SW, Smith RA.** Beyond randomized controlled trials: organized mammographic screening substantially reduces breast carcinoma mortality. Cancer. 2001;91:1724-31. [PMID: 11335897]

102. **Gøtzsche PC, Olsen O.** Is screening for breast cancer with mammography justifiable? Lancet. 2000;355:129-34. [PMID: 10675181]

103. **Rajkumar SV, Hartmann LC.** Screening mammography in women aged 40-49 years. Medicine (Baltimore). 1999;78:410-6. [PMID: 10575423]

104. **Moss S.** A trial to study the effect on breast cancer mortality of annual mammographic screening in women starting at age 40. Trial Steering Group. J Med Screen. 1999;6:144-8. [PMID: 10572845]

105. **Ng EH, Ng FC, Tan PH, Low SC, Chiang G, Tan KP, et al.** Results of intermediate measures from a population-based, randomized trial of mammographic screening prevalence and detection of breast carcinoma among Asian women: the Singapore Breast Screening Project. Cancer. 1998;82:1521-8. [PMID: 9554530]

106. **Hakama M, Pukkala E, Heikkilä M, Kallio M.** Effectiveness of the public health policy for breast cancer screening in Finland: population based cohort study. BMJ. 1997;314:864-7. [PMID: 9093096]

107. **Hakama M, Pukkala E, Söderman B, Day N.** Implementation of screening as a public health policy: issues in design and evaluation. J Med Screen. 1999;6: 209-16. [PMID: 10693068]

108. **Berglund G, Nilsson P, Eriksson KF, Nilsson JA, Hedblad B, Kristenson H, et al.** Long-term outcome of the Malmö preventive project: mortality and cardiovascular morbidity. J Intern Med. 2000;247:19-29. [PMID: 10672127]

109. **Verbeek AL, Hendriks JH, Holland R, Mravunac M, Sturmans F, Day NE.** Reduction of breast cancer mortality through mass screening with modern mammography. First results of the Nijmegen project, 1975-1981. Lancet. 1984; 1:1222-4. [PMID: 6144933]

110. **Chamberlain J, Coleman D, Ellman R, Moss S.** Verification of the cause of death in the trial of early detection of breast cancer. UK Trial of Early Detection of Breast Cancer Group. Trial Co-ordinating Centre. Br J Cancer. 1991;64: 1151-6. [PMID: 1764379]

111. **Collette HJ, de Waard F, Rombach JJ, Collette C, Day NE.** Further evidence of benefits of a (non-randomised) breast cancer screening programme: the DOM project. J Epidemiol Community Health. 1992;46:382-6. [PMID: 1431712]

112. **Moher D, Pham B, Jones A, Cook DJ, Jadad AR, Moher M, et al.** Does quality of reports of randomised trials affect estimates of intervention efficacy reported in meta-analyses? Lancet. 1998;352:609-13. [PMID: 9746022]

113. **Schulz KF, Chalmers I, Hayes RJ, Altman DG.** Empirical evidence of bias. Dimensions of methodological quality associated with estimates of treatment effects in controlled trials. JAMA. 1995;273:408-12. [PMID: 7823387]

114. **Prorok PC, Hankey BF, Bundy BN.** Concepts and problems in the evaluation of screening programs. J Chronic Dis. 1981;34:159-71. [PMID: 7014584]

115. **Schulz KF, Grimes DA, Altman DG, Hayes RJ.** Blinding and exclusions after allocation in randomised controlled trials: survey of published parallel group trials in obstetrics and gynaecology. BMJ. 1996;312:742-4. [PMID: 8605459]

116. **Johansen HK, Gotzsche PC.** Problems in the design and reporting of trials of antifungal agents encountered during meta-analysis. JAMA. 1999;282:1752-9. [PMID: 10568648]

117. **Bailar JC 3rd.** Mammography: a contrary view. Ann Intern Med. 1976;84: 77-84. [PMID: 1106292]

118. **Skrabanek P.** Mass mammography. The time for reappraisal. Int J Technol Assess Health Care. 1989;5:423-30. [PMID: 10303911]

119. **Schmidt JG.** The epidemiology of mass breast cancer screening—a plea for a valid measure of benefit. J Clin Epidemiol. 1990;43:215-25. [PMID: 2107280]

120. **Tarone RE.** The excess of patients with advanced breast cancer in young women screened with mammography in the Canadian National Breast Screening Study. Cancer. 1995;75:997-1003. [PMID: 7842421]

121. **Sutton AJ, Abams KR, Jones DR, et al.** Methods for Meta-Analysis in Medical Research. Chichester, United Kingdom: J Wiley; 2000.

122. **Habbema JD, van Oortmarssen GJ, van Putten DJ, Lubbe JT, van der Maas PJ.** Age-specific reduction in breast cancer mortality by screening: an analysis of the results of the Health Insurance Plan of Greater New York study. J Natl Cancer Inst. 1986;77:317-20. [PMID: 3461193]

123. **Shapiro S, Venet W, Strax P, Venet L, Roeser R.** Selection, follow-up, and analysis in the Health Insurance Plan Study: a randomized trial with breast cancer screening. Natl Cancer Inst Monogr. 1985;67:65-74. [PMID: 4047153]

124. **Frisell J, Lidbrink E.** The Stockholm Mammographic Screening Trial: Risks and benefits in age group 40-49 years. J Natl Cancer Inst Monogr. 1997;49-51. [PMID: 9709275]

125. **Frisell J, Eklund G, Hellström L, Lidbrink E, Rutqvist LE, Somell A.** Randomized study of mammography screening–preliminary report on mortality in the Stockholm trial. Breast Cancer Res Treat. 1991;18:49-56. [PMID: 1854979]

126. **Alexander FE.** The Edinburgh Randomized Trial of Breast Cancer Screening. J Natl Cancer Inst Monogr. 1997:31-5. [PMID: 9709272]

127. **Alexander FE, Anderson TJ, Brown HK, Forrest AP, Hepburn W, Kirkpatrick AE, et al.** The Edinburgh randomised trial of breast cancer screening: results after 10 years of follow-up. Br J Cancer. 1994;70:542-8. [PMID: 8080744]

128. **Roberts MM, Alexander FE, Anderson TJ, Chetty U, Donnan PT, Forrest P, et al.** Edinburgh trial of screening for breast cancer: mortality at seven years. Lancet. 1990;335:241-6. [PMID: 1967717]

Key Points

Colorectal cancer

❏ There is good evidence for the efficacy of screening all men and women 50 years of age or older for colorectal cancer.

❏ There is good evidence that periodic fecal occult blood testing (FOBT) reduces mortality from colorectal cancer, and there is fair evidence that sigmoidoscopy alone or in combination with FOBT reduces mortality.

❏ There is no direct evidence that colonoscopy reduces mortality; however, its integral role in all other strategies supports its efficacy.

❏ There is no direct evidence that double-contract barium enema is effective in reducing mortality, and it is less sensitive than colonoscopy. There is insufficient evidence regarding the newer screening modalities (e.g., computed tomographic colography).

Screening for Colorectal Cancer in Adults at Average Risk: A Summary of the Evidence for the U.S. Preventive Services Task Force

Michael Pignone, MD, MPH; Melissa Rich, MD; Steven M. Teutsch, MD, MPH; Alfred O. Berg, MD, MPH; and Kathleen N. Lohr, PhD

Purpose: To assess the effectiveness of different colorectal cancer screening tests for adults at average risk.

Data Sources: Recent systematic reviews; *Guide to Clinical Preventive Services*, 2nd edition; and focused searches of MEDLINE from 1966 through September 2001. The authors also conducted hand searches, reviewed bibliographies, and consulted context experts to ensure completeness.

Study Selection: When available, the most recent high-quality systematic review was used to identify relevant articles. This review was then supplemented with a MEDLINE search for more recent articles.

Data Extraction: One reviewer abstracted information from the final set of studies into evidence tables, and a second reviewer checked the tables for accuracy. Discrepancies were resolved by consensus.

Data Synthesis: For average-risk adults older than 50 years of age, evidence from multiple well-conducted randomized trials supported the effectiveness of fecal occult blood testing in reducing colorectal cancer incidence and mortality rates compared with no screening. Data from well-conducted case–control studies supported the effectiveness of sigmoidoscopy and possibly colonoscopy in reducing colon cancer incidence and mortality rates. A nonrandomized, controlled trial examining colorectal cancer mortality rates and randomized trials examining diagnostic yield supported the use of fecal occult blood testing plus sigmoidoscopy. The effectiveness of barium enema is unclear. Data are insufficient to support a definitive determination of the most effective screening strategy.

Conclusions: Colorectal cancer screening reduces death from colorectal cancer and can decrease the incidence of disease through removal of adenomatous polyps. Several available screening options seem to be effective, but the single best screening approach cannot be determined because data are insufficient.

The U.S. Preventive Services Task Force (USPSTF) last considered its recommendations regarding colorectal cancer screening in 1996 (1). At that time, the available evidence included one randomized, controlled trial showing that fecal occult blood testing (FOBT) reduced mortality rates (2); a case–control study showing that persons having sigmoidoscopy were less likely to die of colorectal cancer (3); and one nonrandomized, controlled trial of FOBT combined with rigid sigmoidoscopy that suggested some benefit from the two tests together (4). On the basis of this evidence, the USPSTF recommended screening for colorectal cancer with FOBT, sigmoidoscopy, or both (a grade B recommendation) but did not recommend for or against other means of screening (digital rectal examination, double-contrast barium enema, or colonoscopy) because the available evidence was insufficient. (See the companion article in this issue for a description of the USPSTF classification of recommendations.) The Task Force also recommended that FOBT be performed yearly but did not specify an interval for sigmoidoscopy.

Since 1996, important new evidence has emerged regarding the effectiveness of colorectal cancer screening. We performed an updated systematic review to help the USPSTF evaluate new evidence on the effectiveness of different colorectal cancer screening tests as it updated its previous recommendation. We examined the evidence concerning the effectiveness of screening in adults older than 50 years of age who are at average risk for colorectal cancer. The effectiveness, accuracy, and adverse effects of digital rectal examination (with or without a single office-based FOBT),

traditional three-card FOBT (hereafter referred to as FOBT), sigmoidoscopy, FOBT with sigmoidoscopy, double-contrast barium enema, and colonoscopy were examined. Other tests or combinations of tests have not been well evaluated and are not discussed here. A more detailed report of our review can be found on the Web site of the U.S. Agency for Healthcare Research and Quality (www.ahrq.gov/clinic/uspstfix.htm) (5). The USPSTF's updated recommendations for colorectal cancer screening recommendations can be found in the companion article in this issue (6).

METHODS

To identify the relevant literature, we used the *Guide to Clinical Preventive Services*, 2nd edition (1); existing systematic reviews; focused MEDLINE literature searches from 1966 through September 2001; and hand searches of key articles. When available, systematic reviews were used to identify older relevant studies. Literature searches were used to identify newer studies. Detailed descriptions of the literature searches can be found in the Appendix (available at www.annals.org).

To identify relevant studies, one reviewer examined the abstracts of the articles identified in the initial search. A second reviewer examined the excluded articles. Disagreements about inclusion were resolved by consensus. Two reviewers examined the full text of the remaining articles to determine final eligibility. We used evidence from randomized, controlled trials or observational studies that measured patient outcomes, particularly changes in colorectal cancer mortality rates and incidence. When such data were not available, we included indirect information on the accuracy of screening tests. Details about study inclusion are available in the Appendix (available at www.annals.org). We rated the quality of the included articles by using the criteria developed by the USPSTF Methods group (7), which are described in the accompanying article in this issue (6). We used the final set of eligible articles to create evidence tables and a draft report. The draft report was extensively peer reviewed by the USPSTF, experts in the field, governmental agencies, and nongovernmental organizations.

Role of the Funding Source

This evidence report was funded through a contract to the Research Triangle Institute–University of North Carolina Evidence-based Practice Center from the Agency for Healthcare Research and Quality. Staff of the funding source contributed to the study design, reviewed draft and final manuscripts, and made editing suggestions.

RESULTS

Our general search identified 719 articles published since 1995 on colorectal cancer screening. We retained 19 of these articles in our final document. Specific searches from 1966 through 2001 for articles about the accuracy of barium enema and complications of screening yielded 621 and 839 articles, respectively. After review, we retained 13 articles about barium enema and 19 articles about complications of screening. We also included 15 articles identified from the previous USPSTF review or from hand searches of other articles. **Table 1** summarizes our findings.

Digital Rectal Examination
Effectiveness

A case–control study from the Kaiser Permanente Medical Care Program in northern California examined the effect of screening with digital rectal examination on death from colorectal cancer (8). The investigators identified patients 45 years of age and older who died of distal rectal cancer between 1971 and 1986 and selected matched controls from the patient membership. They examined medical records to determine whether the patients and controls had undergone screening digital rectal examination within a year of cancer diagnosis. Investigators found no difference between groups after controlling for potential confounders, although the confidence interval was wide (odds ratio, 0.96 [95% CI, 0.56 to 1.7]).

Accuracy

The potential sensitivity of screening digital rectal examination is low; fewer than 10% of cases of colorectal cancer are within reach of the examining finger (28). The specificity of positive results on digital rectal examination has not been examined in outpatients at average risk for colorectal cancer.

In-Office Fecal Occult Blood Testing after Digital Rectal Examination
Effectiveness

No studies have examined the effect of a single in-office FOBT after digital rectal examination on colorectal cancer incidence or mortality rates.

Accuracy

A single in-office FOBT is likely to be less sensitive than the traditional three-card FOBT performed at home because only one sample is taken (9). In a large study from Japan, Yamamoto and Nakama (10) found that the first test card detected only 58% of cancer found after a three-card test. The single in-office FOBT may be less specific than a properly performed three-card FOBT because the in-office test does not allow degradation of the vegetable peroxidases that sometimes produce false-positive results (9). In addition, the potential trauma from the in-office examination itself may also result in lower specificity (9). Two studies of poor to fair quality that used existing data to retrospectively compare the specificity of the single in-office FOBT and the three-card home FOBT (11, 12) found little difference in specificity between the two groups. However, the validity of these studies is limited because neither could ensure that similar patient samples received each test.

Fecal Occult Blood Testing
Effectiveness

In addition to an older randomized trial performed in Minnesota (2), which was available to the USPSTF in 1996, two newer randomized, controlled trials have examined the effectiveness of biennial FOBT for reducing death from colorectal cancer (13, 14). These more recent trials, from the United Kingdom (13) and Denmark (14), found 15% and 18% reductions in mortality rates, respectively, with biennial testing. Neither trial used slides that were rehydrated before development (**Table 2**).

The Minnesota trial compared annual and biennial testing with no screening and rehydrated most test cards (83%). Cumulative colorectal cancer mortality rates after 18 years of follow-up were 33% (CI, 17% to 49%) lower among persons randomly assigned to undergo annual FOBT than in a control group that was not offered screening (absolute rates, 9.5 deaths per 1000 participants vs. 14.1 deaths per 1000 participants; difference, 4.6 deaths per 1000 participants) (2). Biennial screening, which did not show a reduction in mortality rates at 13-year follow-up, produced a 21% (CI, 3% to 38%) reduction in mortality rate at 18 years (15). The 18-year follow-up also showed that the incidence of colorectal cancer decreased by 20% (CI, 10% to 30%) and 17% (CI, 6% to 27%) in the groups screened annually and biennially, respectively, compared with controls (16). Because of differences in hydration, test frequency, duration, and effect size, the results of these trials could not be combined in a meta-analysis.

Table 1. **Characteristics of Screening Tests for Colorectal Cancer***

Screening Strategy for CRC	Effectiveness in Reducing Incidence of and Death from CRC	Evidence Grade†	Ability To Detect Cancer	Evidence Grade†
Digital rectal examination	Case–control study found no difference in mortality rates; OR, 0.96 [0.56–1.7] (8)	Level II—poor	Pathologic data suggest <10% of CRC is within reach of examining finger	
Office FOBT (one card)	Unknown		Only 58% of cancer cases are detected on the first of three cards, suggesting lower sensitivity than three-card testing (10)	Level III—fair
Home FOBT (three cards), unrehydrated	Biennial testing: 2 trials found mortality reductions of 15% [1%–26%] (13) and 18% [1%–32%] (14)	Level I—good	One-time sensitivity 30%–40% Unrehydrated FOBT finds about 25% of cancer cases (9)	
Home FOBT (three cards), rehydrated	Annual testing: 33% [13–50] reduction in mortality (2); 20% [10%–30%] reduction in cancer incidence (16) Biennial testing: 21% [3%–38%] reduction in mortality (15); 17% [6%–27%] reduction in cancer incidence (16)	Level I—good	Single-test accuracy 50% [30%–70%] for cancer, 24% [19%–29%] for advanced neoplasms (17) Over 13 years, rehydrated FOBT finds 50% of cancer cases (2)	Level III—good
Sigmoidoscopy	Small RCT found decreased CRC mortality rates with screening; RR, 0.50 [0.10–2.72] (18) Case–control studies suggest a 59% [31%–75%] reduction in mortality rate within reach of scope (3)	Level I—fair Level II—good	One-time screening detects 68%–78% of advanced neoplasia (17, 20)	Level III—good
Combined FOBT and sigmoidoscopy	Nonrandomized trial found a 43% reduction in mortality rate when FOBT was added to rigid sigmoidoscopy; RR, 0.57 [0.56–1.19] (4)	Level I—fair to poor	One-time screening detects 76% of advanced neoplasia (17) Increased yield when sigmoidoscopy is added to FOBT (21–23)	Level III—good
Double-contrast barium enema	Unknown		Sensitivity of one-time test for cancer or large polyps 48% [24%–67%] (24)	Level III—fair
Colonoscopy	Case–control study found an OR of 0.43 [0.30–0.63] for death from CRC; CRC incidence decreased by 40%–60% (26)	Level II—fair	Sensitivity for large adenomas >90%; sensitivity for cancer probably higher (27)	Level III—good

* CRC = colorectal cancer; FOBT = fecal occult blood test; NA = not applicable (see text); OR = odds ratio; RCT = randomized, controlled trial; RR = relative risk. Numbers in square brackets are 95% CIs; numbers in parentheses are reference numbers.
† Level I = evidence from one or more controlled trials; level II = evidence from cohort or case–control studies; level III = evidence from diagnostic accuracy studies or case series. For each level, the investigators have assigned a quality score based on methods described in reference 7.

Accuracy

A systematic review from 1997 found that the sensitivity of a single unrehydrated FOBT for cancer was approximately 40%; its specificity seems to range from 96% to 98%. Rehydration was found to increase sensitivity to between 50% and 60% but decreased specificity to 90% (9, 29). In a recent study, Lieberman and colleagues (17) found that the sensitivity of rehydrated FOBT for cancer was 50% (CI, 30% to 70%). For advanced neoplasia (cancer and polyps that are large, villous, or dysplastic), sensitivity was 24% (CI, 19% to 29%) and specificity was 94% (CI, 93% to 95%).

In the annual screening arm of the 13-year Minnesota trial, which primarily used rehydrated test cards and had a high initial rate of participation (approximately 90%), 49% of patients who developed colorectal cancer were identified through screening. Thirty-eight percent of all patients had had at least one colonoscopy (2). Biennial screening detected 39% of patients with cancer in the intervention group, and 28% of patients required colonoscopy. Compared with the Minnesota trial, the two European trials were population-based, lasted 8 to 10 years, used only biennial testing, and had lower participation rates (60% to 70% of patients completed the first screen-

ing). Screening detected 27% of patients in the intervention group who developed colorectal cancer, and only 5% of patients had colonoscopy (13, 14).

Adverse Effects

Fecal occult blood testing itself has few adverse effects, but false-positive results lead to further tests, such as colonoscopy, during which adverse effects may occur. The specific adverse effects of colonoscopy are described later in this review. Theoretically, a previously negative result on FOBT could falsely reassure patients and lead to delayed response to the development of colorectal symptoms if cancer were to develop, but this concern has not been evaluated empirically.

Sigmoidoscopy
Effectiveness

Thiis-Evensen and coworkers (18) performed a small randomized trial of sigmoidoscopy screening in Norway. In 1983, 799 men and women who were 50 to 59 years of age and were drawn from a population registry were randomly assigned to receive screening flexible sigmoidoscopy (400 patients) or no screening (399 patients). Eighty-one percent of those offered flexible sigmoidoscopy accepted.

Table 1—Continued

Chance of False-Positive Results	Evidence Grade†	Adverse Effects	Evidence Grade†
Unknown		No direct adverse effects known	
Little difference compared with three-card testing (11, 12)	Level III—poor	No direct adverse effects known	
Single-test specificity 96%–98%	Level III—good	No direct adverse effects known	
5%–10% of patients will require colonoscopy over 10 years of biennial testing (9)			
Single–test specificity 90%	Level III—good	Inconvenience, adverse events resulting from follow-up tests after positive results	
Over 10 to 13 years, 38% of patients tested annually and 28% tested biennially with rehydrated FOBT required colonoscopy (2)			
NA		Perforation rate for diagnostic examinations <1 in 10 000; bleeding in 2.5% of patients after diagnostic studies, 5.5% after procedures with polypectomy (19)	Level III—good
NA		Sum of adverse effects from each test alone	
One-time specificity, 85% [82%–88%] (24)	Level III—fair	Perforation rate 1 in 25 000 in a study with screening and symptomatic patients (25)	Level III—poor
NA		Diagnostic procedures: perforation rate 1 in 2000 Polypectomy: perforation rate 1 in 500–1000; bleeding rate 1 in 100–500; mortality rate 1 in 20 000 (5)	Level III—fair to good

All patients found to have polyps on sigmoidoscopy underwent immediate diagnostic colonoscopy and had surveillance examinations 2 and 6 years later. Over the 13 years of the trial, two cases of colorectal cancer were diagnosed in the intervention group and 10 were diagnosed in the control group (relative risk for colorectal cancer, 0.2 [CI, 0.03 to 0.95]). One person who was assigned to the intervention group but never had sigmoidoscopy died of colorectal cancer, as did three controls (relative risk, 0.50 [CI, 0.10 to 2.72]). Overall mortality rate was higher in the intervention group than in the control group (14% vs. 9%; relative risk, 1.57 [CI, 1.03 to 2.40]), mostly because of an excess of cardiovascular deaths. No clear relationship emerged between excess deaths and any procedure-related complications.

Two ongoing randomized trials using flexible sigmoidoscopy will report their initial results within 5 years. One trial in the United Kingdom is examining the effect of screening with sigmoidoscopy once per lifetime (19), and a second trial in the United States is examining sigmoidoscopy screening every 5 years in patients who are assumed to be receiving FOBT as part of usual care (30).

Two older, well-designed case–control studies that provide other important information on the effectiveness of sigmoidoscopy screening were available to the USPSTF in 1996. Using data from the Kaiser Permanente Medical Care Program in northern California, Selby and associates (3) found that rigid sigmoidoscopy had been performed in 9% of persons who died of colorectal cancer occurring within 20 cm of the anus and in 24% of persons who did not die of cancer occurring within 20 cm of the anus. The adjusted odds ratio of 0.41 (CI, 0.25 to 0.69) suggested that sigmoidoscopy screening reduced the risk for death by 59% for cancer within reach of the rigid sigmoidoscope.

The investigators noted that the adjusted odds ratio was 0.96 for proximal colon cancer that was beyond the reach of the sigmoidoscope (3). This finding added support to the hypothesis that the reduced risk for death from cancer within reach of the rigid sigmoidoscope could be attributed to screening rather than to confounding factors. The risk reduction associated with sigmoidoscopy screening did not diminish during the first 9 to 10 years after the test was performed. The study by Selby and associates mostly used rigid sigmoidoscopes. However, in another case–control study supporting the effectiveness of sigmoidoscopy, 75% of the examinations were performed with a flexible instrument (31).

Accuracy

Two recent studies have examined the sensitivity of screening sigmoidoscopy for cancer or advanced adenomas

Table 2. Trials of Fecal Occult Blood Testing

Trial Characteristics	Trial (Reference)		
	Minnesota (2)	United Kingdom (13)	Denmark (14)
Frequency of testing	Annual and biennial	Biennial	Biennial
Participants, *n*	>45 000 men and women	>150 000 men and women	>60 000 men and women
Age, *y*	50–80	45–74	45–74
Duration of follow-up, *y*	18 (annual and biennial)	8	10
Hydration of slides	Yes (83%)	No	No
Participation rate, %*	90 (annual and biennial)	60	67
Patients requiring colonoscopy, %	38 (annual); 28 (biennial)	5	5
Positive predictive value, %	1.9 (annual); 2.7 (biennial)†	10–12	8–18
Relative risk reduction for death from colorectal cancer [95% CI], %	33 [17–49] (annual); 21 [3–38] (biennial)	15 [1–26]	18 [1–32]
Absolute risk reduction for death from colorectal cancer per 1000 participants	4.6 (annual); 2.9 (biennial)	0.8	1.4

* Participation was defined as completion of at least one test.
† Mostly rehydrated slides (83%).

in healthy patients, using colonoscopy as the criterion standard. They found that sigmoidoscopy would identify 70% to 80% of patients with advanced adenomas or cancer (17, 20). Sigmoidoscopy can produce false-positive results by detecting hyperplastic polyps that do not have malignant potential or adenomatous polyps that are unlikely to become malignant during the patient's lifetime. Because studies of diagnostic accuracy cannot measure whether small or large adenomas that are identified and removed would have become cancer, it is not possible to classify such findings in terms of accuracy in detecting cancer. In practice, most investigators consider all adenomas to be "true positives" regardless of whether they would ever progress to cancer. Comparison of the specificity of sigmoidoscopy with that of nonendoscopic screening methods, such as FOBT and barium enema, is therefore difficult.

Adverse Effects

Estimates of bowel perforations from sigmoidoscopy have generally been in the range of 1 to 2 or fewer per 10 000 examinations, particularly since the introduction of the flexible sigmoidoscope (32). Atkin and colleagues (19) recently reported initial results from a trial of sigmoidoscopy screening in which experienced endoscopists performed sigmoidoscopy in 1235 asymptomatic adults 55 to 64 years of age. Two hundred eighty-eight patients had polyps removed during the examination. Adverse effects, including pain, anxiety, or any degree of bleeding, were assessed by a written questionnaire immediately after the test and by a mailed questionnaire 3 months later. Of all patients, 3.2% (40 of 1235) reported bleeding, 16 of 288 (5.5%) after polypectomy and 24 of 947 (2.5%) after diagnostic studies. One patient required hospital admission, and no patients required a transfusion. Fourteen percent of patients reported moderate pain, and 0.4% reported severe pain. More than 25% of patients reported gas or flatus. No

perforations were reported, but one patient died of peritonitis after a complicated open surgical procedure to remove a severely dysplastic adenoma. A recent study of endoscopic complications from the Mayo Clinic in Arizona identified two perforations in 49 501 sigmoidoscopy procedures (33).

Fecal Occult Blood Test and Sigmoidoscopy
Effectiveness

Currently, no randomized trials that examine death from colorectal cancer as an end point have compared FOBT alone or sigmoidoscopy alone with a strategy of performing both tests. In 1992, Winawer and coworkers (4) conducted a nonrandomized trial of more than 12 000 first-time attendees at a preventive health clinic in New York. This trial was available to the USPSTF in 1996. The control group received rigid sigmoidoscopy at the first visit, and all study participants were invited to return for annual reexamination with rigid sigmoidoscopy. Patients in the intervention group received rigid sigmoidoscopy and were also asked to complete Hemoccult (Beckman Coulter, Fullerton, California) FOBT cards. Patients who had adenomas larger than 3 mm on sigmoidoscopy or who had positive results on FOBT underwent full colonic examination with barium enema and colonoscopy. The control group received rigid sigmoidoscopy at the first visit, and participants were invited to return for annual reexamination. Few patients continued to participate after the first examination (20% had FOBT at year 2, 15% at year 3). Incidence of colorectal cancer and death were assessed over a 9-year period, and follow-up data were available for 97% of patients.

Demographic and clinical data suggest that the groups were comparable, despite the absence of randomization. More cases of colorectal cancer were detected on initial examination in intervention patients than in control patients (4.5 per 1000 participants vs. 2.5 per 1000 participants). Incidence rates (cancer detected after the initial examination) were similar between groups (0.9 per 1000 person-years in each group). Incidence of death from colorectal cancer was 0.36 per 1000 patient-years in the intervention group and 0.63 per 1000 patient-years among controls (relative risk, 0.56 [CI, 0.25 to 1.19]).

Fecal occult blood testing combined with rigid sigmoidoscopy seems to increase the yield of initial screening and may reduce mortality rates. Because rigid sigmoidoscopy is no longer used for screening, the generalizability of these results to the use of FOBT plus flexible sigmoidoscopy is unclear. Whether the incremental yield of combined screening will change after additional rounds of testing also remains uncertain.

Accuracy

Recent randomized trials from Europe examined the additional diagnostic yield of performing sigmoidoscopy plus FOBT at one point in time for patients who were not already part of an ongoing screening program (21–23). In each study, adding sigmoidoscopy to FOBT increased the identification of significant adenomas or cancer by a factor of two or more. Adding FOBT to sigmoidoscopy did not seem to identify any additional significant lesions. Winawer and coworkers (4), however, found an increased yield from adding FOBT to rigid sigmoidoscopy. In each study, data were limited to a single round of testing. The additional yield of this strategy may be lower after the first round of testing, but the impact of this strategy on mortality rates has not been fully evaluated.

Adverse Effects

The adverse effects of FOBT plus sigmoidoscopy are equal to the adverse effects of each test alone.

Double-Contrast Barium Enema
Effectiveness

We identified no published studies that examined the effectiveness of double-contrast barium enema in reducing incidence of or death from colorectal cancer. Several studies have examined the accuracy of double-contrast barium enema for diagnosing colorectal cancer or adenomatous polyps (24, 34–43). Most are of methodologically poor quality, however, because they examined patients with symptoms or did not prospectively collect blinded data.

The National Polyp Study is a randomized trial of different intervals of surveillance after polypectomy (examinations at 1 and 3 years vs. at 3 years only). In a substudy of this trial, Winawer and colleagues (24) compared the accuracy of double-contrast barium enema with that of colonoscopy. The sensitivity of double-contrast barium enema was 32% (CI, 25% to 39%) for polyps smaller than 0.5 cm; 53% (CI, 40% to 66%) for polyps 0.6 to 1 cm; and 48% (CI, 24% to 67%) for polyps larger than 1 cm, including two cases of cancerous polyps. Results of double-contrast barium enema were positive in 83 of 470 patients

in whom colonoscopy detected no polyps (specificity, 85% [CI, 82% to 88%]).

Winawer and colleagues (24) examined patients who previously had colonoscopy and removal of all polyps. Their results, therefore, may have limited generalizability for screening because screening largely involves persons who have not had recent colonoscopic examination and polypectomy and therefore may be more likely to have large polyps or tumors. However, the low sensitivity for large polyps and tumors reported by Winawer and colleagues is cause for concern and may limit the potential effectiveness of screening with double-contrast barium enema.

Adverse Effects

The estimated risk for perforation during barium enema is low. Kewenter and Brevinge (44) found that no perforations or other complications occurred among 1987 screening patients undergoing barium enema as part of a screening work-up. Blakeborough and associates (25) surveyed radiologists in the United Kingdom about complications of barium enema during a 3-year period (1992 through 1994). All examinations were included, regardless of the indication for the procedure. Important complications of any type occurred in 1 in 10 000 examinations. Perforation occurred in 1 of 25 000 examinations, and death occurred in 1 in 55 000 examinations, although it is not clear whether all deaths were procedure related.

Colonoscopy
Effectiveness

The ability of colonoscopy to prevent colorectal cancer or death has not been measured in a screening trial. The National Polyp Study estimated that 76% to 90% of cancer could be prevented by regular colonoscopic surveillance examinations, based on comparison with historic controls (45). However, these results should be interpreted with caution. The comparison groups were not from the same underlying population, which could introduce bias. In addition, all trial participants had polyps detected and removed, limiting generalizability of the results to the average screening population.

Müller and Sonnenberg (26), in a case–control study at Veterans Affairs hospitals, found that patients with a diagnosis of colorectal cancer were less likely to have had previous colonoscopy. The odds ratios for disease incidence were 0.47 (CI, 0.37 to 0.58) for colon cancer and 0.61 (CI, 0.48 to 0.77) for rectal cancer. For death from colorectal cancer, the odds ratio was also lower for patients with previous colonoscopy (odds ratio, 0.43 [CI, 0.30 to 0.63]).

Accuracy

Because colonoscopy is commonly used as the criterion standard examination, it is difficult to calculate its sensitivity. Using tandem colonoscopic examinations, Rex and colleagues (27) found single-test sensitivity to be 90% for large adenomas and 75% for small adenomas (<1 cm); sensitivity for cancer probably exceeds 90%.

Recent identification of flat lesions that can be missed on regular colonoscopy suggests that some histologic variants do not progress through the typical adenoma–carcinoma development sequence and thus may not be easily detectable in the precancerous phase (46). If flat lesions account for 10% of all adenomas, sensitivity of all endoscopic screening methods may be lower than previously thought.

The specificity of colonoscopy with biopsy is generally reported to be 99% or 100%, but this assumes that all detected adenomas represent true-positive results. As with sigmoidoscopy, most detected adenomas, especially small adenomas, will never develop into cancer. If detection of an adenoma that will not become cancer is considered a false-positive result that subjects a patient to risk without benefit, then the actual specificity of colonoscopy would be much lower.

Adverse Effects

Colonoscopy, which uses sedation and requires skilled support personnel, is more expensive and has a higher risk for procedural complications than other screening tests, particularly when polypectomy is performed. Use of conscious sedation adds the risk for complications attributable to the sedative agent. In our systematic review of studies examining the principal complications of colonoscopy (5), we focused on hemorrhage and perforation but noted the less frequent complications of death, infections, sedation-related events, and chemical colitis. Two recent studies examined the incidence of complications from colonoscopy performed in screening populations. Lieberman and associates (17), in a study in patients in Veterans Affairs medical centers, found that 10 of 3121 patients (0.3%) had major complications during or immediately after the procedures. Of these 10 patients, 6 had bleeding that required hospitalization and 1 each had a stroke, myocardial infarction, Fournier gangrene, and thrombophlebitis. Three other patients died within 1 month, probably of causes unrelated to the procedure. In a study of employees of a large corporation, Imperiale and coworkers (20) found that among 1994 persons 50 years of age and older who underwent colonoscopy, 1 (0.05%) had a perforation that did not require surgery and 3 (0.15%) had bleeding that required emergency department visits but not admission or surgery.

Apart from these two screening studies, most of the studies examining colonoscopy complications are retrospective reviews of endoscopy records from U.S. university hospitals that recorded only immediate complications and included a mixture of screening and diagnostic procedures (17, 20, 33, 47–61). A prospective study that also included a patient questionnaire administered 10 days after the pro-

cedure identified several additional important complications that occurred outside the hospital, suggesting that hospital record review alone may underestimate actual complication rates (47).

Despite these limitations, these studies provide a useful approximation of the complication rates that can be expected from colonoscopy. For diagnostic procedures, perforation rates were low (0.029% to 0.61%). Bleeding was not reported in enough studies to generate an estimate of its frequency. For therapeutic procedures, complication rates were higher (perforations, 0.07% to 0.72%; bleeding, 0.2% to 2.67%). Deaths occurred infrequently; reported rates ranged from 1 in 30 000 persons to 1 in 3000 persons. Mortality rates were higher in studies that included older patients and more symptomatic patients. The rate of screening-related death may be on the lower end of this range; one cost-effectiveness analysis estimated it to be 1 per 20 000 patients (29). Other clinically relevant complications were reported too infrequently and measured too inconsistently to allow accurate estimation of their true incidence.

DISCUSSION

Our systematic review supports the effectiveness of screening as a means of reducing death from colorectal cancer. For biennial FOBT, three high-quality randomized, controlled trials have shown disease-specific reductions in mortality rate of 15% to 21% over 8 to 13 years. Annual FOBT with rehydrated slides seems to be more effective in reducing mortality rates (33% in one trial). Case–control studies have shown that sigmoidoscopy and possibly colonoscopy are also associated with decreased death from colorectal cancer. The combined strategy of FOBT and sigmoidoscopy was supported by one nonrandomized trial that showed a borderline statistically significant reduction in mortality rates (43%) when FOBT was added to rigid sigmoidoscopy (4). This strategy was also supported by indirect evidence showing increased yield with both tests compared with FOBT alone. Double-contrast barium enema has not been studied as extensively as other screening methods; further data are required in screening populations.

Although strong direct and indirect evidence supports colorectal cancer screening, no trials have directly compared different screening strategies by using colorectal cancer incidence or mortality rates as the end point of interest. Some groups believe that recent evidence showing the superior single-test accuracy of colonoscopy proves its broader superiority and have recommended it as the procedure of choice for screening. However, these analyses have not always considered differences in yield over time, complications, and real-world performance, which may not always favor colonoscopy (62, 63). One solution to these problems would be to perform a trial of colonoscopy, but such a trial would be expensive, particularly if colonoscopy were compared with other screening methods rather than with no screening, and would require many years of follow-up. In the face of good general evidence supporting screening but uncertainty about the most effective screening method, providers and patients may benefit from discussing pros and cons and from incorporating patients' preferences into decisions about how to screen (64).

Several areas of colorectal cancer screening and prevention warrant additional research. There is a critical need to learn more about adherence to screening among informed patients. Furthermore, we need better data on the real-world complication rates of colonoscopic screening and polypectomy, including whether complications become more or less likely as procedure volume increases. Double-contrast barium enema should be studied in a screening population. The accuracy of novel screening techniques, including virtual colonoscopy and genetic stool tests (or other novel noninvasive tests), should be evaluated in screening populations.

Additional means of prevention, including chemopreventive agents (such as nonsteroidal anti-inflammatory drugs, calcium, or estrogen), also warrant further study. Behavioral factors, including physical activity, dietary fat intake, dietary fiber intake, and fruit and vegetable consumption, seem to be related to colorectal cancer incidence. Further research would clarify whether these relationships are causal or the result of uncontrolled confounding.

Despite its apparent effectiveness, colorectal cancer screening is currently underused by age-eligible adults because of patient-, provider-, and system-specific barriers (65). Effective colon cancer screening requires ongoing efforts to ensure test ordering and adherence. Screening with FOBT, for example, may require offering annual testing to 500 to 1000 people for 10 years to prevent one death from colorectal cancer (2). Although this level of effort may seem inefficient or low in yield, the potential benefit is large and the costs per person are small. To achieve high rates of screening in real-world settings rather than in trials, which focused strictly on one aspect of preventive care, colorectal cancer screening must be integrated with other care needs, including other preventive services.

Several strategies have been shown to be effective in raising screening rates in primary care settings over the short term, including reminder systems, patient decision aids, and special screening clinics (66). Further research is needed to determine whether such systems can maintain their effect over time and to identify novel means of reaching persons at risk who currently are not served or are underserved by the existing health care system.

APPENDIX: SEARCH STRATEGIES

To update the evidence on screening for colorectal cancer, we performed three separate literature searches using MEDLINE: one general update from January 1995 to December 2001 and two focused searches for evidence related to barium enema and

complications of screening that used search dates from 1966 through December 2001. All searches were limited to "human" subjects.

For the general search, we combined the MeSH headings "colorectal neoplasms" or "occult blood" or "sigmoidoscopy" or "colonoscopy" with the term *mass screening*. This search produced 719 results, 19 of which we retained in the final document. To identify articles on the use of barium enema, we combined the exploded MeSH terms "colorectal neoplasms" and "barium sulfate" and "enema," which yielded 621 results. We retained 13 articles in our final data set. For studies about the complications of screening, we combined the exploded MeSH terms "colonoscopy/ae [adverse effects] and sigmoidoscopy/ae [adverse effects]," "intestinal perforation," "intraoperative complications," "postoperative complications," or "gastrointestinal hemorrhage," with a search combining the test names and the keyword "complications." Our search yielded 839 articles, 16 of which we retained. In addition to these searches, we used peer review and hand searching of the bibliographies of included articles and other systematic reviews, as well as articles from the 1996 document. This yielded an additional 15 references for our final document.

Appendix Table. **Eligibility Criteria***

Test	Type of Studies Included
Digital rectal examination	Diagnostic accuracy studies, observational studies
FOBT	RCTs
Sigmoidoscopy	RCTs, observational studies
FOBT plus sigmoidoscopy	Controlled trials, observational studies, diagnostic accuracy studies
Barium enema	Diagnostic accuracy studies
Colonoscopy	Observational studies, diagnostic accuracy studies
Adverse effects (any test)	Case series, observational studies, RCTs

* FOBT = fecal occult blood test; RCT = randomized, controlled trial.

We developed eligibility criteria to guide decisions about inclusion of articles. In general, we sought to identify and include the highest quality evidence available. The Appendix Table shows the criteria for each specific topic.

From University of North Carolina, Chapel Hill, and Research Triangle Institute, Research Triangle Park, North Carolina; Merck & Co., Inc., West Point, Pennsylvania; and University of Washington, Seattle, Washington.

Disclaimer: The authors of this article are responsible for its contents, including any clinical or treatment recommendations. No statement in this article should be construed as an official position of the U.S. Agency for Healthcare Research and Quality, the U.S. Department of Health and Human Services, or Merck & Co., Inc.

Acknowledgments: The authors thank David Atkins, MD, MPH, Agency for Healthcare Research and Quality, and Eve Shapiro, managing editor of the U.S. Preventive Services Task Force (under contract to the Agency for Healthcare Research and Quality). They also thank the staff of the Research Triangle Institute–University of North Carolina Evidence-based Practice Center; Sonya Sutton, BSPH, Sheila White, and Loraine Monroe, Research Triangle Institute; and Carol Krasnov, University of North Carolina at Chapel Hill Cecil G. Sheps Center for Health Services Research.

Grant Support: This study was developed by the Research Triangle Institute–University of North Carolina Evidence-based Practice Center under contract to the Agency for Healthcare Research and Quality (contract no. 290-97-0011), Rockville, Maryland.

Requests for Reprints: Reprints are available from the AHRQ Web site at www.preventiveservices.ahrq.gov and in print through the AHRQ Publications Clearinghouse (800-358-9295).

Current author addresses are available at www.annals.org.

Current Author Addresses: Dr. Pignone: University of North Carolina at Chapel Hill, Department of Medicine and Cecil Sheps Center for Health Services Research, 5039 Old Clinic Building, CB #7110, Chapel Hill, NC 27599.
Dr. Teutsch: Merck & Co., Inc., 770 Sumneytown Pike, West Point, PA WP399-169.
Dr. Rich: University of North Carolina at Chapel Hill, 724 Burnett Womack, CB 7080, Chapel Hill, NC 27599.
Dr. Berg: University of Washington, Department of Family Medicine, C-408 Health Sciences, Box 356390, Seattle, WA 98195.
Dr. Lohr: Research Triangle Institute, 3040 Cornwallis Road, Research Triangle Park, NC 27709-2194.

References

1. Guide to Clinical Preventive Services. 2nd ed. U.S. Preventive Services Task Force. Alexandria, VA: International Medical Publishing; 1996.

2. **Mandel JS, Bond JH, Church TR, Snover DC, Bradley GM, Schuman LM, et al.** Reducing mortality from colorectal cancer by screening for fecal occult blood. Minnesota Colon Cancer Control Study. N Engl J Med. 1993;328:1365-71. [PMID: 8474513]

3. **Selby JV, Friedman GD, Quesenberry CP Jr, Weiss NS.** A case-control study of screening sigmoidoscopy and mortality from colorectal cancer. N Engl J Med. 1992;326:653-7. [PMID: 1736103]

4. **Winawer SJ, Flehinger BJ, Schottenfeld D, Miller DG.** Screening for colorectal cancer with fecal occult blood testing and sigmoidoscopy. J Natl Cancer Inst. 1993;85:1311-8. [PMID: 8340943]

5. **Pignone MP, Rich M, Teutsch SM, Berg AO, Lohr KN.** Screening for Colorectal Cancer in Adults. Systematic Evidence Review No. 7. AHRQ publication no. 02-S003. Rockville, MD: Agency for Healthcare Research and Quality; 2002.

6. Screening for colorectal cancer: recommendations and rationale. U.S. Preventive Services Task Force. Ann Intern Med. 2002;137:129-131.

7. **Harris RP, Helfand M, Woolf SH, Lohr KN, Mulrow CD, Teutsch SM, et al.** Current methods of the US Preventive Services Task Force: a review of the process. Am J Prev Med. 2001;20:21-35. [PMID: 11306229]

8. **Herrinton LJ, Selby JV, Friedman GD, Quesenberry CP, Weiss NS.** Case-control study of digital-rectal screening in relation to mortality from cancer of the distal rectum. Am J Epidemiol. 1995;142:961-4. [PMID: 7572977]

9. **Ransohoff DF, Lang CA.** Screening for colorectal cancer with the fecal occult blood test: a background paper. American College of Physicians. Ann Intern Med. 1997;126:811-22. [PMID: 9148658]

10. **Yamamoto M, Nakama H.** Cost-effectiveness analysis of immunochemical occult blood screening for colorectal cancer among three fecal sampling methods. Hepatogastroenterology. 2000;47:396-9. [PMID: 10791199]

11. **Eisner MS, Lewis JH.** Diagnostic yield of a positive fecal occult blood test found on digital rectal examination. Does the finger count? Arch Intern Med. 1991;151:2180-4. [PMID: 1953220]

12. **Bini EJ, Rajapaksa RC, Weinshel EH.** The findings and impact of nonrehydrated guaiac examination of the rectum (FINGER) study: a comparison of 2 methods of screening for colorectal cancer in asymptomatic average-risk patients.

Arch Intern Med. 1999;159:2022-6. [PMID: 10510987]

13. **Hardcastle JD, Chamberlain JO, Robinson MH, Moss SM, Amar SS, Balfour TW, et al.** Randomised controlled trial of faecal-occult-blood screening for colorectal cancer. Lancet. 1996;348:1472-7. [PMID: 8942775]

14. **Kronborg O, Fenger C, Olsen J, Jørgensen OD, Søndergaard O.** Randomised study of screening for colorectal cancer with faecal-occult-blood test. Lancet. 1996;348:1467-71. [PMID: 8942774]

15. **Mandel JS, Church TR, Ederer F, Bond JH.** Colorectal cancer mortality: effectiveness of biennial screening for fecal occult blood. J Natl Cancer Inst. 1999;91:434-7. [PMID: 10070942]

16. **Mandel JS, Church TR, Bond JH, Ederer F, Geisser MS, Mongin SJ, et al.** The effect of fecal occult-blood screening on the incidence of colorectal cancer. N Engl J Med. 2000;343:1603-7. [PMID: 11096167]

17. **Lieberman DA, Weiss DG, Bond JH, Ahnen DJ, Garewal H, Chejfec G.** Use of colonoscopy to screen asymptomatic adults for colorectal cancer. Veterans Affairs Cooperative Study Group 380. N Engl J Med. 2000;343:162-8. [PMID: 10900274]

18. **Thiis-Evensen E, Hoff GS, Sauar J, Langmark F, Majak BM, Vatn MH.** Population-based surveillance by colonoscopy: effect on the incidence of colorectal cancer. Telemark Polyp Study I. Scand J Gastroenterol. 1999;34:414-20. [PMID: 10365903]

19. **Atkin WS, Hart A, Edwards R, McIntyre P, Aubrey R, Wardle J, et al.** Uptake, yield of neoplasia, and adverse effects of flexible sigmoidoscopy screening. Gut. 1998;42:560-5. [PMID: 9616321]

20. **Imperiale TF, Wagner DR, Lin CY, Larkin GN, Rogge JD, Ransohoff DF.** Risk of advanced proximal neoplasms in asymptomatic adults according to the distal colorectal findings. N Engl J Med. 2000;343:169-74. [PMID: 10900275]

21. **Verne JE, Aubrey R, Love SB, Talbot IC, Northover JM.** Population based randomized study of uptake and yield of screening by flexible sigmoidoscopy compared with screening by faecal occult blood testing. BMJ. 1998;317:182-5. [PMID: 9665902]

22. **Berry DP, Clarke P, Hardcastle JD, Vellacott KD.** Randomized trial of the addition of flexible sigmoidoscopy to faecal occult blood testing for colorectal neoplasia population screening. Br J Surg. 1997;84:1274-6. [PMID: 9313712]

23. **Rasmussen M, Kronborg O, Fenger C, Jørgensen OD.** Possible advantages and drawbacks of adding flexible sigmoidoscopy to hemoccult-II in screening for colorectal cancer. A randomized study. Scand J Gastroenterol. 1999;34:73-8. [PMID: 10048736]

24. **Winawer SJ, Stewart ET, Zauber AG, Bond JH, Ansel H, Waye JD, et al.** A comparison of colonoscopy and double-contrast barium enema for surveillance after polypectomy. National Polyp Study Work Group. N Engl J Med. 2000; 342:1766-72. [PMID: 10852998]

25. **Blakeborough A, Sheridan MB, Chapman AH.** Complications of barium enema examinations: a survey of UK Consultant Radiologists 1992 to 1994. Clin Radiol. 1997;52:142-8. [PMID: 9043049]

26. **Müller AD, Sonnenberg A.** Protection by endoscopy against death from colorectal cancer. A case-control study among veterans. Arch Intern Med. 1995; 155:1741-8. [PMID: 7654107]

27. **Rex DK, Cutler CS, Lemmel GT, Rahmani EY, Clark DW, Helper DJ, et al.** Colonoscopic miss rates of adenomas determined by back-to-back colonoscopies. Gastroenterology. 1997;112:24-8. [PMID: 8978338]

28. **Winawer SJ, Fletcher RH, Miller L, Godlee F, Stolar MH, Mulrow CD, et al.** Colorectal cancer screening: clinical guidelines and rationale. Gastroenterology. 1997;112:594-642. [PMID: 9024315]

29. **Wagner J, Tunis S, Brown M, Ching A, Almeida R.** Cost-effectiveness of colorectal cancer screening in average-risk adults. In: Young G, Rozen P, Levin B, eds. Prevention and Early Detection of Colorectal Cancer. London: Saunders; 1996:321-56.

30. **Kramer BS, Gohagan J, Prorok PC, Smart C.** A National Cancer Institute sponsored screening trial for prostatic, lung, colorectal, and ovarian cancers. Cancer. 1993;71:589-93. [PMID: 8420681]

31. **Newcomb PA, Norfleet RG, Storer BE, Surawicz TS, Marcus PM.** Screening sigmoidoscopy and colorectal cancer mortality. J Natl Cancer Inst. 1992;84: 1572-5. [PMID: 1404450]

32. **Nelson RL, Abcarian H, Prasad ML.** Iatrogenic perforation of the colon and rectum. Dis Colon Rectum. 1982;25:305-8. [PMID: 7083975]

33. **Anderson ML, Pasha TM, Leighton JA.** Endoscopic perforation of the

colon: lessons from a 10-year study. Am J Gastroenterol. 2000;95:3418-22. [PMID: 11151871]

34. Ott DJ, Scharling ES, Chen YM, Wu WC, Gelfand DW. Barium enema examination: sensitivity in detecting colonic polyps and carcinomas. South Med J. 1989;82:197-200. [PMID: 2644698]

35. Rex DK, Rahmani EY, Haseman JH, Lemmel GT, Kaster S, Buckley JS. Relative sensitivity of colonoscopy and barium enema for detection of colorectal cancer in clinical practice. Gastroenterology. 1997;112:17-23. [PMID: 8978337]

36. Johnson CD, Carlson HC, Taylor WF, Weiland LP. Barium enemas of carcinoma of the colon: sensitivity of double- and single-contrast studies. AJR Am J Roentgenol. 1983;140:1143-9. [PMID: 6602483]

37. Bloomfield JA. Reliability of barium enema in detecting colonic neoplasia. Med J Aust. 1981;1:631-3. [PMID: 7254054]

38. Teefey SA, Carlson HC. The fluoroscopic barium enema in colonic polyp detection. AJR Am J Roentgenol. 1983;141:1279-81. [PMID: 6606327]

39. Brady AP, Stevenson GW, Stevenson I. Colorectal cancer overlooked at barium enema examination and colonoscopy: a continuing perceptual problem. Radiology. 1994;192:373-8. [PMID: 8029400]

40. Strøm E, Larsen JL. Colon cancer at barium enema examination and colonoscopy: a study from the county of Hordaland, Norway. Radiology. 1999; 211:211-4. [PMID: 10189473]

41. Brekkan A, Kjartansson O, Tulinius H, Sigvaldason H. Diagnostic sensitivity of X-ray examination of the large bowel in colorectal cancer. Gastrointest Radiol. 1983;8:363-5. [PMID: 6642154]

42. Glick S, Wagner JL, Johnson CD. Cost-effectiveness of double-contrast barium enema in screening for colorectal cancer. AJR Am J Roentgenol. 1998; 170:629-36. [PMID: 9490943]

43. Myllylä V, Päivänsalo M, Laitinen S. Sensitivity of single and double contrast barium enema in the detection of colorectal carcinoma. ROFO Fortschr Geb Rontgenstr Nuklearmed. 1984;140:393-7. [PMID: 6425161]

44. Kewenter J, Brevinge H. Endoscopic and surgical complications of work-up in screening for colorectal cancer. Dis Colon Rectum. 1996;39:676-80. [PMID: 8646956]

45. Winawer SJ, Zauber AG, Ho MN, O'Brien MJ, Gottlieb LS, Sternberg SS, et al. Prevention of colorectal cancer by colonoscopic polypectomy. The National Polyp Study Workgroup. N Engl J Med. 1993;329:1977-81. [PMID: 8247072]

46. Rembacken BJ, Fujii T, Cairns A, Dixon MF, Yoshida S, Chalmers DM, et al. Flat and depressed colonic neoplasms: a prospective study of 1000 colonoscopies in the UK. Lancet. 2000;355:1211-4. [PMID: 10770302]

47. Newcomer MK, Shaw MJ, Williams DM, Jowell PS. Unplanned work absence following outpatient colonoscopy. J Clin Gastroenterol. 1999;29:76-8. [PMID: 10405238]

48. Eckardt VF, Kanzler G, Schmitt T, Eckardt AJ, Bernhard G. Complications and adverse effects of colonoscopy with selective sedation. Gastrointest Endosc. 1999;49:560-65. [PMID: 10228252]

49. Zubarik R, Fleischer DE, Mastropietro C, Lopez J, Carroll J, Benjamin S, et al. Prospective analysis of complications 30 days after outpatient colonoscopy. Gastrointest Endosc. 1999;50:322-8. [PMID: 10462650]

50. Wexner SD, Forde KA, Sellers G, Geron N, Lopes A, Weiss EG, et al. How well can surgeons perform colonoscopy?. Surg Endosc. 1998;12:1410-4. [PMID: 9822468]

51. Farley DR, Bannon MP, Zietlow SP, Pemberton JH, Ilstrup DM, Larson DR. Management of colonoscopic perforations. Mayo Clin Proc. 1997;72:729-33. [PMID: 9276600]

52. Foliente RL, Chang AC, Youssef AI, Ford LJ, Condon SC, Chen YK. Endoscopic cecal perforation: mechanisms of injury. Am J Gastroenterol. 1996; 91:705-8. [PMID: 8677933]

53. Gibbs DH, Opelka FG, Beck DE, Hicks TC, Timmcke AE, Gathright JB Jr. Postpolypectomy colonic hemorrhage. Dis Colon Rectum. 1996;39:806-10. [PMID: 8674375]

54. Ure T, Dehghan K, Vernava AM 3rd, Longo WE, Andrus CA, Daniel GL. Colonoscopy in the elderly. Low risk, high yield. Surg Endosc. 1995;9:505-8. [PMID: 7676371]

55. Lo AY, Beaton HL. Selective management of colonoscopic perforations. J Am Coll Surg. 1994;179:333-7. [PMID: 8069431]

56. Rosen L, Bub DS, Reed JF 3rd, Nastasee SA. Hemorrhage following colonoscopic polypectomy. Dis Colon Rectum. 1993;36:1126-31. [PMID: 8253009]

57. DiPrima RE, Barkin JS, Blinder M, Goldberg RI, Phillips RS. Age as a risk factor in colonoscopy: fact versus fiction. Am J Gastroenterol. 1988;83:123-5. [PMID: 3341334]

58. Nivatvongs S. Complications in colonoscopic polypectomy: lessons to learn from an experience with 1576 polyps. Am Surg. 1988;54:61-3. [PMID: 3341645]

59. Brynitz S, Kjaergård H, Struckmann J. Perforations from colonoscopy during diagnosis and treatment of polyps. Ann Chir Gynaecol. 1986;75:142-5. [PMID: 3740781]

60. Webb WA, McDaniel L, Jones L. Experience with 1000 colonoscopic polypectomies. Ann Surg. 1985;201:626-32. [PMID: 3873221]

61. Macrae FA, Tan KG, Williams CB. Towards safer colonoscopy: a report on the complications of 5000 diagnostic or therapeutic colonoscopies. Gut. 1983; 24:376-83. [PMID: 6601604]

62. Rex DK, Johnson DA, Lieberman DA, Burt RW, Sonnenberg A. Colorectal cancer prevention 2000: screening recommendations of the American College of Gastroenterology. American College of Gastroenterology. Am J Gastroenterol. 2000;95:868-77. [PMID: 10763931]

63. Podolsky DK. Going the distance—the case for true colorectal-cancer screening [Editorial]. N Engl J Med. 2000;343:207-8. [PMID: 10900282]

64. Woolf SH. The best screening test for colorectal cancer—a personal choice [Editorial]. N Engl J Med. 2000;343:1641-3. [PMID: 11096175]

65. Vernon SW. Participation in colorectal cancer screening: a review. J Natl Cancer Inst. 1997;89:1406-22. [PMID: 9326910]

66. Balas EA, Weingarten S, Garb CT, Blumenthal D, Boren SA, Brown GD. Improving preventive care by prompting physicians. Arch Intern Med. 2000;160: 301-8. [PMID: 10668831]

Prostate cancer

❏ There is no direct evidence that prostate cancer screening decreases mortality.

❏ There is good evidence that prostate-specific antigen (PSA) screening can detect early-stage cancer but inconclusive evidence that early detection improves health outcomes.

❏ The large discrepancy between prostate cancer diagnoses and deaths indicates that some, and probably most, tumors detected by screening are clinically unimportant.

❏ Screening for prostate cancer with PSA is associated with frequent false-positives, which leads to unnecessary biopsies and patient anxiety and increases the risk for complications.

Screening for Prostate Cancer: An Update of the Evidence for the U.S. Preventive Services Task Force

Russell Harris, MD, MPH, and Kathleen N. Lohr, PhD

Background: In U.S. men, prostate cancer is the most common noncutaneous cancer and the second leading cause of cancer death. Screening for prostate cancer is controversial.

Purpose: To examine for the U.S. Preventive Services Task Force the evidence of benefits and harms of screening and earlier treatment.

Data Sources: MEDLINE and the Cochrane Library, experts, and bibliographies of reviews.

Study Selection: Researchers developed eight questions representing a logical chain between screening and reduced mortality, along with eligibility criteria for admissible evidence for each question. Admissible evidence was obtained by searching the data sources.

Data Extraction: Two reviewers abstracted relevant information using standardized abstraction forms and graded article quality according to Task Force criteria.

Data Synthesis: No conclusive direct evidence shows that screening reduces prostate cancer mortality. Some screening tests can detect prostate cancer at an earlier stage than clinical detection. One study provides good evidence that radical prostatectomy reduces disease-specific mortality for men with localized prostate cancer detected clinically. No study has examined the additional benefit of earlier treatment after detection by screening. Men with a life expectancy of fewer than 10 years are unlikely to benefit from screening even under favorable assumptions. Each treatment is associated with several well-documented potential harms.

Conclusions: Although potential harms of screening for prostate cancer can be established, the presence or magnitude of potential benefits cannot. Therefore, the net benefit of screening cannot be determined.

The American Cancer Society estimates that 189 000 men will receive a diagnosis of prostate cancer in 2002 and that 30 200 men will die of the disease (1). Many more men receive a diagnosis of prostate cancer than die of it (lifetime risk, about 1 in 6 vs. about 1 in 29). Among types of cancer, only lung cancer kills more men each year. The cause of prostate cancer is unknown, and the best-documented risk factors (age, ethnicity, and family history) are not modifiable. The burden of prostate cancer falls disproportionately on men who are older or black. The median age at diagnosis is approximately 71 years, and the median age at death is 78 years (2). More than 75% of all cases of prostate cancer are diagnosed in men older than 65 years of age, and 90% of deaths occur in this age group (2, 3). Incidence is approximately 60% higher and mortality rate is twofold higher in black men than in white men (2). Asian-American men and Hispanic men have lower incidence rates than non-Hispanic white persons (3).

Although approaches to primary prevention of prostate cancer are being tested, to date none are known to be effective. The most common strategy for reducing the burden of prostate cancer is screening, but screening remains controversial. Many studies on this topic have been published since 1996, when the U.S. Preventive Services Task Force (USPSTF) last examined prostate screening (4). To assist the USPSTF in updating its recommendation, the Research Triangle Institute–University of North Carolina Evidence-based Practice Center performed a systematic review of the evidence on screening for prostate cancer.

METHODS

Using USPSTF methods (5), we developed an analytic framework and eight key questions to guide our literature search. Because we found no direct evidence connecting screening and reduced mortality, we searched for indirect evidence on the yield of screening, the efficacy and harms of various forms of treatment for early prostate cancer, and the costs and cost-effectiveness of screening. We developed eligibility criteria for selecting relevant evidence to answer the key questions (Table 1). We examined the critical literature from the 1996 USPSTF review and used search terms consistent with the eligibility criteria to search the MEDLINE database and Cochrane Library for English-language reviews and relevant studies published between 1 January 1994 and 15 September 2002.

The first author and at least one trained assistant reviewed abstracts and articles to find those that met the eligibility criteria. For these studies, the two reviewers abstracted relevant information using standardized abstraction forms. We graded the quality of all included articles according to USPSTF criteria (5). The authors worked closely with two members of the USPSTF throughout the review and periodically presented reports to the full USPSTF. We distributed a draft of the systematic evidence review to experts in the field and relevant professional organizations and federal agencies for broad-based external peer review and made revisions based on the feedback. We then revised the full systematic evidence review into this manuscript. A more complete account of the methods of this review can be found in the Appendix (available at

Table 1. Key Questions, Inclusion Criteria, and Articles Meeting Criteria*

Key Question	Inclusion Criteria	Articles Meeting Criteria, *n*
All	Published from 1 January 1994 to 15 September 2002 English language MEDLINE, Cochrane Human participants	
1. Efficacy of screening (direct evidence)	RCT; case–control study; or ecologic evidence directly connecting screening with health outcomes	1 RCT 2 case–control 15 ecologic
2. Yield of screening	Unselected population without prostate cancer Screening test offered to all Work-up offered to all with positive results on screening tests Screening test compared with a valid reference standard	35
3. Efficacy of radical prostatectomy	RCT; clinically localized disease Follow-up ≥2 years ≥75% of patients followed	1
4. Efficacy of radiation therapy	Health outcomes	0
5. Efficacy of androgen deprivation therapy		2
6. Efficacy of watchful waiting		1
7. Harms of treatment	Patient self-report Use of valid measurement instrument Follow-up from pretreatment to at least 12 months post-treatment *or* Comparison with similar untreated control group at least 12 months post-treatment	32
8. Costs and cost-effectiveness of treatment	Valid assessment of costs of screening and treatment Assess direct and indirect costs Cost-effectiveness, cost-benefit, cost-utility Modeling studies	2

* RCT = randomized, controlled trial.

www.annals.org). The complete systematic evidence review is available on the Web site of the Agency for Healthcare Research and Quality (www.ahrq.gov) (6).

This evidence report was funded through a contract to the Research Triangle Institute–University of North Carolina Evidence-based Practice Center from the Agency for Healthcare Research and Quality. Staff of the funding agency and members of the USPSTF contributed to the study design, reviewed draft and final manuscripts, and made editing suggestions.

RESULTS
Direct Evidence That Screening Reduces Mortality
Randomized, Controlled Trials

Labrie and colleagues (7) completed the first randomized, controlled trial (RCT) of prostate cancer screening with more than 46 000 men. At the end of 8 years of follow-up, approximately 23% of the invited group and 6.5% of the not-invited group had been screened with prostate-specific antigen (PSA) testing and digital rectal examination (DRE). Prostate cancer death rates did not differ between groups (4.6 vs. 4.8 deaths per 1000 persons, respectively).

Two other RCTs of prostate cancer screening, both initiated in 1994, are ongoing: the U.S. National Cancer Institute Prostate, Lung, Colorectal, and Ovary Trial and the European Randomized Study of Screening for Prostate Cancer. Neither study will have data on mortality for several more years.

Case–Control Studies

Three well-conducted, nested case–control studies (two since 1994) examined the relationship between chart review documentation of DRE and advanced prostate cancer or death from prostate cancer. Two studies found no relationship (8, 9). The third study found that men who died of prostate cancer had fewer DREs in the years before diagnosis (odds ratio indicating a protective effect of DRE, 0.51 [95% CI, 0.31 to 0.84]) (10).

Why results from these otherwise similar studies differ is not clear. The three studies depended on large databases and on individual medical records. They defined cases slightly differently and used different approaches to differentiate screening DRE from diagnostic DRE. Because such studies are complex in design, we were not able to determine whether one method was more accurate than another (11). All three studies were small, and all were consistent with a reduction in prostate cancer mortality of up to 50% with DRE.

We found no case–control studies of PSA screening. This can be explained, at least in part, by the fact that insufficient time has elapsed since the introduction of PSA as a screening test in the late 1980s. Such studies are under way (12).

Ecologic Studies

Around 1987, use of PSA screening began to increase rapidly in the United States. Important trends in prostate cancer incidence and mortality also occurred at that time. Although incidence rates had been slowly increasing for some years before 1987, data from the U.S. Surveillance, Epidemiology, and End Results program showed a dramatic increase in age-adjusted prostate cancer incidence—20% per year—from 1989 to 1992. The rates then decreased at 10.8% per year (13), stabilizing after 1994 (14). Most of the increase in incidence was seen in localized or regional disease. Incidence of distant-stage disease at diagnosis showed little initial increase and then began to decline; annual decline for white men was 17.9% after 1991 (15).

Disease-specific mortality rates paralleled trends in prostate cancer incidence (15, 16). In the late 1980s, the average annual percentage increase rose from 0.7% to 3.1% for white men and from 1.6% to 3.2% for black men. In 1991, prostate cancer mortality rates for white men began to decline (21.6% decrease from 1991 to 1999); in 1993, rates for black men followed suit (16.0% decrease from 1993 to 1999) (14). Mortality rates decreased in all age groups at about the same time. Analyses of trends in prostate cancer incidence and mortality in Olmsted County, Minnesota (17), and in Canada (18, 19) have shown similar results.

Ecologic evidence is difficult to interpret. Although screening probably explains trends in incidence of prostate cancer (20), trends in mortality are more difficult to understand. Some aspects of the trends (for example, a decline in distant-stage disease) are consistent with screening, but other aspects (for example, the short time between increased screening and decreased mortality) (21) are not as consistent with our current view of the natural history of prostate cancer. The argument that the decline in mortality can be attributed to PSA screening would be stronger if it could be shown that the decline was largest in areas with more screening. To date, data on this issue are conflicting (19, 22–27).

Other possible explanations for decreased mortality include "attribution bias" and improved treatment. Attribution bias suggests that some deaths are mistakenly attributed to prostate cancer. If the percentage of deaths so attributed is stable, then the prostate cancer mortality rate would be expected to increase and decrease in close approximation with the incidence of prostate cancer in the population (16).

Changes in prostate cancer treatment during the late 1980s and early 1990s included higher rates of radical prostatectomy, development of luteinizing hormone–releasing hormone (LHRH) agonists (allowing improved androgen deprivation therapy without castration), and refinements in radiation therapy. Such changes may explain the reduction in prostate cancer mortality. A recent study by Bartsch and coworkers (27), for example, documented a greater reduction in prostate cancer mortality in the Austrian state of Tyrol, which had instituted a free PSA screening program, compared with the rest of Austria. This finding could be a consequence of the screening program, changes in treatment that accompanied the screening program, misattribution of cause of death, or some combination of the three.

Accuracy of Screening

Three problems complicate any attempt to determine the accuracy of screening tests for prostate cancer. First, research has yet to clarify which tumors screening should target. Second, the reference standard (prostate biopsy) for diagnosing prostate cancer after positive results on a screening test is imperfect. Third, few studies perform biopsy on men with negative results on screening tests.

Prostate cancer is a heterogeneous tumor. Different cases of prostate cancer have widely varying growth rates and potential for causing death. Ideally, prostate cancer screening would target only tumors that would cause clinically important disease. Currently available prognostic markers can distinguish a small number of men with excellent prognosis for long-term survival and a small number of men with poor prognosis for long-term survival (28). However, they cannot help us correctly categorize the prognosis of those in the middle category, which includes most men with prostate cancer (29–33). Since research has not yet clearly defined the characteristics of clinically important prostate cancer, we do not know what the specific target of screening should be.

The usual reference standard used in prostate cancer screening studies, transrectal needle biopsy of the prostate, is imperfect for two reasons. First, it misses some cases of cancer; 10% to 30% of men who have negative results on an initial series of biopsies have cancer on repeated biopsy series (34–39). Thus, some men categorized as not having cancer actually have it, falsely lowering the test's measured sensitivity. Second, in clinical practice and research, a "biopsy" is actually four to six (or more) biopsies. Many biopsy specimens are obtained, most from normal-appearing areas of the prostate. An analysis of this practice concluded that up to 25% of apparently PSA-detected tumors and more than 25% of apparently DRE-detected tumors were likely to have been detected by serendipity, that is, as an incidental finding on a blind biopsy (40). Thus, some men who are categorized as having cancer detected by screening actually have serendipity-detected cancer. This error falsely increases sensitivity.

In addition to problems of the accuracy of the reference standard, few studies perform biopsy on men who have negative results on screening tests. This reduces our ability to determine the number of false-negative screening tests and to calculate sensitivity. Most studies use several noninvasive tests together, measuring the sensitivity of one test against the combined findings of all tests. The extent to which these combined tests actually detect all important cancer is unknown. This bias probably leads to an overestimate of sensitivity.

Screening Methods

Prostate-Specific Antigen Testing

An analysis from the Physicians' Health Study avoided some of the bias of the problematic reference standard by using longitudinal follow-up instead of biopsy (41). In this study, which used a PSA cut-point of 4.0 ng/mL or higher, the sensitivity for detecting cancer appearing within 2 years after screening was 73.2%. Although the study calculated sensitivity separately for aggressive (that is, extracapsular or higher grade) and nonaggressive (that is, intracapsular and lower grade) cancer (sensitivity, 91% vs. 56%), it is not clear that these categories correspond to clinically important and clinically unimportant tumors. Among men who did not receive a diagnosis of prostate cancer in those 2 years, 14.6% had an initial PSA level of 4.0 ng/mL or greater, corresponding to a specificity of 85.4%.

Other studies have provided similar estimates of sensitivity and specificity for PSA level with a cut-point of 4.0 ng/mL (42–44). Specificity for PSA screening is lower among men with larger prostate glands, including the large number of older men with benign prostatic hyperplasia. One study of four carefully chosen samples found that the likelihood ratios for various PSA levels were much lower among men with benign prostatic hyperplasia than among men without benign prostatic hyperplasia (45). Thus, the PSA test is not as accurate in detecting cancer in men with benign prostatic hyperplasia as in those without.

Because of the reduced specificity in older men with benign prostatic hyperplasia, some experts have proposed that the PSA cut-point be adjusted for age, with higher cut-points for older men and lower cut-points for younger men (46). Such a strategy increases sensitivity and lowers specificity in younger men, while the reverse is true in older men. Experts disagree about whether this strategy would improve health outcomes (47, 48).

Some experts have also proposed decreasing the cut-point defining an abnormal PSA level from 4.0 ng/mL to 3.0 ng/mL (or even 2.6 ng/mL) for all men (44, 49, 50). This approach results in more biopsies and more cancer detected (49, 51–55). Because of the uncertainty about the definition of clinical importance, the value of this increased detection is unknown.

In the serum, PSA circulates in two forms: free and complexed with such molecules as α_1-antichymotrypsin. Men with prostate cancer tend to have a lower percentage of free PSA than men without prostate cancer (56, 57). In research, the percentage of free PSA (or a similar test measuring the level of complexed PSA) (58–62) has mainly been used to increase the specificity of screening by distinguishing between men with PSA levels of 4.0 ng/mL to 9.9 ng/mL who should undergo biopsy and those who should not (52, 63–70). Different studies have suggested different cut-points for percentage of free PSA; a lower cut-point avoids more biopsies but also misses more cancer. High cut-points (for example, 25%) would avoid about 20% of biopsies, and the probability of cancer at that cut-point is about 8% (66). In practice, it is not clear whether this probability would be low enough for men and their physicians to forgo biopsy (71).

Men with prostate cancer have a greater increase in PSA level over time than men without cancer (72). It is unclear, however, whether examining the annual rate of change in PSA level (PSA velocity) improves health outcomes or reduces unnecessary biopsies (47, 73). Because of intraindividual variation, PSA velocity is useful only in men who have three or more tests of PSA level over a period of 1 to 3 years (47, 74, 75).

Digital Rectal Examination

It is more difficult to detect cancer with DRE than with PSA. A meta-analysis examining studies of DRE in unselected samples screened by both PSA and DRE found a sensitivity of 59% (64% for the four best studies) (76). Digital rectal examination detects cancer in some men with PSA levels below 4.0 ng/mL (positive predictive value, about 10% according to one large study [63]) or even 3.0 ng/mL, but the tumors were usually small and well differentiated (77). Digital rectal examination has limited reproducibility (78).

Yield of Large Screening Programs

Using six studies of screening with a single PSA test or with PSA and DRE among large, previously unscreened samples, we were able to estimate the yield of a new screening program among men in different age groups (79) who had not previously been screened (7, 44, 49, 63, 64, 79–83). The **Figure** gives estimates of positive test results and cases of cancer detected after screening with PSA alone or screening with PSA and DRE among men in their 60s. Men in their 50s have fewer positive test results and cases of cancer detected, while men in their 70s have more.

The percentage of participants with a PSA level of 4.0 ng/mL or higher ranged from about 4% (79) among men in their 50s to about 27% (64) among men in their 70s. The percentage of men who had a PSA level of 4.0 ng/mL or higher or abnormal results on DRE ranged from 15% among younger men to 40% among older men (79). Few other screening tests have such a high percentage of positive results (63, 64, 81, 82).

In the screening studies, some men with abnormal results on screening tests did not undergo biopsy. If we assume that biopsy is performed on all men with an abnor-

Figure. Estimated yield of screening with prostate-specific antigen (*PSA*) testing or with PSA testing and digital rectal examination (*DRE*).

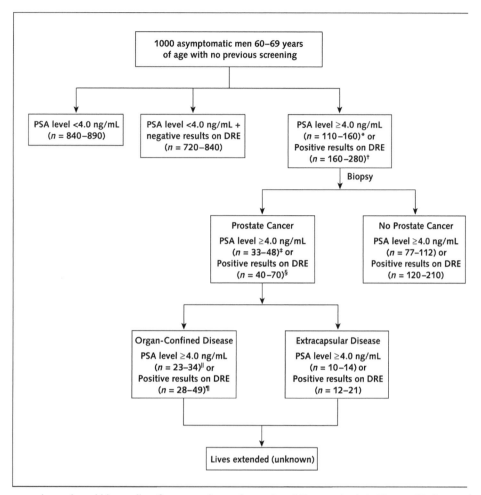

The number of cancer cases detected would be smaller after repeated annual screening. * For men in their 50s, $n = 50$; for men in their 70s, $n = 270$. † For men in their 50s, $n = 150$; for men in their 70s, $n = 400$. ‡ For men in their 50s, $n = 17$; for men in their 70s, $n = 90$. § For men in their 50s, $n = 30$; for men in their 70s, $n = 100$. ||For men in their 50s, $n = 12$; for men in their 70s, $n = 63$. ¶ For men in their 50s, $n = 21$; for men in their 70s, $n = 70$. In all footnotes, numbers are approximate.

mal result on a screening test and that the rate of cancer detection is the same as for men who undergo study biopsy, we estimate that the percentage of all men screened who would have prostate cancer detected would range from approximately 1.5% (PSA screening alone for men in their 50s) (81) to 10% (PSA and DRE screening for men in their 70s) (44).

The **Figure** gives general percentages from all studies. In these six studies, biopsies detected cancer in approximately 30% of men with a PSA level of 4.0 ng/mL or higher and in 20% to 27% of men with a PSA level of 4.0 ng/mL or higher or an abnormal result on DRE (7, 49, 79, 80, 83). The probability of prostate cancer with a PSA level of 2.5 ng/mL to 4.0 ng/mL and negative results on DRE is also about 20% (51). Although the studies found that 60% to 70% of screen-detected cancer is organ confined (7, 49, 80, 82, 83), they do not provide information about the number of lives extended by detecting either organ-confined or extracapsular tumors.

Yield with Different Screening Intervals

Rates of positive results and cancer detection decrease on screening a year after the initial screening round (7, 49, 80, 83–85). In one study, approximately 26% of men with a PSA level of 4.0 ng/mL or greater had prostate cancer after the first round of screening and approximately 6.2% had cancer after subsequent rounds (7). Other studies have concluded that annual screening confers little gain compared with intervals of at least 2 years (86), especially for the 70% of the population with PSA levels of 2.0 ng/mL or less (41, 87).

Effectiveness of Current Treatments for Localized Disease
Radical Prostatectomy

Since 1991, radical prostatectomy has been the most common treatment for clinically localized prostate cancer. It is the initial treatment for more than one third of patients with new diagnoses, most commonly men 75 years of age or younger (2). The procedure is usually performed with curative intent in men who have a life expectancy of at least 10 years.

One well-conducted RCT compared radical prostatectomy with "watchful waiting" (in which treatment is not given initially but is reserved for progressive or symptomatic disease) among men with clinically detected prostate cancer (88). About 75% of the men in this study had palpable cancerous tumors, few of which were the size usually detected by PSA screening (73, 84, 89). After 8 years of follow-up, 7.1% of the radical prostatectomy group had died of prostate cancer compared with 13.6% of men in the watchful waiting group (relative hazard, 0.50 [CI, 0.27 to 0.91]). The absolute difference in prostate cancer mortality was 6.6% (CI, 2.1% to 11.1%) (number needed to treat for benefit, 17). The groups did not differ in all-cause mortality.

No other well-conducted RCT has compared any other treatment with radical prostatectomy for clinically localized prostate cancer. One ongoing RCT, the Prostatectomy Intervention versus Observation Trial in the United States, will publish results in the future (90, 91).

One observational study that used internal controls and data from the Surveillance, Epidemiology, and End Results program provided information on the effectiveness of radical prostatectomy relative to other treatments (92). For men with well-differentiated cancer, 10-year disease-specific survival did not differ between the radical prostatectomy group and the age-matched radiation or watchful waiting groups. Disease-specific survival was slightly higher for the radical prostatectomy group in men with moderately differentiated tumors (radical prostatectomy group, 87%; radiation group, 76%; watchful waiting group, 77%) and was much higher for men with poorly differentiated cancer (radical prostatectomy group, 67%; radiation group, 53%; watchful waiting group, 45%). Other cohort studies without controls have found similar survival rates after radical prostatectomy (33, 93–97).

Radiation Therapy

Radiation therapy is the second most commonly used treatment for nonmetastatic prostate cancer and is the most common treatment for men 70 to 80 years of age (2). The two common types of radiation therapy reviewed here are external-beam radiation therapy (EBRT) and brachytherapy, the insertion of radioactive pellets directly into prostate tissue.

No well-conducted RCT with clinical outcomes compares EBRT with any other therapy for clinically localized prostate cancer. In the large cohort study discussed earlier (92), 10-year disease-specific survival rates in the EBRT group were similar to those in the watchful waiting group for men with well-differentiated and moderately differentiated tumors but were higher for men with poorly differentiated cancer (92).

Brachytherapy is most often used alone for men with well or moderately differentiated intracapsular prostate cancer or in combination with EBRT for men with more aggressive cancer. No RCT with clinical outcomes compared brachytherapy with any other treatment for prostate cancer. Two observational studies involving 100 or more patients with clinically localized prostate cancer found high survival rates for patients treated with radioactive gold or iodine seeds (98, 99).

Androgen Deprivation Therapy

The traditional approach to androgen deprivation therapy has been surgical bilateral orchiectomy. A newer approach uses LHRH agonists (for example, goserelin or leuprolide), a group of drugs that stimulate the release of luteinizing hormone from the pituitary gland. Paradoxically, when used clinically, LHRH agonists result in down-regulation of pituitary receptors, thus markedly reducing the level of testosterone production to that of a castrated man. Luteinizing hormone–releasing hormone agonists have been used clinically since the late 1980s.

Two well-conducted RCTs compared clinical outcomes between men with clinically localized prostate cancer who were treated with androgen deprivation therapy (with orchiectomy [100] or estramustine [101]) and men treated with EBRT. Androgen deprivation therapy either increased overall survival (100) or reduced clinical recurrence (101); outcomes improved primarily among men who had lymph node involvement.

Four additional RCTs of androgen deprivation therapy (with LHRH agonists) as an adjuvant to EBRT or radical prostatectomy for locally advanced prostate cancer found statistically significant improved overall survival (10% to 20% absolute difference) in men who received androgen deprivation therapy (102–108). Another RCT of immediate versus deferred androgen deprivation therapy (with orchiectomy or LHRH agonists) and no other treatment found improved survival (8% absolute difference) for the immediate therapy group in men who had a new diagnosis of locally advanced prostate cancer (109).

Watchful Waiting

The term *watchful waiting* implies that no treatment is given initially but that the patient is followed for evidence of progressive or symptomatic disease, for which treatment might be offered. Because the only well-conducted RCT that compares watchful waiting and more aggressive treatment examined men with prostate cancer detected clinically rather than by screening (88), the best information about the outcomes of watchful waiting comes from observational studies of men who, for various reasons, were not treated for prostate cancer. These studies also provide information about the natural history of the disease.

Four well-conducted retrospective cohort studies (29, 30, 110, 111) and one pooled analysis of six other cohort studies (28) provide information about survival with untreated prostate cancer. Men with well-differentiated, clin-

Table 2. Harms of Treatment*

Treatment	Men with Reduced Sexual Function	Men with Urinary Problems	Men with Bowel Problems	Men with Other Symptoms
	←———————————————— % ————————————————→			
Radical prostatectomy	20–70	15–50		
External-beam radiation therapy	20–45	2–16	6–25	
Brachytherapy	36†	6–12†	18†	
Androgen deprivation therapy (LHRH agonists)	40–70			Breast swelling: 5–25 Hot flashes: 50–60

* Values are percentages of men treated who had side effects at least 12 months after treatment. LHRH = luteinizing hormone–releasing hormone.
† These findings are less certain than other entries because they are based on less or inferior evidence.

ically localized prostate cancer have excellent long-term survival, with little or no reduction in survival compared with similar men without prostate cancer. Men with poorly differentiated cancer have reduced survival. In one study, 10-year survival was 17% in men with poorly differentiated cancer and 47% in age-matched controls without prostate cancer (92).

Because most prostate cancer detected today by screening is moderately differentiated, survival of men with this type of tumor is important to the debate about screening. On the standard histologic grading system for prostate cancer, these men have tumors with Gleason scores of 5 to 7. Gleason scores range from 2 to 10; lower scores indicate well-differentiated patterns, and higher scores indicate more poorly differentiated tumors.

The most detailed analysis of men with untreated, clinically localized, moderately differentiated cancer found that 15-year prostate cancer–specific survival rates ranged from 30% (Gleason score of 7 in men 50 to 59 years of age) to 94% (Gleason score of 5 in men 50 to 59 years of age) (29, 110). Men in their 70s had survival rates similar to those of men in their 50s for tumors with a Gleason score of 5 but much better survival for tumors with a Gleason score of 7 (58% vs. 30%). Because men in this study received their diagnoses in the pre-PSA era, survival would probably be even better in similar men receiving diagnoses today given the "lead time" added by earlier detection.

Harms of Treatment

Because harms of treatment are experienced by the men themselves, and because men may have problems that are similar to treatment harms but are not attributable to treatment, we prioritized evidence that measured patients' perceptions of their own function. For comparison, we used an untreated group or the same men examined before and at least 12 months after treatment.

Radical Prostatectomy

Thirty-day mortality rates after radical prostatectomy range from 0.3% to 1% for most men and may be higher for men older than 80 years of age (112–116). The pri-

mary long-term adverse effects of radical prostatectomy include erectile dysfunction and urinary incontinence (**Table 2**). At least 20%, perhaps as many as 70%, of men have worsened sexual function as a result of radical prostatectomy (114, 117–135). Fifteen percent to 50% of men who had a radical prostatectomy had some urinary problems 1 year later (112, 114, 117, 119, 121, 123, 126, 127, 131, 132, 135–138). Current evidence is mixed about the extent to which, outside of excellent academic centers (95, 124), the newer nerve-sparing procedure reduces complication rates.

Radiation Therapy

Twenty percent to 45% of men with no erectile dysfunction and 2% to 16% of men with no urinary incontinence before EBRT developed dysfunction 12 to 24 months afterward (**Table 2**) (117, 123, 126–131, 135, 137, 139–146). Six percent to 25% of men who had no bowel dysfunction before EBRT reported marked problems 12 or more months afterward (117, 123, 125, 126, 130, 131, 135, 137, 140, 142, 144–147). The evidence is mixed about whether newer techniques, including three-dimensional conformal EBRT, reduce the frequency of urinary or bowel side effects.

Compared with EBRT or radical prostatectomy, fewer high-quality studies of the harms of brachytherapy have been completed. Our estimates are therefore less precise for this treatment. Among men who were potent before treatment, about 21% are impotent and 36% have decreased erectile function 3 years after brachytherapy (148, 149). A majority of men will have distressing urinary symptoms in the first months after brachytherapy, and 6% to 12% will have such symptoms 1 year later. Up to 25% of men will have some lack of urinary control 12 months after brachytherapy (120, 149–151). Approximately 18% of men will have diarrhea 1 year later (120), and 19% will have some persistent rectal bleeding 12 to 28 months later (152).

Androgen Deprivation Therapy

We focused on the harms of LHRH agonists because the effectiveness studies we reviewed primarily used this type of androgen deprivation therapy. No study has examined reports from the same patients beginning before androgen deprivation therapy and extending for at least 1 year. Our best information comes from two large national studies (153–155) and a systematic review (156, 157). Compared with untreated men, 40% to 70% of men who were sexually active before treatment were not sexually active afterward (**Table 2**). Five percent to 25% of men had breast swelling, and 50% to 60% had hot flashes. Mean scores on quality-of-life indices are lower for men treated with androgen deprivation therapy (154). One RCT of LHRH adjuvant therapy found similar results (107). Potential long-term complications of LHRH therapy include lack of vitality, anemia, and osteoporosis (155, 158, 159). The frequency and severity of these complications are not yet clear.

Quality of Life

Litwin and colleagues (129) compared overall quality-of-life scores among controls and men with prostate cancer within treatment groups. Although they found the same differences in specific symptoms as noted earlier, they found no differences among groups (either among treatment groups or between men with and without prostate cancer) in overall quality of life.

Cost-Effectiveness of Screening

Given the uncertainties about the existence and magnitude of benefits, the cost-effectiveness of screening for prostate cancer has been difficult to calculate. A 1993 decision analysis, which made optimistic assumptions about benefit from screening and early treatment, found little or no benefit for men with well-differentiated tumors (160). For men with moderately or poorly differentiated cancer, screening and early treatment could offer as much as 3.5 years of improvement in quality-adjusted life expectancy, again using the most optimistic assumptions. Even with optimistic assumptions, however, men 75 years of age and older were not likely to benefit from screening and aggressive treatment. One major reason is that any benefits of screening are expected to accrue some years in the future, after many men in this age group have died of some other condition. Two subsequent decision analyses have reached the same conclusions (161, 162).

In 1995, Barry and coworkers (163) published a cost-effectiveness analysis using favorable screening assumptions. The marginal cost-effectiveness of screening men 65 years of age with PSA and DRE, without adjustment for quality of life and without discounting benefits, was between $12 500 and $15 000 per life-year saved. Changing only a few assumptions, however, quickly increased the marginal cost-effectiveness ratio to above $100 000 per life-year saved. This ratio would be even less favorable if a decrement in quality of life associated with the harms of treatment were considered. In 1997, these investigators updated their model with newer data and further assumptions favorable to screening; findings were similar (164).

DISCUSSION

Prostate-specific antigen testing and, to a lesser extent, DRE can detect prostate cancer at an earlier stage than it could be detected clinically. A major problem in considering the utility of screening, however, is the heterogeneity of prostate cancer itself. The large discrepancy between prostate cancer diagnoses and deaths indicates that some and probably most tumors detected by screening are clinically unimportant. Because precise evidence regarding the prognosis of prostate cancer of various types is lacking, researchers have not been able to define the most appropriate targets of screening, that is, the types of cancer that will cause clinical symptoms and death and that can be treated better if detected earlier.

The efficacy of various types of treatment for clinically localized prostate cancer, and especially for the types of localized prostate cancer detected by screening, is largely unknown. Although one RCT found that radical prostatectomy reduced prostate cancer mortality compared with watchful waiting among men with symptomatic localized cancer, the magnitude of any additional benefit of detection and earlier treatment due to screening is still unknown. We lack direct evidence that EBRT, brachytherapy, or androgen deprivation therapy is effective for clinically localized cancer. Each treatment for prostate cancer is associated with various potential harms, including sexual, urinary, and bowel dysfunction.

The costs of a screening program for prostate cancer are potentially high. If treatment is extremely efficacious, then the cost-effectiveness of screening men 50 to 69 years of age may be reasonable; if treatment is less efficacious, the results may be net harm and high costs. Assuming that any potential benefit to screening accrues only after some years, men with a life expectancy of fewer than 10 years are unlikely to benefit. Because prostate cancer incidence and mortality rates are higher among black men, beneficial screening could have a larger absolute benefit in this ethnic group than in white men. The same uncertainties about screening, however, would apply.

Two RCTs of screening are in progress. Because of the problem of screening in control groups, however, some experts fear that even these trials may not provide a definitive answer about screening efficacy. If these trials find a reduction in prostate cancer mortality, further research will be required to determine whether the benefits outweigh the harms and costs for individuals or as a general policy. Research can help by developing new screening and treatment approaches that minimize harms and costs. If the trials show no benefit, research on other approaches to disease control, such as chemoprevention, will be necessary. In the interim, the efficacy of screening for prostate cancer remains uncertain.

From University of North Carolina at Chapel Hill, Chapel Hill, and Research Triangle Institute, Research Triangle Park, North Carolina.

Disclaimer: The authors of this article are responsible for its contents, including any clinical or treatment recommendations. No statement in this article should be construed as an official position of the U.S. Agency for Healthcare Research and Quality or the U.S. Department of Health and Human Services.

Acknowledgments: The authors acknowledge the continuing support of David Atkins, MD, MPH, and the guidance and feedback of Cynthia D. Mulrow, MD, MPH, University of Texas at San Antonio, Paul S. Frame, MD, Cohocton, New York, and other members of the USPSTF.

They thank the staff of the Research Triangle Institute–University of North Carolina Evidence-based Practice Center, including Audrina J. Bunton, BA, Linda Lux, MPA, and Sonya Sutton, BSPH, for substantive and editorial work and Loraine Monroe for secretarial assistance. They also thank Rainer Beck, MD, Paul Godley, MD, MPH, and Kenneth Fink, MD, MPH, for assistance in reviewing articles. In addition, they thank the staff from the University of North Carolina at Chapel Hill and the Cecil G. Sheps Center for Health Services Research, including Timothy S. Carey, MD, MPH, Anne Jackman, MSW, Lynn Whitener, MSLS, DrPH, and Carol Krasnov. They also thank the peer reviewers of the complete systematic evidence review: Michael Barry, MD, Medical Practices Evaluation Center, Boston, Massachusetts; John W. Feightner, MD, MSC, Canadian Task Force on Preventive Health Care, London, Ontario, Canada; Theodore Ganiats, MD, University of California at San Diego, La Jolla, California; Marc B. Garnick, MD, Beth Israel Deaconess Medical Center, Boston, Massachusetts; Richard Hoffman, MD, MPH, Albuquerque Veterans Affairs Medical Center, Albuquerque, New Mexico; Barnett Kramer, MD, National Institutes of Health, Bethesda, Maryland; David Lush, MD, Medical College of Pennsylvania, Philadelphia, Pennsylvania; Curtis Mettlin, MD, Roswell Park Cancer Institute, Buffalo, New York; and Ian M. Thompson Jr., MD, University of Texas Health Sciences Center at San Antonio, San Antonio, Texas.

Grant Support: This study was conducted by the Research Triangle Institute–University of North Carolina Evidence-based Practice Center under contract to the Agency for Healthcare Research and Quality, Rockville, Maryland (contract no. 290-97-0011, task order 3).

Requests for Single Reprints: Reprints are available from the Agency for Healthcare Research and Quality Web site (www.ahrq.gov/clinic/uspstffix.htm) or the Agency for Healthcare Research and Quality Publications Clearinghouse.

Current author addresses, the Appendix, Appendix Table, and Appendix Figures are available at www.annals.org.

References

1. Jemal A, Thomas A, Murray T, Thun M. Cancer statistics, 2002. CA Cancer J Clin. 2002;52:23-47. [PMID: 11814064]

2. Stanford JL, Stephenson RA, Coyle LM, Cerhan J, Correa R, Eley JW, et al. Prostate Cancer Trends 1973-1995. SEER Program, National Cancer Institute. 1999. NIH publication no. 99-4543. Accessed at http://seer.cancer.gov/publications/prostate/ on 14 October 2002.

3. Ross RK, Schottenfeld D. Prostate Cancer. In: Schottenfeld D, Fraumeni JF Jr, eds. Cancer Epidemiology and Prevention. 2nd ed. New York: Oxford Univ Pr; 1996:1180-206.

4. Guide to Clinical Preventive Servicezs. 2nd ed. United States Preventive Services Task Force. Alexandria, VA: International Medical Publishing; 1996:119-34.

5. Harris RP, Helfand M, Woolf SH, Lohr KN, Mulrow CD, Teutsch SM, et al. Current methods of the US Preventive Services Task Force: a review of the process. Am J Prev Med. 2001;20:21-35. [PMID: 11306229]

6. Harris R, Lohr K, Beck R, Fink K, Godley P, Bunton A. Screening for Prostate Cancer. A Systematic Evidence Review No. 16 (Prepared by the Re-

search Triangle Institute–University of North Carolina Evidence-based Practice Center under Contract No. 280-97-0011). Rockville, MD: Agency for Healthcare Research and Quality; 2002. www.ahrq.gov/clinic.serfiles.htm.

7. Labrie F, Candas B, Dupont A, Cusan L, Gomez JL, Suburu RE, et al. Screening decreases prostate cancer death: first analysis of the 1988 Quebec prospective randomized controlled trial. Prostate. 1999;38:83-91. [PMID: 9973093]

8. Friedman GD, Hiatt RA, Quesenberry CP Jr, Selby JV. Case-control study of screening for prostatic cancer by digital rectal examinations. Lancet. 1991;337:1526-9. [PMID: 1675379]

9. Richert-Boe KE, Humphrey LL, Glass AG, Weiss NS. Screening digital rectal examination and prostate cancer mortality: a case-control study. J Med Screen. 1998;5:99-103. [PMID: 9718529]

10. Jacobsen SJ, Bergstralh EJ, Katusic SK, Guess HA, Darby CH, Silverstein MD, et al. Screening digital rectal examination and prostate cancer mortality: a population-based case-control study. Urology. 1998;52:173-9. [PMID: 9697778]

11. Concato J. What is a screening test? Misclassification bias in observational studies of screening for cancer. J Gen Intern Med. 1997;12:607-12. [PMID: 9346456]

12. Concato J, Peduzzi P, Kamina A, Horwitz RI. A nested case-control study of the effectiveness of screening for prostate cancer: research design. J Clin Epidemiol. 2001;54:558-64. [PMID: 11377115]

13. Hankey BF, Feuer EJ, Clegg LX, Hayes RB, Legler JM, Prorok PC, et al. Cancer surveillance series: interpreting trends in prostate cancer—part I: Evidence of the effects of screening in recent prostate cancer incidence, mortality, and survival rates. J Natl Cancer Inst. 1999;91:1017-24. [PMID: 10379964]

14. Ries L, Eisner M, Kosary C, Hankey B, Miller B, Clegg L, et al. SEER Cancer Statistics Review, 1973-1999. National Cancer Institute. 2002. Accessed at http://seer.cancer.gov/csr/1973_1999/ on 11 August 2002.

15. Tarone RE, Chu KC, Brawley OW. Implications of stage-specific survival rates in assessing recent declines in prostate cancer mortality rates. Epidemiology. 2000;11:167-70. [PMID: 11021614]

16. Feuer EJ, Merrill RM, Hankey BF. Cancer surveillance series: interpreting trends in prostate cancer—part II: cause of death misclassification and the recent rise and fall in prostate cancer mortality. J Natl Cancer Inst. 1999; 91:1025-32. [PMID: 10379965]

17. Roberts RO, Bergstralh EJ, Katusic SK, Lieber MM, Jacobsen SJ. Decline in prostate cancer mortality from 1980 to 1997, and an update on incidence trends in Olmsted County, Minnesota. J Urol. 1999;161:529-33. [PMID: 9915441]

18. Meyer F, Moore L, Bairati I, Fradet Y. Downward trend in prostate cancer mortality in Quebec and Canada. J Urol. 1999;161:1189-91. [PMID: 10081867]

19. Oliver SE, May MT, Gunnell D. International trends in prostate-cancer mortality in the "PSA ERA." Int J Cancer. 2001;92:893-8. [PMID: 11351313]

20. Legler JM, Feuer EJ, Potosky AL, Merrill RM, Kramer BS. The role of prostate-specific antigen (PSA) testing patterns in the recent prostate cancer incidence decline in the United States. Cancer Causes Control. 1998;9:519-27. [PMID: 9934717]

21. Etzioni R, Legler JM, Feuer EJ, Merrill RM, Cronin KA, Hankey BF. Cancer surveillance series: interpreting trends in prostate cancer—part III: Quantifying the link between population prostate-specific antigen testing and recent declines in prostate cancer mortality. J Natl Cancer Inst. 1999;91:1033-9. [PMID: 10379966]

22. Brawley OW. Prostate carcinoma incidence and patient mortality: the effects of screening and early detection. Cancer. 1997;80:1857-63. [PMID: 9351560]

23. Lu-Yao G, Albertsen PC, Stanford JL, Stukel TA, Walker-Corkery ES, Barry MJ. Natural experiment examining impact of aggressive screening and treatment on prostate cancer mortality in two fixed cohorts from Seattle area and Connecticut. BMJ. 2002;325:740-5. [PMID: 12364300]

24. Oliver SE, Gunnell D, Donovan JL. Comparison of trends in prostate-cancer mortality in England and Wales and the USA [Letter]. Lancet. 2000;355:1788-9. [PMID: 10832832]

25. Crocetti E, Ciatto S, Zappa M. Prostate cancer: different incidence but not mortality trends within two areas of Tuscany, Italy [Letter]. J Natl Cancer Inst. 2001;93:876-7. [PMID: 11390538]

26. Bartsch G, Horninger W, Klocker H, Oberaigner W, Severi G, Robertson C, et al. Decrease in prostate cancer mortality following introduction of prostate

specific antigen (PSA) screening in the Federal State of Tyrol, Austria. J Urol. 2000;163:88.

27. Bartsch G, Horninger W, Klocker H, Reissigl A, Oberaigner W, Schönitzer D, et al. Prostate cancer mortality after introduction of prostate-specific antigen mass screening in the Federal State of Tyrol, Austria. Urology. 2001;58:417-24. [PMID: 11549491]

28. Chodak GW, Thisted RA, Gerber GS, Johansson JE, Adolfsson J, Jones GW, et al. Results of conservative management of clinically localized prostate cancer. N Engl J Med. 1994;330:242-8. [PMID: 8272085]

29. Albertsen PC, Hanley JA, Gleason DF, Barry MJ. Competing risk analysis of men aged 55 to 74 years at diagnosis managed conservatively for clinically localized prostate cancer. JAMA. 1998;280:975-80. [PMID: 9749479]

30. Johansson JE, Holmberg L, Johansson S, Bergström R, Adami HO. Fifteen-year survival in prostate cancer. A prospective, population-based study in Sweden. JAMA. 1997;277:467-71. [PMID: 9020270]

31. Woolf SH. Defining clinically insignificant prostate cancer [Letter]. JAMA. 1996;276:28-9. [PMID: 8667530]

32. Roach M, Lu J, Pilepich MV, Asbell SO, Mohiuddin M, Terry R, et al. Four prognostic groups predict long-term survival from prostate cancer following radiotherapy alone on Radiation Therapy Oncology Group clinical trials. Int J Radiat Oncol Biol Phys. 2000;47:609-15. [PMID: 10837943]

33. Pound CR, Partin AW, Eisenberger MA, Chan DW, Pearson JD, Walsh PC. Natural history of progression after PSA elevation following radical prostatectomy. JAMA. 1999;281:1591-7. [PMID: 10235151]

34. Keetch DW, Catalona WJ, Smith DS. Serial prostatic biopsies in men with persistently elevated serum prostate specific antigen values. J Urol. 1994;151:1571-4. [PMID: 7514690]

35. Stewart CS, Leibovich BC, Weaver AL, Lieber MM. Prostate cancer diagnosis using a saturation needle biopsy technique after previous negative sextant biopsies. J Urol. 2001;166:86-91. [PMID: 11435830]

36. Djavan B, Zlotta A, Remzi M, Ghawidel K, Basharkhah A, Schulman CC, et al. Optimal predictors of prostate cancer on repeat prostate biopsy: a prospective study of 1,051 men. J Urol. 2000;163:1144-8; discussion 1148-9. [PMID: 10737484]

37. Rabbani F, Stroumbakis N, Kava BR, Cookson MS, Fair WR. Incidence and clinical significance of false-negative sextant prostate biopsies. J Urol. 1998; 159:1247-50. [PMID: 9507846]

38. Levine MA, Ittman M, Melamed J, Lepor H. Two consecutive sets of transrectal ultrasound guided sextant biopsies of the prostate for the detection of prostate cancer. J Urol. 1998;159:471-5; discussion 475-6. [PMID: 9649265]

39. Terris MK. Sensitivity and specificity of sextant biopsies in the detection of prostate cancer: preliminary report. Urology. 1999;54:486-9. [PMID: 10475359]

40. McNaughton Collins M, Ransohoff DF, Barry MJ. Early detection of prostate cancer. Serendipity strikes again. JAMA. 1997;278:1516-9. [PMID: 9363972]

41. Gann PH, Hennekens CH, Stampfer MJ. A prospective evaluation of plasma prostate-specific antigen for detection of prostatic cancer. JAMA. 1995; 273:289-94. [PMID: 7529341]

42. Mettlin C, Murphy GP, Babaian RJ, Chesley A, Kane RA, Littrup PJ, et al. The results of a five-year early prostate cancer detection intervention. Investigators of the American Cancer Society National Prostate Cancer Detection Project. Cancer. 1996;77:150-9. [PMID: 8630923]

43. Jacobsen SJ, Bergstralh EJ, Guess HA, Katusic SK, Klee GG, Oesterling JE, et al. Predictive properties of serum-prostate-specific antigen testing in a community-based setting. Arch Intern Med. 1996;156:2462-8. [PMID: 8944739]

44. Schröder FH, van der Cruijsen-Koeter I, de Koning HJ, Vis AN, Hoedemaeker RF, Kranse R. Prostate cancer detection at low prostate specific antigen. J Urol. 2000;163:806-12. [PMID: 10687982]

45. Meigs JB, Barry MJ, Oesterling JE, Jacobsen SJ. Interpreting results of prostate-specific antigen testing for early detection of prostate cancer. J Gen Intern Med. 1996;11:505-12. [PMID: 8905498]

46. Oesterling JE, Jacobsen SJ, Chute CG, Guess HA, Girman CJ, Panser LA, et al. Serum prostate-specific antigen in a community-based population of healthy men. Establishment of age-specific reference ranges. JAMA. 1993;270:860-4. [PMID: 7688054]

47. Mettlin C, Littrup PJ, Kane RA, Murphy GP, Lee F, Chesley A, et al. Relative sensitivity and specificity of serum prostate specific antigen (PSA) level compared with age-referenced PSA, PSA density, and PSA change. Data from the American Cancer Society National Prostate Cancer Detection Project. Cancer. 1994;74:1615-20. [PMID: 7520352]

48. Catalona WJ, Southwick PC, Slawin KM, Partin AW, Brawer MK, Flanigan RC, et al. Comparison of percent free PSA, PSA density, and age-specific PSA cutoffs for prostate cancer detection and staging. Urology. 2000;56:255-60. [PMID: 10925089]

49. Labrie F, Dupont A, Suburu R, Cusan L, Tremblay M, Gomez JL, et al. Serum prostate specific antigen as pre-screening test for prostate cancer. J Urol. 1992;147:846-51; discussion 851-2. [PMID: 1371560]

50. Catalona WJ, Hudson MA, Scardino PT, Richie JP, Ahmann FR, Flanigan RC, et al. Selection of optimal prostate specific antigen cutoffs for early detection of prostate cancer: receiver operating characteristic curves. J Urol. 1994;152:2037-42. [PMID: 7525995]

51. Babaian RJ, Fritsche H, Ayala A, Bhadkamkar V, Johnston DA, Naccarato W, et al. Performance of a neural network in detecting prostate cancer in the prostate-specific antigen reflex range of 2.5 to 4.0 ng/mL. Urology. 2000;56:1000-6. [PMID: 11113747]

52. Catalona WJ, Smith DS, Ornstein DK. Prostate cancer detection in men with serum PSA concentrations of 2.6 to 4.0 ng/mL and benign prostate examination. Enhancement of specificity with free PSA measurements. JAMA. 1997;277:1452-5. [PMID: 9145717]

53. Schröder F, Tribukait B, Böcking A, DeVere White R, Koss L, Lieber M, et al. Clinical utility of cellular DNA measurements in prostate carcinoma. Consensus Conference on Diagnosis and Prognostic Parameters in Localized Prostate Cancer. Stockholm, Sweden, May 12-13, 1993. Scand J Urol Nephrol Suppl. 1994;162:51-63. [PMID: 7529429]

54. Lodding P, Aus G, Bergdahl S, Frösing R, Lilja H, Pihl CG, et al. Characteristics of screening detected prostate cancer in men 50 to 66 years old with 3 to 4 ng./ml. Prostate specific antigen. J Urol. 1998;159:899-903. [PMID: 9474178]

55. Babaian RJ, Johnston DA, Naccarato W, Ayala A, Bhadkamkar VA, Fritsche HA Jr. The incidence of prostate cancer in a screening population with a serum prostate specific antigen between 2.5 and 4.0 ng/ml: relation to biopsy strategy. J Urol. 2001;165:757-60. [PMID: 11176461]

56. Stenman UH, Hakama M, Knekt P, Aromaa A, Teppo L, Leinonen J. Serum concentrations of prostate specific antigen and its complex with alpha 1-antichymotrypsin before diagnosis of prostate cancer. Lancet. 1994;344:1594-8. [PMID: 7527116]

57. Stenman UH, Leinonen J, Alfthan H, Rannikko S, Tuhkanen K, Alfthan O. A complex between prostate-specific antigen and alpha 1-antichymotrypsin is the major form of prostate-specific antigen in serum of patients with prostatic cancer: assay of the complex improves clinical sensitivity for cancer. Cancer Res. 1991;51:222-6. [PMID: 1703033]

58. Finne P, Zhang WM, Auvinen A, Leinonen J, Määttänen L, Rannikko S, et al. Use of the complex between prostate specific antigen and alpha 1-protease inhibitor for screening prostate cancer. J Urol. 2000;164:1956-60. [PMID: 11061890]

59. Brawer MK. Screening and early detection of prostate cancer will decrease morbidity and mortality from prostate cancer: the argument for. Eur Urol. 1996; 29(Suppl 2):19-23. [PMID: 8717456]

60. Okegawa T, Noda H, Nutahara K, Higashihara E. Comparisons of the various combinations of free, complexed, and total prostate-specific antigen for the detection of prostate cancer. Eur Urol. 2000;38:380-7. [PMID: 11025374]

61. Lein M, Jung K, Elgeti U, Petras T, Stephan C, Brux B, et al. Comparison of the clinical validity of free prostate-specific antigen, alpha-1 antichymotrypsin-bound prostate-specific antigen and complexed prostate-specific antigen in prostate cancer diagnosis. Eur Urol. 2001;39:57-64. [PMID: 11173940]

62. Mitchell ID, Croal BL, Dickie A, Cohen NP, Ross I. A prospective study to evaluate the role of complexed prostate specific antigen and free/total prostate specific antigen ratio for the diagnosis of prostate cancer. J Urol. 2001;165:1549-53. [PMID: 11342915]

63. Catalona WJ, Richie JP, Ahmann FR, Hudson MA, Scardino PT, Flanigan RC, et al. Comparison of digital rectal examination and serum prostate specific antigen in the early detection of prostate cancer: results of a multicenter clinical trial of 6,630 men. J Urol. 1994;151:1283-90. [PMID: 7512659]

64. Richie JP, Catalona WJ, Ahmann FR, Hudson MA, Scardino PT, Flanigan

RC, et al. Effect of patient age on early detection of prostate cancer with serum prostate-specific antigen and digital rectal examination. Urology. 1993;42:365-74. [PMID: 7692657]

65. Mettlin C, Chesley AE, Murphy GP, Bartsch G, Toi A, Bahnson R, et al. Association of free PSA percent, total PSA, age, and gland volume in the detection of prostate cancer. Prostate. 1999;39:153-8. [PMID: 10334103]

66. Catalona WJ, Partin AW, Slawin KM, Brawer MK, Flanigan RC, Patel A, et al. Use of the percentage of free prostate-specific antigen to enhance differentiation of prostate cancer from benign prostatic disease: a prospective multicenter clinical trial. JAMA. 1998;279:1542-7. [PMID: 9605898]

67. Reissigl A, Klocker H, Pointner J, Fink K, Horninger W, Ennemoser O, et al. Usefulness of the ratio free/total prostate-specific antigen in addition to total PSA levels in prostate cancer screening. Urology. 1996;48:62-6. [PMID: 8973702]

68. Bangma CH, Kranse R, Blijenberg BG, Schröder FH. The value of screening tests in the detection of prostate cancer. Part II: Retrospective analysis of free/total prostate-specific analysis ratio, age-specific reference ranges, and PSA density. Urology. 1995;46:779-84. [PMID: 7502415]

69. Catalona WJ, Smith DS, Wolfert RL, Wang TJ, Rittenhouse HG, Ratliff TL, et al. Evaluation of percentage of free serum prostate-specific antigen to improve specificity of prostate cancer screening. JAMA. 1995;274:1214-20. [PMID: 7563511]

70. Bangma CH, Blijenberg BG, Schröder FH. Prostate-specific antigen: its clinical use and application in screening for prostate cancer. Scand J Clin Lab Invest Suppl. 1995;221:35-44. [PMID: 7544483]

71. Hoffman RM, Clanon DL, Littenberg B, Frank JJ, Peirce JC. Using the free-to-total prostate-specific antigen ratio to detect prostate cancer in men with nonspecific elevations of prostate-specific antigen levels. J Gen Intern Med. 2000; 15:739-48. [PMID: 11089718]

72. Carter HB, Pearson JD, Metter EJ, Brant LJ, Chan DW, Andres R, et al. Longitudinal evaluation of prostate-specific antigen levels in men with and without prostate disease. JAMA. 1992;267:2215-20. [PMID: 1372942]

73. Smith DS, Catalona WJ. Rate of change in serum prostate specific antigen levels as a method for prostate cancer detection. J Urol. 1994;152:1163-7. [PMID: 7520949]

74. Morote J, Raventós CX, Lorente JA, Enbabo G, López M, de Torres I. Intraindividual variations of total and percent free serum prostatic-specific antigen levels in patients with normal digital rectal examination. Eur Urol. 1999;36: 111-5. [PMID: 10420031]

75. Littrup PJ, Kane RA, Mettlin CJ, Murphy GP, Lee F, Toi A, et al. Cost-effective prostate cancer detection. Reduction of low-yield biopsies. Investigators of the American Cancer Society National Prostate Cancer Detection Project. Cancer. 1994;74:3146-58. [PMID: 7526969]

76. Hoogendam A, Buntinx F, de Vet HC. The diagnostic value of digital rectal examination in primary care screening for prostate cancer: a meta-analysis. Fam Pract. 1999;16:621-6. [PMID: 10625141]

77. Schröder FH, van der Maas P, Beemsterboer P, Kruger AB, Hoedemaeker R, Rietbergen J, et al. Evaluation of the digital rectal examination as a screening test for prostate cancer. Rotterdam section of the European Randomized Study of Screening for Prostate Cancer. J Natl Cancer Inst. 1998;90:1817-23. [PMID: 9839522]

78. Smith DS, Catalona WJ. Interexaminer variability of digital rectal examination in detecting prostate cancer. Urology. 1995;45:70-4. [PMID: 7529449]

79. Määttänen L, Auvinen A, Stenman UH, Rannikko S, Tammela T, Aro J, et al. European randomized study of prostate cancer screening: first-year results of the Finnish trial. Br J Cancer. 1999;79:1210-4. [PMID: 10098761]

80. Labrie F, Candas B, Cusan L, Gomez JL, Diamond P, Suburu R, et al. Diagnosis of advanced or noncurable prostate cancer can be practically eliminated by prostate-specific antigen. Urology. 1996;47:212-7. [PMID: 8607237]

81. Horninger W, Reissigl A, Rogatsch H, Volgger H, Studen M, Klocker H, et al. Prostate cancer screening in the Tyrol, Austria: experience and results. Eur J Cancer. 2000;36:1322-35. [PMID: 10882875]

82. Martín E, Luján M, Sánchez E, Herrero A, Páez A, Berenguer A. Final results of a screening campaign for prostate cancer. Eur Urol. 1999;35:26-31. [PMID: 9933791]

83. Labrie F, Dupont A, Suburu R, Cusan L, Gomez JL, Koutsilieris M, et al. Optimized strategy for detection of early stage, curable prostate cancer: role of

prescreening with prostate-specific antigen. Clin Invest Med. 1993;16:425-39. [PMID: 7516831]

84. Hoedemaeker RF, van der Kwast TH, Boer R, de Koning HJ, Roobol M, Vis AN, et al. Pathologic features of prostate cancer found at population-based screening with a four-year interval. J Natl Cancer Inst. 2001;93:1153-8. [PMID: 11481387]

85. Smith DS, Catalona WJ, Herschman JD. Longitudinal screening for prostate cancer with prostate-specific antigen. JAMA. 1996;276:1309-15. [PMID: 8861989]

86. Ross KS, Carter HB, Pearson JD, Guess HA. Comparative efficiency of prostate-specific antigen screening strategies for prostate cancer detection. JAMA. 2000;284:1399-405. [PMID: 10989402]

87. Carter HB, Epstein JI, Chan DW, Fozard JL, Pearson JD. Recommended prostate-specific antigen testing intervals for the detection of curable prostate cancer. JAMA. 1997;277:1456-60. [PMID: 9145718]

88. Holmberg L, Bill-Axelson A, Helgesen F, Salo JO, Folmerz P, Häggman M, et al. A randomized trial comparing radical prostatectomy with watchful waiting in early prostate cancer. N Engl J Med. 2002;347:781-9. [PMID: 12226148]

89. Smith DS, Catalona WJ. The nature of prostate cancer detected through prostate specific antigen based screening. J Urol. 1994;152:1732-6. [PMID: 7523720]

90. Moon TD, Brawer MK, Wilt TJ. Prostate Intervention Versus Observation Trial (PIVOT): a randomized trial comparing radical prostatectomy with palliative expectant management for treatment of clinically localized prostate cancer. PIVOT Planning Committee. J Natl Cancer Inst Monogr. 1995;(19):69-71. [PMID: 7577210]

91. Norlén BJ. Swedish randomized trial of radical prostatectomy versus watchful waiting. Can J Oncol. 1994;4(Suppl 1):38-40. [PMID: 8853488]

92. Lu-Yao GL, Yao SL. Population-based study of long-term survival in patients with clinically localised prostate cancer. Lancet. 1997;349:906-10. [PMID: 9093251]

93. Zincke H, Bergstralh EJ, Blute ML, Myers RP, Barrett DM, Lieber MM, et al. Radical prostatectomy for clinically localized prostate cancer: long-term results of 1,143 patients from a single institution. J Clin Oncol. 1994;12:2254-63. [PMID: 7964940]

94. Zincke H, Oesterling JE, Blute ML, Bergstralh EJ, Myers RP, Barrett DM. Long-term (15 years) results after radical prostatectomy for clinically localized (stage T2c or lower) prostate cancer. J Urol. 1994;152:1850-7. [PMID: 7523733]

95. Walsh PC, Partin AW, Epstein JI. Cancer control and quality of life following anatomical radical retropubic prostatectomy: results at 10 years. J Urol. 1994; 152:1831-6. [PMID: 7523730]

96. Paulson DF. Impact of radical prostatectomy in the management of clinically localized disease. J Urol. 1994;152:1826-30. [PMID: 7523729]

97. Gerber GS, Thisted RA, Scardino PT, Frohmuller HG, Schroeder FH, Paulson DF, et al. Results of radical prostatectomy in men with clinically localized prostate cancer. JAMA. 1996;276:615-9. [PMID: 8773633]

98. Hochstetler JA, Kreder KJ, Brown CK, Loening SA. Survival of patients with localized prostate cancer treated with percutaneous transperineal placement of radioactive gold seeds: stages A2, B, and C. Prostate. 1995;26:316-24. [PMID: 7784271]

99. Schellhammer PF, Moriarty R, Bostwick D, Kuban D. Fifteen-year minimum follow-up of a prostate brachytherapy series: comparing the past with the present. Urology. 2000;56:436-9. [PMID: 10962309]

100. Granfors T, Modig H, Damber JE, Tomic R. Combined orchiectomy and external radiotherapy versus radiotherapy alone for nonmetastatic prostate cancer with or without pelvic lymph node involvement: a prospective randomized study. J Urol. 1998;159:2030-4. [PMID: 9598512]

101. Schmidt JD, Gibbons RP, Murphy GP, Bartolucci A. Evaluation of adjuvant estramustine phosphate, cyclophosphamide, and observation only for node-positive patients following radical prostatectomy and definitive irradiation. Investigators of the National Prostate Cancer Project. Prostate. 1996;28:51-7. [PMID: 8545281]

102. Bolla M, Gonzalez D, Warde P, Dubois JB, Mirimanoff RO, Storme G, et al. Improved survival in patients with locally advanced prostate cancer treated

with radiotherapy and goserelin. N Engl J Med. 1997;337:295-300. [PMID: 9233866]

103. Bolla M, Collette L, Blank L, Warde P, Dubois JB, Mirimanoff RO, et al. Long-term results with immediate androgen suppression and external irradiation in patients with locally advanced prostate cancer (an EORTC study): a phase III randomised trial. Lancet. 2002;360:103-6. [PMID: 12126818]

104. Corn BW, Winter K, Pilepich MV. Does androgen suppression enhance the efficacy of postoperative irradiation? A secondary analysis of RTOG 85-31. Radiation Therapy Oncology Group. Urology. 1999;54:495-502. [PMID: 10475361]

105. Pilepich MV, Buzydlowski JW, John MJ, Rubin P, McGowan DG, Marcial VA. Phase II trial of hormonal cytoreduction with megestrol and diethylstilbestrol in conjunction with radiotherapy for carcinoma of the prostate: outcome results of RTOG 83-07. Int J Radiat Oncol Biol Phys. 1995;32:175-80. [PMID: 7721614]

106. Pilepich MV, Caplan R, Byhardt RW, Lawton CA, Gallagher MJ, Mesic JB, et al. Phase III trial of androgen suppression using goserelin in unfavorable-prognosis carcinoma of the prostate treated with definitive radiotherapy: report of Radiation Therapy Oncology Group Protocol 85-31. J Clin Oncol. 1997;15:1013-21. [PMID: 9060541]

107. Messing EM, Manola J, Sarosdy M, Wilding G, Crawford ED, Trump D. Immediate hormonal therapy compared with observation after radical prostatectomy and pelvic lymphadenectomy in men with node-positive prostate cancer. N Engl J Med. 1999;341:1781-8. [PMID: 10588962]

108. Pilepich MV, Winter K, John MJ, Mesic JB, Sause W, Rubin P, et al. Phase III radiation therapy oncology group (RTOG) trial 86-10 of androgen deprivation adjuvant to definitive radiotherapy in locally advanced carcinoma of the prostate. Int J Radiat Oncol Biol Phys. 2001;50:1243-52. [PMID: 11483335]

109. Immediate versus deferred treatment for advanced prostatic cancer: initial results of the Medical Research Council Trial. The Medical Research Council Prostate Cancer Working Party Investigators Group. Br J Urol. 1997;79:235-46. [PMID: 9052476]

110. Albertsen PC, Fryback DG, Storer BE, Kolon TF, Fine J. Long-term survival among men with conservatively treated localized prostate cancer. JAMA. 1995;274:626-31. [PMID: 7637143]

111. Sandblom G, Dufmats M, Varenhorst E. Long-term survival in a Swedish population-based cohort of men with prostate cancer. Urology. 2000;56:442-7. [PMID: 10962312]

112. Begg CB, Riedel ER, Bach PB, Kattan MW, Schrag D, Warren JL, et al. Variations in morbidity after radical prostatectomy. N Engl J Med. 2002;346:1138-44. [PMID: 11948274]

113. Wilt TJ, Cowper DC, Gammack JK, Going DR, Nugent S, Borowsky SJ. An evaluation of radical prostatectomy at Veterans Affairs Medical Centers: time trends and geographic variation in utilization and outcomes. Med Care. 1999;37:1046-56. [PMID: 10524371]

114. Steineck G, Helgesen F, Adolfsson J, Dickman PW, Johansson JE, Norlén BJ, et al. Quality of life after radical prostatectomy or watchful waiting. N Engl J Med. 2002;347:790-6. [PMID: 12226149]

115. Lu-Yao GL, McLerran D, Wasson J, Wennberg JE. An assessment of radical prostatectomy. Time trends, geographic variation, and outcomes. The Prostate Patient Outcomes Research Team. JAMA. 1993;269:2633-6. [PMID: 8487445]

116. Optenberg SA, Wojcik BE, Thompson IM. Morbidity and mortality following radical prostatectomy: a national analysis of Civilian Health and Medical Program of the Uniformed Services beneficiaries. J Urol. 1995;153:1870-2. [PMID: 7752336]

117. Schwartz K, Bunner S, Bearer R, Severson RK. Complications from treatment for prostate carcinoma among men in the Detroit area. Cancer. 2002;95:82-9. [PMID: 12115320]

118. Robinson JW, Dufour MS, Fung TS. Erectile functioning of men treated for prostate carcinoma. Cancer. 1997;79:538-44. [PMID: 9028365]

119. Litwin MS. Editorial comments. J Urol. 2000;163:1806-7.

120. Krupski T, Petroni GR, Bissonette EA, Theodorescu D. Quality-of-life comparison of radical prostatectomy and interstitial brachytherapy in the treatment of clinically localized prostate cancer. Urology. 2000;55:736-42. [PMID: 10792092]

121. Stanford JL, Feng Z, Hamilton AS, Gilliland FD, Stephenson RA, Eley JW, et al. Urinary and sexual function after radical prostatectomy for clinically localized prostate cancer: the Prostate Cancer Outcomes Study. JAMA. 2000;283:354-60. [PMID: 10647798]

122. Litwin MS, Flanders SC, Pasta DJ, Stoddard ML, Lubeck DP, Henning JM. Sexual function and bother after radical prostatectomy or radiation for prostate cancer: multivariate quality-of-life analysis from CaPSURE. Cancer of the Prostate Strategic Urologic Research Endeavor. Urology. 1999;54:503-8. [PMID: 10475362]

123. Talcott JA, Rieker P, Clark JA, Propert KJ, Weeks JC, Beard CJ, et al. Patient-reported symptoms after primary therapy for early prostate cancer: results of a prospective cohort study. J Clin Oncol. 1998;16:275-83. [PMID: 9440753]

124. Talcott JA, Rieker P, Propert KJ, Clark JA, Wishnow KI, Loughlin KR, et al. Patient-reported impotence and incontinence after nerve-sparing radical prostatectomy. J Natl Cancer Inst. 1997;89:1117-23. [PMID: 9262249]

125. Helgason AR, Adolfsson J, Dickman P, Arver S, Fredrikson M, Steineck G. Factors associated with waning sexual function among elderly men and prostate cancer patients. J Urol. 1997;158:155-9. [PMID: 9186344]

126. Shrader-Bogen CL, Kjellberg JL, McPherson CP, Murray CL. Quality of life and treatment outcomes: prostate carcinoma patients' perspectives after prostatectomy or radiation therapy. Cancer. 1997;79:1977-86. [PMID: 9149026]

127. Fosså SD, Woehre H, Kurth KH, Hetherington J, Bakke H, Rustad DA, et al. Influence of urological morbidity on quality of life in patients with prostate cancer. Eur Urol. 1997;31(Suppl 3):3-8. [PMID: 9101208]

128. Helgason AR, Adolfsson J, Dickman P, Fredrikson M, Arver S, Steineck G. Waning sexual function—the most important disease-specific distress for patients with prostate cancer. Br J Cancer. 1996;73:1417-21. [PMID: 8645589]

129. Litwin MS, Hays RD, Fink A, Ganz PA, Leake B, Leach GE, et al. Quality-of-life outcomes in men treated for localized prostate cancer. JAMA. 1995;273:129-35. [PMID: 7799493]

130. Potosky AL, Legler J, Albertsen PC, Stanford JL, Gilliland FD, Hamilton AS, et al. Health outcomes after prostatectomy or radiotherapy for prostate cancer: results from the Prostate Cancer Outcomes Study. J Natl Cancer Inst. 2000;92:1582-92. [PMID: 11018094]

131. Litwin MS. Health-related quality of life after treatment for localized prostate cancer. Cancer Supplement. 1995;75:2000-3.

132. Walsh PC, Marschke P, Ricker D, Burnett AL. Patient-reported urinary continence and sexual function after anatomic radical prostatectomy. Urology. 2000;55:58-61. [PMID: 10654895]

133. Litwin MS, Melmed GY, Nakazon T. Life after radical prostatectomy: a longitudinal study. J Urol. 2001;166:587-92. [PMID: 11458073]

134. Siegel T, Moul JW, Spevak M, Alvord WG, Costabile RA. The development of erectile dysfunction in men treated for prostate cancer. J Urol. 2001;165:430-5. [PMID: 11176390]

135. Madalinska JB, Essink-Bot ML, de Koning HJ, Kirkels WJ, van der Maas PJ, Schröder FH. Health-related quality-of-life effects of radical prostatectomy and primary radiotherapy for screen-detected or clinically diagnosed localized prostate cancer. J Clin Oncol. 2001;19:1619-28. [PMID: 11250990]

136. Olsson LE, Salomon L, Nadu A, Hoznek A, Cicco A, Saint F, et al. Prospective patient-reported continence after laparoscopic radical prostatectomy. Urology. 2001;58:570-2. [PMID: 11597541]

137. Adolfsson J, Helgason AR, Dickman P, Steineck G. Urinary and bowel symptoms in men with and without prostate cancer: results from an observational study in the Stockholm area. Eur Urol. 1998;33:11-6. [PMID: 9471035]

138. Litwin MS, Pasta DJ, Yu J, Stoddard ML, Flanders SC. Urinary function and bother after radical prostatectomy or radiation for prostate cancer: a longitudinal, multivariate quality of life analysis from the Cancer of the Prostate Strategic Urologic Research Endeavor. J Urol. 2000;164:1973-7. [PMID: 11061894]

139. Fransson P, Widmark A. Self-assessed sexual function after pelvic irradiation for prostate carcinoma. Comparison with an age-matched control group. Cancer. 1996;78:1066-78. [PMID: 8780545]

140. Fowler FJ Jr, Barry MJ, Lu-Yao G, Wasson JH, Bin L. Outcomes of external-beam radiation therapy for prostate cancer: a study of Medicare beneficiaries in three surveillance, epidemiology, and end results areas. J Clin Oncol. 1996;14:2258-65. [PMID: 8708715]

141. Roach M 3rd, Chinn DM, Holland J, Clarke M. A pilot survey of sexual function and quality of life following 3D conformal radiotherapy for clinically

localized prostate cancer. Int J Radiat Oncol Biol Phys. 1996;35:869-74. [PMID: 8751394]

142. **Hamilton AS, Stanford JL, Gilliland FD, Albertsen PC, Stephenson RA, Hoffman RM, et al.** Health outcomes after external-beam radiation therapy for clinically localized prostate cancer: results from the Prostate Cancer Outcomes Study. J Clin Oncol. 2001;19:2517-26. [PMID: 11331331]

143. **Chen CT, Valicenti RK, Lu J, Derose T, Dicker AP, Strup SE, et al.** Does hormonal therapy influence sexual function in men receiving 3D conformal radiation therapy for prostate cancer? Int J Radiat Oncol Biol Phys. 2001;50:591-5. [PMID: 11395224]

144. **Fransson P, Damber JE, Tomic R, Modig H, Nyberg G, Widmark A.** Quality of life and symptoms in a randomized trial of radiotherapy versus deferred treatment of localized prostate carcinoma. Cancer. 2001;92:3111-9. [PMID: 11753990]

145. **Beard CJ, Propert KJ, Rieker PP, Clark JA, Kaplan I, Kantoff PW, et al.** Complications after treatment with external-beam irradiation in early-stage prostate cancer patients: a prospective multiinstitutional outcomes study. J Clin Oncol. 1997;15:223-9. [PMID: 8996146]

146. **Widmark A, Fransson P, Tavelin B.** Self-assessment questionnaire for evaluating urinary and intestinal late side effects after pelvic radiotherapy in patients with prostate cancer compared with an age-matched control population. Cancer. 1994;74:2520-32. [PMID: 7923010]

147. **Nguyen LN, Pollack A, Zagars GK.** Late effects after radiotherapy for prostate cancer in a randomized dose-response study: results of a self-assessment questionnaire. Urology. 1998;51:991-7. [PMID: 9609638]

148. **Stock RG, Kao J, Stone NN.** Penile erectile function after permanent radioactive seed implantation for treatment of prostate cancer. J Urol. 2001;165: 436-9. [PMID: 11176391]

149. **Fulmer BR, Bissonette EA, Petroni GR, Theodorescu D.** Prospective assessment of voiding and sexual function after treatment for localized prostate carcinoma: comparison of radical prostatectomy to hormonobrachytherapy with and without external beam radiotherapy. Cancer. 2001;91:2046-55. [PMID: 11391584]

150. **Gelblum DY, Potters L, Ashley R, Waldbaum R, Wang XH, Leibel S.** Urinary morbidity following ultrasound-guided transperineal prostate seed implantation. Int J Radiat Oncol Biol Phys. 1999;45:59-67. [PMID: 10477007]

151. **Brandeis JM, Litwin MS, Burnison CM, Reiter RE.** Quality of life outcomes after brachytherapy for early stage prostate cancer. J Urol. 2000;163:851-7. [PMID: 10687991]

152. **Hu K, Wallner K.** Clinical course of rectal bleeding following I-125 prostate brachytherapy. Int J Radiat Oncol Biol Phys. 1998;41:263-5. [PMID: 9607339]

153. **Potosky AL, Knopf K, Clegg LX, Albertsen PC, Stanford JL, Hamilton AS, et al.** Quality-of-life outcomes after primary androgen deprivation therapy:

results from the Prostate Cancer Outcomes Study. J Clin Oncol. 2001;19:3750-7. [PMID: 11533098]

154. **Fowler FJ Jr, McNaughton Collins M, Walker Corkery E, Elliott DB, Barry MJ.** The impact of androgen deprivation on quality of life after radical prostatectomy for prostate carcinoma. Cancer. 2002;95:287-95. [PMID: 12124828]

155. **Potosky AL, Reeve BB, Clegg LX, Hoffman RM, Stephenson RA, Albertsen PC, et al.** Quality of life following localized prostate cancer treated initially with androgen deprivation therapy or no therapy. J Natl Cancer Inst. 2002;94: 430-7. [PMID: 11904315]

156. **Seidenfeld J, Samson DJ, Hasselblad V, Aronson N, Albertsen PC, Bennett CL, et al.** Single-therapy androgen suppression in men with advanced prostate cancer: a systematic review and meta-analysis. Ann Intern Med. 2000;132: 566-77. [PMID: 10744594]

157. **Aronson N, Seidenfeld J, Samson DJ, Albertson PC, Bayoumi AM, Bennett C, et al.** Relative effectiveness and cost-effectiveness of methods of androgen suppression in the treatment of advanced prostate cancer. Evidence Report/Technology Assessment No. 4. AHCPR publication no. 99-E0012. Rockville, MD: Agency for Health Care Policy and Research; 1999.

158. **Strum SB, McDermed JE, Scholz MC, Johnson H, Tisman G.** Anaemia associated with androgen deprivation in patients with prostate cancer receiving combined hormone blockade. Br J Urol. 1997;79:933-41. [PMID: 9202563]

159. **Daniell HW, Dunn SR, Ferguson DW, Lomas G, Niazi Z, Stratte PT.** Progressive osteoporosis during androgen deprivation therapy for prostate cancer. J Urol. 2000;163:181-6. [PMID: 10604342]

160. **Fleming C, Wasson JH, Albertsen PC, Barry MJ, Wennberg JE.** A decision analysis of alternative treatment strategies for clinically localized prostate cancer. Prostate Patient Outcomes Research Team. JAMA. 1993;269:2650-8. [PMID: 8487449]

161. **Krahn MD, Mahoney JE, Eckman MH, Trachtenberg J, Pauker SG, Detsky AS.** Screening for prostate cancer. A decision analytic view. JAMA. 1994; 272:773-80. [PMID: 7521400]

162. **Kattan MW, Cowen ME, Miles BJ.** A decision analysis for treatment of clinically localized prostate cancer. J Gen Intern Med. 1997;12:299-305. [PMID: 9159699]

163. **Barry MJ, Fleming C, Coley CM, Wasson JH, Fahs MC, Oesterling JE.** Should Medicare provide reimbursement for prostate-specific antigen testing for early detection of prostate cancer? Part IV: Estimating the risks and benefits of an early detection program. Urology. 1995;46:445-61. [PMID: 7571211]

164. **Coley CM, Barry MJ, Fleming C, Fahs MC, Mulley AG.** Early detection of prostate cancer. Part II: Estimating the risks, benefits, and costs. American College of Physicians. Ann Intern Med. 1997;126:468-79. [PMID: 9072935]

APPENDIX

This appendix documents procedures that the Research Triangle Institute–University of North Carolina Evidence-based Practice Center (EPC) staff used to develop this report on screening for prostate cancer. During preparation of the evidence report, we collaborated with two current members of the USPSTF who served as liaisons to the EPC topic team. We first document the analytic framework and key questions developed at the beginning of the review. We then describe the inclusion and exclusion criteria for admissible evidence, our strategy for literature search and synthesis, and our approach to developing the final summary of the evidence.

Analytic Framework and Key Questions

The analytic framework (**Appendix Figure 1**) describes the relationship between screening and treating patients in a clinical setting and reduced morbidity or mortality from prostate cancer. We examined one overarching question (key question 1, linking screening and ultimate health outcomes) and eight additional questions pertaining to specific links in the analytic framework. The key questions were as follows: 1) What are the health outcomes (both type and magnitude) of screening a defined population for prostate cancer compared with not screening? 2) What is the yield of screening for prostate cancer (that is, accuracy and reliability of screening tests, prevalence of undetected cancer in various populations)? 3–6) What are the health outcomes associated with treating clinically localized prostate cancer with radical prostatectomy, external-beam radiation therapy or brachytherapy, androgen deprivation, or watchful waiting? 7) What harms are associated with these treatments of clinically localized prostate cancer? 8) What costs are associated with screening for and early treatment of prostate cancer? Have studies modeled the potential benefits of screening? What is the cost-effectiveness of screening for prostate cancer? 9) What harms are associated with screening for prostate cancer?

Because we found little evidence about key question 9, the harms of screening (one article with inconclusive results), we did not discuss this issue in our article.

Eligibility Criteria for Admissible Evidence

The EPC staff and USPSTF liaisons developed eligibility criteria for selecting relevant evidence to answer the key questions (**Appendix Table**). We first searched for evidence from RCTs for the efficacy of screening. Because we found no well-conducted and well-analyzed RCT of screening, we then examined case–control and ecologic evidence regarding the overarching key question (key question 1).

For key question 2, concerning the operating characteristics of screening tests, we examined well-conducted systematic reviews and individual studies that started with a primary care or unselected sample without prostate cancer and that compared the findings of one or more screening tests with an adequate reference standard. We also examined evidence of the yield of screening from well-conducted screening programs. For key questions 3 through 6, concerning the effectiveness of various therapies, we required evidence from RCTs. For key questions 7 and 9, concerning the harms of screening or treatment, we required either

RCTs or well-controlled studies that included patient reports and the use of a valid measurement instrument. Finally, for key question 8, we searched for evidence of the costs and cost-effectiveness of screening, including models of potential benefits, that considered all appropriate costs and estimates of effectiveness supported by reasonable assumptions based on good evidence.

Literature Search Strategy and Synthesis

The analytic framework and key questions guided our literature searches. We examined the critical literature described in the review published by the USPSTF in 1996 (4) and searched the reference lists of systematic reviews (including Cochrane Library reviews) published since 1993. We then used our eligibility criteria to develop search terms and searched the MEDLINE database for relevant English-language articles that used human subjects and were published between 1 January 1994 and 15 September 2002. We especially looked for articles involving patients whose experience was clearly generalizable to a primary care U.S. population.

The search strategy and results are given in the **Appendix Table** and in **Appendix Figures 2** through **5**. All searches started with the term *prostate neoplasm* and then proceeded by adding further terms as shown in the **Appendix Table**. The first author reviewed abstracts of all articles found in the searches to determine which met eligibility criteria. Other EPC authors of the full systematic evidence review reviewed all abstracts excluded by the first reviewer. We retrieved the full text of all articles not excluded by both reviewers (**Appendix Table**).

One reviewer then compared the full text of all retrieved articles against the eligibility criteria and discussed all excluded articles with one of the other reviewers. We included any article that either reviewer judged had met eligibility criteria (**Appendix Table**). Three of the authors of the systematic evidence review then divided the articles and abstracted data from them, entering the relevant data into predesigned evidence tables (see Appendix B to the systematic evidence review "Screening for Prostate Cancer," available on the Agency for Healthcare Research and Quality Web site [www.ahrq.gov]). The author who abstracted the articles also graded them using USPSTF criteria (5). The first author read all articles, checked the grading, and discussed crucial ones with a second reviewer. The authors also discussed key articles with the USPSTF liaisons.

Development of the Final Systematic Evidence Review

We presented an initial work plan, including a provisional analytic framework and key questions, to the entire Task Force in September 2000; we also presented interim reports on results of the literature search and the early results of the synthesis of information in December 2000 and March 2001. A draft of the systematic evidence review was submitted for broad-based external peer review in May 2001; the peer review involved experts in the field, representatives of relevant professional organizations, and representatives of organizations and federal agencies that serve as liaisons to the USPSTF. We revised the evidence review as appropriate after receiving peer review comments. The Task Force reviewed all information and voted on a recommendation in June 2001, revising the recommendation and rationale statement in the spring of 2002 after review by involved professional associations and agencies. We then updated the searches, finalized the review, and shortened it for publication.

From University of North Carolina at Chapel Hill, Chapel Hill, and Research Triangle Institute, Research Triangle Park, North Carolina.

Current Author Addresses: Dr. Harris: Cecil G. Sheps Center for Health Services Research, CB# 7590, University of North Carolina School of Medicine, 725 Airport Road, Chapel Hill, NC 27599-7590. Dr. Lohr: Research Triangle Institute, PO Box 12194, 3040 Cornwallis Road, Research Triangle Park, NC 27709-2194.

Appendix Figure 1. **Analytic framework for screening for prostate cancer.**

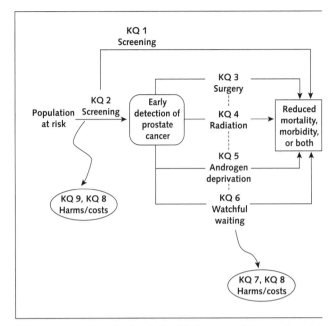

Arrows represent steps in the chain of logic connecting screening with reduced morbidity or mortality from prostate cancer. KQ = key question.

Appendix Table. **Eligibility Criteria, Search Strategy, and Results of Searches***

Key Question	Inclusion Criteria	Search Terms Used	Articles Identified for Abstract Review	Articles Retained for Full Review
			n	
1. Efficacy of screening in reducing mortality from prostate cancer	RCT or case–control study *or*	"Prostate neoplasms" "Mass screening" "RCT" "Case–control"	100	RCT: 1 Case–control: 2
	Surveillance (ecologic) study of prostate cancer incidence, morbidity, or mortality over time	"Prostate neoplasms" "Incidence" "Mortality" "Trends" "Surveillance"	1399	Ecologic: 15
2. Yield of screening tests	Unselected sample without prostate cancer	"Prostate neoplasms"	1905	35
	Screening test used for all Result of screening test compared with a valid reference standard	"Mass screening" "DRE, PSA" "Diagnosis" "Sensitivity/specificity" "Predictive value" "Reproducibility" "Screening programs"		
3–6. Health outcomes of treatment	RCT ≤2 years of follow-up ≤75% of patients followed Health outcomes	"Prostate neoplasms" "Therapeutics" "Treatment" "Surgery" "Prostatectomy" "Radiation" "Brachytherapy" "RCT"	656	KQ 3: 1 KQ 4: 0 KQ 5: 2 KQ 6: 1
7. Harms of treatment	Unselected sample with prostate cancer Treated group compared with valid comparison group Randomized trial or adjustment for confounders Not metastatic cancer Valid measures of harms ≤75% of patients followed ≤1 year of follow-up	"Prostate neoplasms" "Therapeutics" "Treatment" "Surgery" "Prostatectomy" "Radiation" "Adverse effects" "Side effects" "Impotence" "Urinary incontinence" "Quality of life"	923	32
8. Costs/cost-effectiveness of screening	Costs of screening Costs of treatment Cost-effectiveness, cost-utility Modeling studies	"Costs and cost analysis" "Cost–benefit" "Cost-effectiveness"	84	2
9. Harms of screening	Unselected sample Screened group compared with unscreened group Randomized trial or adjustment for confounders Reliable measure of adverse effects	"Prostate neoplasms" "Mass screening" "Adverse effects" "Anxiety, depression" "Labeling" "Quality of life"	94	1

* DRE = digital rectal examination; KQ = key question; PSA = prostate-specific antigen; RCT = randomized, controlled trial.

Appendix Figure 2. **Selection of articles based on key question 1.**

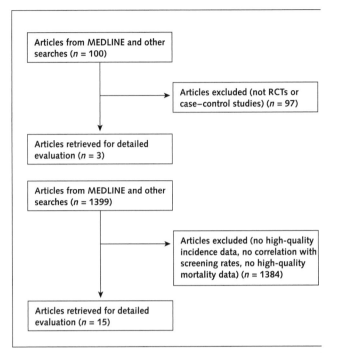

Top. Direct evidence of screening efficacy. **Bottom.** Ecologic studies of screening efficacy. RCT = randomized, controlled trial.

Appendix Figure 3. **Selection of articles based on key question 2.**

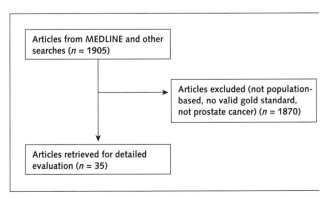

Arrows represent steps in the chain of logic connecting screening with reduced morbidity or mortality from prostate cancer.

Appendix Figure 4. **Selection of articles based on key questions 3 through 6 (*top*) and top question 7 (*bottom*).**

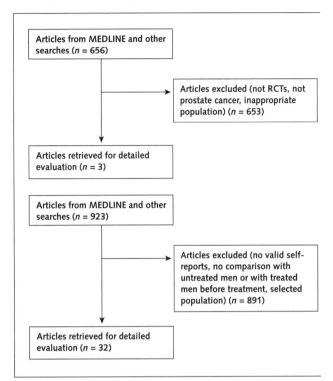

Key questions 3 through 6 address health outcomes of treatment; key question 7 addresses harms of treatment. RCT = randomized, controlled trial.

Appendix 5. **Selection of articles based on key questions 8 (*top*) and 9 (*bottom*).**

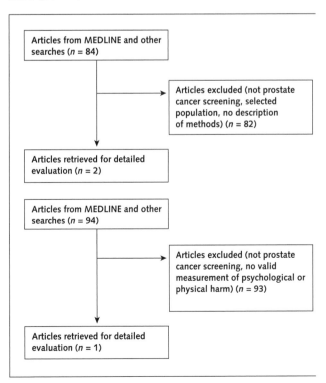

Key question 8 addresses costs and cost-effectiveness of screening, and key question 9 deals with the harms of screening.

Hypertension

❏ Screening for hypertension is a wise strategy only if follow-up and treatment are effective and efficient.

❏ All adults being seen in a clinician's office should be screened for hypertension.

❏ The trend towards newer and more expensive (but not more effective) medications threatens the cost-effectiveness of screening for hypertension.

❏ The most benefit from treating hypertension is seen in reduced morbidity and mortality from strokes and congestive heart failure and all-cause mortality.

Screening for Hypertension

Scott Luria, MD, and Benjamin Littenberg, MD

Publisher's Note: This article has been specially written for *Screening for Diseases*. It has not been previously published.

The rationale for any screening program requires an unbroken chain of requirements to be met in order to achieve significant gains in health. First, the disease must be an important and common cause of morbidity and mortality. Second, the disease must be detectable at a treatable, pre-symptomatic stage. Third, early treatment must be available, effective, and have a beneficial impact beyond the alternative of waiting for symptoms to occur. Finally, the cost-effectiveness of the screening policy must compare favorably with other uses of scarce health care resources. We review here the state of knowledge on how well screening for high blood pressure meets these requirements.

IS HYPERTENSION IMPORTANT?

Prevalence

In spite of years of focus by medical and public health workers, hypertension remains common in the United States. Results from the Third National Health and Nutrition Examination Survey showed that 24% of the adult population, and 32.4% of blacks, had blood pressure greater than 140/90. Prevalence varied from 1% in white women under 30 to 80% for elderly black women. Over one third of the hypertensive population were unaware of their condition, and only 24% of patients had achieved control (1).

Natural History and Impact

The risks of stroke, myocardial infarction, and renal dysfunction increase with even mildly elevated blood pressures (2, 3). High blood pressure contributes to a large percentage of deaths in the United States (4). The higher the pressure, especially when other risk factors are present, the higher is the incidence of heart disease, stroke, and death. Even among normotensive individuals, an increase in blood pressure is associated with an increase in the rate of cardiovascular complications (5). A prolonged 10 mm Hg reduction in diastolic blood pressure from usual levels is associated with 56% less stroke and 37% less coronary heart disease. Hypertension increases the hazard for developing congestive heart failure by 2- to 6-fold, and for atrial fibrillation by 1.5-fold (6, 7). Blood pressures over 210/120 are associated with a 22-fold increase in risk of end-stage renal disease in men compared with controls with blood pressures less than 120/80 (8).

Conclusion: Hypertension is Important

Hypertension is common; is a significant risk factor for stroke, coronary artery disease, and renal disease; and is still underdetected and undertreated. It is certainly important enough to warrant major efforts at control.

IS HYPERTENSION DETECTABLE?

Hypertension is usually asymptomatic. Waiting for symptoms to appear is not acceptable because the initial clinical complaint is often stroke, renal failure, myocardial infarction, or sudden death. Blood pressure may be determined by direct cannulation of an artery or noninvasively by sphygmomanometry, which may be performed intermittently during clinical encounters or during a structured mass screening program. Recently, continuous ambulatory sphygmomanometry has become available.

Sphygmomanometry

The test characteristics of routine sphygmomanometry are not precisely known because there is no obvious reference criterion to use for comparison. Especially in the elderly and obese, cuff pressures tend to overestimate "true" arterial pressures as measured by arterial cannulation (9, 10). However, most of what is known about the natural history of hypertension (e.g., the Framingham study) is based on cuff pressures taken under conditions that approximate a medical clinic or doctor's office. Therefore indirect sphygmomanometry is an appropriate method for estimating prognosis and monitoring therapy. In a certain sense, there is no standard to compare to at all; arterial hypertension by sphygmomanometry in the doctor's office essentially is the definition of the condition. Community standards of care are based on this definition.

Although sphygmomanometry may be the gold standard process, individual sphygmomanometers may be wanting. Reviews have shown that 24% to 70% of aneroid and 2% to 8% of mercury sphygmomanometers deviate more than 3 mm from standards. The recent push to eliminate mercury sphygmomanometers because of their toxicity risk increases the potential for less accuracy overall in the future (11).

Significant errors in diagnosis (and therefore treatment) are possible if sphygmomanometry is not properly performed and interpreted. Guidelines from the World Health Organization (12) specify that the patient should be seated comfortably for several minutes before pressures are measured, an appropriate size cuff be used, the cuff inflated to a pressure greater than systolic before slowly releasing pressure, and the patient positioned so that the cuff is at the level of the heart. Pressures in both arms should be measured and the higher arm used for future monitoring. The appearance of the Korotkoff sounds (Phase I) indicates systolic pressure. Their disappearance (Phase V) indicates diastolic pressure. The mean of at least two determinations should be recorded. A screening blood pressure over 120/80 mm Hg should lead to repeat visits. Hypertension should not be diagnosed unless the blood pressure recorded in the office or clinic is above 140/90 mm Hg on at least three occasions over several weeks.

Unfortunately, these guidelines are not well implemented. Of 114 physicians studied, none completely followed the recommended procedures. The most common errors were failure to allow a resting period, not initially obtaining pressures in both arms and thereupon using the higher arm, using the wrong cuff size, and deflating the cuff at an inappropriate rate (14).

Ambulatory Blood Pressure Monitoring

With ongoing concern about the phenomenon of "office hypertension," the use of ambulatory blood pressure monitoring (with an automated sphygmomanometer that records blood pressure at frequent intervals, typically over 24 hours) is increasing. Of 1187 people with clinical hypertension studied by this method, 19% were found to be normotensive on ambulatory monitoring and did not have an increase in cardiovascular events compared with controls. A systematic review confirmed this phenomenon but noted that the direct costs of universal application could be as high as $6 billion and that nonphysician measurements may yield almost as valid information (15). One small study found conflicting results: that those with isolated office hypertension (not confirmed by ambulatory monitoring) did show deterioration in echocardiographically measured diastolic ventricular function compared with controls (16).

Reference ranges for ambulatory monitoring have yet to be established. As a starting point, a meta-analysis of normotensives found mean pressures to be 118/72 mm Hg, with 95% of observations (± 2 SD) falling within 97 to 139 mm Hg systolic and 57 to 87 mm Hg diastolic (17).

Intra-Arterial Measurement

Direct measurement of intra-arterial blood pressure by introducing a catheter into the bloodstream has the advantage of identifying a subset of patients with falsely elevated cuff pressures (pseudohypertension) (9, 18). However, this invasive procedure is expensive, painful, dangerous, time-consuming, and not generally available outside special facilities. Furthermore, long-term epidemiologic follow-up of hypertension is based on sphygmomanometry, not direct pressure recording. A shift in the diagnostic standard away from sphygmomanometry would weaken our estimates of the sequelae of any given level of blood pressure.

Conclusions: Hypertension is Detectable

Office measurement of blood pressure by sphygmomanometry remains the standard of care, but correct procedures must be followed. Ambulatory monitoring is still a costly and somewhat impractical technology, but evidence is mounting for its validity in identifying a subgroup of hypertensive subjects who may not benefit from treatment. As costs and practicality continue to improve, we look for its more widespread application. Arterial cannulation has little role in screening.

Is Treatment Effective?
Moderate and Severe Hypertension

In contrast to some other screening situations such as cancer, the benefits of treating hypertension are greatest for those with more severe rather than "earlier stage" disease. For patients whose blood pressure exceeds 160/100 mm Hg, treatment can markedly reduce the frequency of complications. In the Veterans Administration Cooperative Study, severe morbidity or mortality occurred in 27 of 70 control patients compared with 2 of 73 treated patients within 24 months ($P < 0.0001$) (19). Most physicians believe that severe hypertension, even without symptoms or signs of end-organ damage, should be treated aggressively (13).

For patients with diastolic blood pressure consistently in the range of 104 to 114 mm Hg, the benefits of treatment are less dramatic but still important. Among male veterans with moderate hypertension, for example, reduction in morbidity and mortality was highly significant: 34 of 110 placebo patients had significant cardiovascular morbidity or mortality compared with 10 of 100 treated patients over 3.3 years ($P < 0.0002$) (20).

Other trials of moderate-to-severe hypertension have been too small to yield statistically significant results but tend to demonstrate benefit among treated hypertensive patients (21). Most guidelines advocate aggressive treatment of moderate hypertension (13). In the Framingham Heart Study, from 1950 to 1989, the rate of antihypertensive medication use increased from 2.3% to 27.7%. The prevalence of systolic blood pressure of at least 160/100 declined from 18.5% to 9.2% among men and from 28.0% to 7.7% among women. This decline was accompanied by reductions in the prevalence of electrocardiographic evidence of left ventricular hypertrophy, from 4.5% to 2.5% among men and from 3.6% to 1.1% among women (22).

A review of randomized trials in moderate hypertension found that a 5- to 6-mm reduction in diastolic blood pressure was associated with a 42% reduction in stroke and a 14% reduction in coronary heart disease and that most of these reductions appeared rapidly (23).

Mild Hypertension

Mild hypertension (usually defined as consistent blood pressures of 140/90 to 159/99 mm Hg) is a more controversial subject. Prospective trials have produced conflicting evidence about the benefits of treating mild elevations of blood pressure. Adverse events are rare in mild hypertension, although they are more common than in normotensive subjects. Therefore large numbers of patients must be studied to measure the effects of lowering the blood pressure. The majority of newly discovered hypertensive patients have blood pressures in the mild range. The trade off between the effectiveness of treatment and its costs and risks is less obviously beneficial for mild hypertension than for moderate or severe hypertension. Therefore, we will more closely examine the evidence for treating mild hypertension.

At least 18 large-scale randomized placebo-controlled trials of mild hypertension treatment have been reported. Although all have limitations and many use differing definitions of hypertension, in general they show a modest beneficial effect of therapy (21, 24, 25). Much of this benefit comes from reduction in strokes and congestive heart failure. The hoped-for impact on coronary deaths has not been consistently demonstrated.

Pooling the results of mild hypertension therapy trials yields a relative reduction in annualized total ("all-cause") mortality of 5% to 12% depending on drug class (25). Assuming an untreated death rate similar to the Multiple Risk Factor Intervention Trial population (about 60 deaths per 10,000 per year), treatment would save about 5 deaths per 10,000 per year. In a group with a higher death rate [e.g., 900 deaths per 10,000 per year in the elderly participants in the European Working Party Study) (26)], about 60 per 10,000 of the treated population would be spared death annually.

The difference between absolute and relative reductions in mortality is an important source of confusion when the baseline rate of death is low, as in mild hypertension (27). With low baseline death rates, even very large relative improvements correspond to quite small changes in absolute mortality. For instance, although reducing the death rate by 12% (in relative terms) seems substantial, the case for intervention seems less compelling when the effect is viewed as an absolute reduction of less than 1 per 1000. We can probably eliminate up to one tenth of deaths in patients with mild hypertension by treating them all. However, for a low-risk individual weighing the benefits and costs of treatment, the absolute effect is more meaningful: to improve his chance of surviving for 5 years from 95.3% to 95.8%, he must be treated for those 5 years and bear the costs and adverse effects of the medications. Over 200 such patients with mild hypertension must be treated for 5 years to prevent one death from hypertension.

Meta-analyses of the other end-points of the randomized trials of treatment in mild hypertension (24, 25) demonstrate a significant decrease in strokes. Other sources of data corroborate the relationship between blood pressure control and stroke. In Rochester, Minnesota, for instance, the incidence of stroke in men dropped about 10 years after control of mild hypertension improved in the community (28).

The impact of treatment of mild hypertension upon coronary artery disease is not as clearly beneficial. The 1997 meta-analysis demonstrated a 28% reduction in coronary heart disease with low-dose diuretics but not with other regimens (25).

Several caveats should be applied to pooled results. The pooled trials often used different definitions of hypertension, different treatment regimens, different control regimens, and different patient populations. Most of these studies tested pharmacologic therapies; the effect of non-drug therapies on prognosis is not well studied.

Despite the uncertainties inherent in the data and in the pooling methods, certain conclusions can be drawn. For instance, with a combined enrollment of over 48,000 subjects with mild hypertension, the 18 trials were able to demonstrate a beneficial impact of therapy upon morbidity and mortality from stroke and congestive heart failure (25).

Various lifestyle modifications have proven useful as complements to drug therapy (and sometimes as effective substitutes) (13). However, many Americans find it difficult to persist in weight loss, alcohol reduction, smoking cessation, dietary changes, and physical activity efforts.

Isolated Systolic Hypertension

Elevated systolic pressure with normal diastolic pressure is associated with advanced age and poor long-term outcomes. A recent review of eight randomized, controlled trials involving almost 16,000 elderly subjects found substantial benefits associated with antihypertensive therapy (29). These included reductions in cardiovascular mortality (16%), stroke (30%), coronary events (23%), and total mortality (10%).

Hypertension in Diabetic Patients

The Joint National Committee on Prevention, Detection, Evaluation, and Treatment of High Blood Pressure recently lowered its treatment threshold for diabetic patients to 130/80. The American Diabetes Association also advises the lower threshold. A cost-effectiveness analysis (30) confirmed the wisdom of this approach. For a typical 60-year-old diabetic person with hypertension, achieving the new, lower blood pressure goal increases life expectancy and actually lowers lifetime medical costs compared with using the old, higher thresholds. The authors conclude that "any incremental treatment for 60-year-olds that costs less than $414 annually and successfully lowers blood pressure from below 140/90 to below 130/85 mm Hg would be cost saving in the long term because of the reduction in attendant costs of future morbidity. The lower treatment goal recommended for high-risk hypertensive patients compares favorably in cost-effectiveness with many other frequently recommended treatment strategies and saves money overall for patients aged 60 years and older."

Conclusions: Treatment Can Be Effective

Although the evidence is clear that treatment of hypertension is efficacious under study conditions, its effectiveness in clinical use is less certain. Enhanced tracking and outreach support yields better follow-up with medical care (31). Lack of insurance or an established relationship with a physician or clinic, but not income, is associated with less follow-up and treatment (32). A study of unionized workers with full access to medical care found that only 12% of hypertensives were controlled, and that duration of medication, rather than physician visits, was associated with control (33).

Treatment of moderate and severe hypertension has

clear-cut benefits. Although the effect is somewhat smaller for mild hypertension, we believe that thoughtful management of these patients results in benefit. This result does not imply that every adult with a diastolic pressure of 90 mm Hg should be started on drug therapy. Rather, we believe that patients with mild hypertension will benefit from assessment of other cardiac risk-factors, long-term follow-up, consideration of nonpharmacologic therapy, and, in selected cases, judicious use of antihypertensive medications.

Treatment of hypertension is effective in lowering blood pressure and reducing morbidity, but many social barriers remain. The original, low-cost therapies with diuretics and beta-blockers continue to show the best results and quality-of-life outcomes (25). The angiotensin-converting enzyme inhibitors have significant renal and cardioprotective effects in select populations and are becoming available generically, which will increase their appeal.

THE DECISION TO SCREEN: BENEFITS, RISKS, AND COSTS

So far, we have concluded that hypertension is important, it is detectable, and that, once detected, treatment is wise for certain populations. These are necessary but not sufficient criteria for a useful screening program. Do the benefits of screening for hypertension outweigh the costs and risks of detection and therapy? Because there are no published controlled trials of screening for hypertension, we must use indirect evidence to answer this question.

Benefits

The benefits of screening for hypertension accrue to those patients who are found to have the condition, are successfully and safely treated, comply with treatment, and are spared stroke, renal failure, premature death, or other complications. Therefore the direct benefits accrue to only a small fraction of the population screened. On the other hand, the indirect benefits are more widely distributed. If fewer people suffer stroke, renal failure, heart disease, and premature death, families and communities are spared loss and more resources may be available to meet other needs.

Risks and Costs

The direct risks of routine sphygmomanometry are nearly nil but do include published reports of nerve injury (34) and an unpublished anecdote of an elderly woman who was unable to deflate the cuff on her automatic home monitoring equipment and suffered significant contusions (35). However, a diagnosis of hypertension has several indirect risks for the patient. First, a normotensive patient may be misdiagnosed on the basis of a spuriously elevated pressure. These patients are subject to the adverse effects of anti-hypertensive therapy with little potential for benefit. The diagnosis of mild hypertension should be based on repeated measures at each of several encounters, with care-

ful attention paid to cuff size and other confounding variables (12, 13, 36).

Treatment of a correctly diagnosed hypertensive patient also includes risks, of which the most important are the adverse effects of drug therapy. Antihypertensive medications cause a plethora of adverse effects ranging from headache and constipation to hemolytic anemia and sudden death. There is evidence that some antihypertensive preparations can have a harmful effect on cardiac risk factors such as cholesterol level (37). In addition, treatment can be expensive. The lifelong direct costs of medications alone can reach tens of thousands of dollars. Especially for mild hypertension, these risks and costs might easily exceed the potential benefits of treatment. However, lower-cost regimens such as a diuretic or a diuretic plus a beta-blocker may actually be more effective in reducing blood pressure than costlier regimens such as calcium channel blockers (38).

Labeling a patient as hypertensive may induce an unwanted change in the patient's behavior (39). There is some evidence that sense of well-being may deteriorate and absenteeism may rise after diagnosis (40). There is controversial but disturbing data that the incomes of labeled hypertensives are lower than their normotensive peers (41).

The search for treatable secondary causes of hypertension can be costly and dangerous. Invasive tests such as intravenous pyelography, renal arteriography, and selective adrenal vein sampling are sometimes advocated for selected patients. These tests have substantial risks, including contrast reactions, nephrotoxicity, local vascular damage, and the ever-present possibility of misinformation (42).

The cost per case detected and treated is probably higher in mass screening programs than in office-based case finding because of the need to deploy the screeners especially for the program. In a primary care office, the marginal cost of obtaining a blood pressure measurement is quite low.

Balancing Risks, Costs and Benefits: Cost-Effectiveness

In 1976, Weinstein and Stason estimated the cost-effectiveness of screening and treating known hypertension (43). The unit of measure for this type of analysis is the dollar cost of changing to a new procedure (the marginal cost) divided by the resultant change in life expectancy (the marginal benefit). The authors modified the value of years of life to account for pain, disability, or other morbidity. The analysis yielded estimates of quality-adjusted life expectancy. For instance, the authors assumed that suffering a stroke is equivalent to losing 1.5 years of healthy life span on average. They also assumed that the treated subject would be better off than an untreated hypertensive but would not attain the full benefit of being naturally normotensive. This "fraction of benefit" analysis was performed before most of the trials of treatment for hypertension had been completed; the efficacy estimates used by Weinstein and Stason were the authors' subjective judgments.

Table 1. Cost-Effectiveness of Screening Asymptomatic Adults for Hypertension

	Men			Women		
	Age 20	**Age 40**	**Age 60**	**Age 20**	**Age 40**	**Age 60**
Average increased life expectancy per screenee						
Measured in years	0.0096	0.0302	0.0544	0.0017	0.0110	0.0293
Measured in days	4	11	20	1	4	11
Cost of management	*Cost-effectiveness ($/QALY)*					
$50/year	4182	2131	1013	8269	3308	1619
$300/year	22,291	16,280	8374	44,412	23,216	12,404
$500/year	49,348	27,599	14,263	73,326	39,143	21,031
$1000/year	99,548	55,897	28,985	145,612	78,960	42,600
$1500/year	149,741	84,195	43,707	217,897	118,776	64,169
$2000/year	199,933	112,492	58,430	290,183	158,593	85,738
$2500/year	250,126	140,790	73,152	362,468	198,409	107,307

QALY = quality-adjusted life-year.
Adapted from Littenberg B. A practice guideline revisited: screening for hypertension. Ann Intern Med. 1995;122:937–9.

Weinstein and Stason found the cost per quality-adjusted life-year (QALY, a measure of life expectancy corrected to account for morbidity) saved by screening depended upon the pretreatment blood pressure, age, and sex. Under their central assumptions (especially that compliance with treatment is imperfect), and allowing the treatment threshold to vary by age, sex, and diastolic pressure, they estimated the marginal cost-effectiveness of community-wide screening to be $20,077/QALY. Case-finding (the testing of patients who present to the provider for other reasons) had lower marginal costs than mass screening because fewer patients are lost to follow-up and the cost of case finding itself is simply added to an existing episode of care. Weinstein and Stason found case-finding to cost $15,818/QALY. Both of these estimates are well within the range of the estimated cost-effectiveness for other widely accepted health interventions.

In 1990, Littenberg et al updated the work of Weinstein and Stason to reflect the results of treatment trials and other information newly available (44). Their analysis found screening to be reasonable over a wide range of assumptions but also found that the cost of drug therapy and the age of the screened populations are major drivers of cost-effectiveness. An update in 1995 expanded the analysis of treatment cost (**Table 1**) (45). Many analysts accept a health intervention as cost-effective if the cost per quality-adjusted life year ($/QALY) is below $50,000 to $75,000. If screening is inexpensive (less than $5 per subject) and therapy can be delivered for less than $500 per year, then screening is probably below this threshold.

We recently obtained retail costs of various treatment regimens from an Internet supplier (www.drugstore.com). A 1-year supply of the generic diuretic hydrochlorothiazide (either 25 or 50 mg per day) is available for about $33. The generic beta-blocker atenolol (100 mg per day) costs $57 per year. Angiotensin conversion enzyme inhibition with generic captopril (50 mg three times per day) costs

$237. Evaluation by a physician with some laboratory work adds about $250, bringing the total cost of treatment to under $500 per year. The annual costs of newer medications can be much higher. The angiotensin receptor blocker Atacand (candesartan 16 mg per day) costs about $511 per year. The calcium channel blocker Vascor (bepridil 300 mg per day) costs $1636. The beta-blocker Betapace (sotalol 120 mg twice a day) costs $3042 per year. If the costs of management (including physician and laboratory services) exceed about $1000 per year, screening becomes prohibitively inefficient for all but the highest-risk subgroups.

Conclusions: Screening Can Be Cost-Effective

Screening for hypertension is a wise strategy only if follow-up and treatment are effective and efficient. The trend towards newer, more expensive (but not more effective) medications threatens the cost-effectiveness of screening for high blood pressure.

FREQUENCY OF SCREENING

Because hypertension is common, measuring blood pressure in previously unscreened adults will frequently reveal new cases of hypertension. Repeat screening, however, has a much lower yield. Because the number of undiagnosed cases in the population is lower after the initial screen, the cost of finding an undiagnosed case goes up. The critical question, therefore, is not just "Should we screen?" but also "How often should we screen?" A rational answer depends in part upon the yield of hypertensive subjects in a previously screened population and the consequences of a delay in treatment. What is the chance that a normotensive (or borderline) subject will develop hypertension during the screening interval? What is the damage done by not treating during that interval? These basic aspects of the natural history of hypertension and the effect of hypertensive therapy are unknown. However, some data are available to help the physician decide how often to measure blood pressure.

In a follow-up study of adult patients seen at the Mayo Clinic (46), blood pressure at initial examination predicted the incidence of subsequent hypertension (defined as greater than 160/100 mm Hg). At 10 years, only 25% of those with diastolic pressures from 85 to 89 mm Hg developed hypertension; less than 5% of those with diastolic blood pressures below 85 mm Hg did so. An observational study in the Netherlands found that patients with a diastolic blood pressure less than 75 mm Hg and no weight gain had little risk for developing hypertension over 18 years (47).

Other investigators have found a positive correlation between initial and subsequent blood pressure in a variety of populations (48–52). At 4 years of follow-up, the reported correlation coefficients have been in the 0.6 range. Therefore long intervals between measurements will allow a substantial fraction of subjects to develop unrecognized hypertension between measures. However, if delays in the diagnosis of hypertension and initiation of therapy are not associated with significant risks, longer screening intervals will not be risky. Subjects with other cardiovascular risk factors (and therefore at higher risk for complications of hypertension) are more likely to benefit from screening and should be screened more often than low-risk subjects.

Though these data are useful, they are inadequate to support a specific conclusion concerning the optimal frequency of screening for hypertension. Patients with very low blood pressures are unlikely to become hypertensive as rapidly as those with pressures nearer the treatment threshold. Subjects with other cardiovascular risks may derive more benefit from more frequent screening.

RECOMMENDATIONS

Hypertension, including mild hypertension, is a common and important cause of morbidity and mortality among adults. The disease is easily detectable, and presymptomatic therapy is available, effective, and has a beneficial impact compared with waiting for symptoms to occur. We believe that the costs and risks of screening for mild hypertension are offset by the benefits gained and offer the following recommendations:

1. Every adult should be screened for hypertension.

2. Because the direct cost of screening for hypertension in a patient who is already visiting the doctor for some other reason (case-finding) is low, we recommend that blood pressure be measured routinely when adults seek care.

3. Patients with a history of borderline elevations in blood pressure or other risk factors for vascular disease (known coronary artery disease, diabetes, previous hypertension, etc.) should have their hypertension identified early and treated aggressively.

4. Because the cost-effectiveness of screening for hypertension (and of treating mild hypertension) can be severely reduced by using an expensive treatment regimen, every effort should be made to manage hypertension with the lowest-cost interventions consonant with good pressure control, patient acceptability, and safety.

References

1. **Burt VL, Whelton P, Roccella EJ, et al.** Prevalence of hypertension in the US adult population: results from the Third National Health and Nutrition Examination Survey, 1988-1991. Hypertension. 1995;25:305-13.

2. **Paul O.** Risks of mild hypertension: a ten-year report. Br Heart J. 1971; (Suppl)33:116-21.

3. **Fujii I, Ueda K, Omae T, et al.** Natural history of borderline hypertension in the Hisayama community, Japan.–I. The relative prognostic importance of transient variability in blood pressure. J Chron Dis. 1984;37:895-902.

4. **Remington RD.** Blood pressure: the population burden. Geriatrics. 1976;31: 48-54.

5. Society of Actuaries and Association of Life Insurance Medical Directors of America. Blood Pressure Study, 1979. Chicago: Society of Actuaries; 1980.

6. **Levy D, Larson MG, Vasan RS, et al.** The progression from hypertension to congestive heart failure. JAMA. 1996;275:1557-62.

7. **Brown MJ, Haydock S.** Pathoaetiology, epidemiology and diagnosis of hypertension. Drugs. 2000;59(Suppl 2):1-12.

8. **Klag MJ, Whelton PK, Randall BL, et al.** Blood pressure and end-stage renal disease in men. N Engl J Med. 1996;334:13-8.

9. **Finnegan TP, Spence JD, Wong DG, Wells GA.** Blood pressure measurement in the elderly. J Hypertens. 1985;3:231-5.

10. **Trout KW, Bertrand CA, Williams MH.** Measurement of blood pressure in obese persons. JAMA. 1956;162:970-1.

11. **O'Brien E.** Replacing the mercury sphygmomanometer requires clinicians to demand better automated devices. Br Med J. 2000;320:815-6.

12. **World Health Organization/International Society of Hypertension.** 1986 Guidelines for the treatment of mild hypertension. J Hypertens. 1986;4:383-6. Revised: WHO Expert Committee on Hypertension Control, Geneva, 24-31 October 1994; http://www.who.int/ncd/cvd/trs862.html.

13. **Chobanian AV, Bakris GL, Black HR, et al.** Joint National Committee on Prevention, Detection, Evaluation, and Treatment of High Blood Pressure. National Heart, Lung, and Blood Institute; National High Blood Pressure Education Program Coordinating Committee. Seventh Report of the Joint National Committee on Prevention, Detection, Evaluation, and Treatment of High Blood Pressure. Hypertension. 2003;42:1206–52.

14. **Bailey RH, Bauer JH.** A review of common errors in the indirect measurement of blood pressure. Sphygmomanometry. Arch Intern Med. 1993;153: 2741-8.

15. **Appel LJ, Stason WB.** Ambulatory blood pressure monitoring and blood pressure self-measurement in the diagnosis and management of hypertension. Ann Intern Med. 1993;118:867-82.

16. **Ferrara LA, Guida L, Pasanisi F, et al.** Isolated office hypertension and end-organ damage. J Hypertens. 1997;15:979-85.

17. **Staessen JA, Fagard RH, Lijnen PJ, et al.** Mean and range of the ambulatory pressure in normotensive subjects from a meta-analysis of 23 studies. Am J Cardiol. 1991;67:723-7.

18. **Littenberg B, Wolfberg C.** Pseudohypertension masquerading as malignant hypertension. Am J Med. 1988;84:539-42.

19. Veterans Administration Cooperative Study Group on Antihypertensive Agents. Effects of treatment on morbidity in hypertension: results in patients with diastolic blood pressures averaging 115 through 129 mm Hg. JAMA. 1967;202: 1028-34.

20. Veterans Administration Cooperative Study Group on Antihypertensive Agents. Effects of treatment on morbidity in hypertension: influence of age, diastolic pressure and prior cardiovascular disease: further analysis of side effects. Circulation. 1972;45:991-1004.

21. **MacMahon SW, Cutler JA, Furberg CD, Payne GH.** The effects of drug

treatment for hypertension on morbidity and mortality from cardiovascular disease: a review of randomized controlled trials. Prog Cardiovasc Dis. 1986; 29(Suppl 1):99-118.

22. **Mosterd A, D'Agostino RB, Silbershatz H, et al.** Trends in the prevalence of hypertension, antihypertensive therapy, and left ventricular hypertrophy from 1950 to 1989. N Engl J Med. 1999;340:1221-7.

23. **Collins R, Peto R, MacMahon S, et al.** Blood pressure, stroke, and coronary heart disease.–Part 2. Short-term reductions in blood pressure: overview of randomised drug trials in their epidemiological context. Lancet. 1990;335:827-38.

24. **Hebert PR, Fiebach NH, Eberlein KA, et al.** The community-based randomized trials of pharmacologic treatment of mild-to-moderate hypertension. Am J Epidemiol. 1988;127:581-90.

25. **Psaty BM, Smith NL, Siscovick DS, et al.** Health outcomes associated with antihypertensive therapies as first-line agents: a systematic review and meta-analysis. JAMA. 1997;277:739-45.

26. **Amery A, Birkenhager W, Brixko P, et al.** Mortality and morbidity results from the European Working Party on high blood pressure in the elderly trial. Lancet. 1985;1:1349-54.

27. **Pickering TG.** Treatment of mild hypertension and the reduction of cardiovascular mortality: the "of" or "by" dilemma. JAMA. 1983;249:399-400.

28. **Garraway WM, Whisnant JP.** The changing pattern of hypertension and the declining incidence of stroke. JAMA. 1987;258:214-7.

29. **Staessen JA, Gasowski J, Wang JG, et al.** Risks of untreated and treated systolic hypertension in the elderly:meta-analysis of outcome trials. Lancet. 2000; 355:865-72.

30. **Elliott WJ, Weir DR, Black HR.** Cost-effectiveness of the lower treatment goal (of JNC VI) for diabetic hypertensive patients. Arch Intern Med. 2000;160: 1277-83.

31. **Krieger J, Collier C, Song L, Martin D.** Linking community-based blood pressure measurement to clinical care: a randomized controlled trial of outreach and tracking by community health workers. Am J Pub Health. 1999;89:856-61.

32. **Moy E, Bartman BA, Weir MR.** Access to hypertensive care: effects of income, insurance, and source of care. Arch Intern Med. 1995;155:1497-502.

33. **Stockwell DH, Madhavan S, Cohen H, et al.** The determinants of hypertension awareness, treatment, and control in an insured population. Am J Pub Health. 1994;84:1768-74.

34. **Lin CC, Jawan B, de Villa MV, et al.** Blood pressure cuff compression injury of the radial nerve. J Clin Anesth. 2001;13:306-8.

35. **Russo CD.** Personal communication, 13 June 1995.

36. **Beevers G, Lip GYH, O'Brien E.** Blood pressure measurement.–Part II. Conventional sphygmomnometry technique of auscultatory blood pressure management. Br Med J. 2001;322:1043-7.

37. **Pollare T, Lithell H, Berne C.** A comparison of the effects of hydrochlorothiazide and captopril on glucose and lipid metabolism in patients with hypertension. N Engl J Med. 1989;321:868-73.

38. **Perry HM Jr, Bingham S, Horney A, et al.** Antihypertensive efficacy of treatment regimens used in Veterans Administration hypertension clinics. Department of Veterans Affairs Cooperative Study Group on Antihypertensive Agents. Hypertension. 1998;31:771-9.

39. **MacDonald LA, Sackett DL, Haynes RB, Taylor DW.** Labelling in hypertension: a review of the behavioural and psychological consequences. J Chron Dis. 1984;37:933-42.

40. **Haynes RB, Sackett DL, Taylor DW, et al.** Increased absenteeism from work after detection and labeling of hypertensive patients. N Engl J Med. 1978; 299:741-4.

41. **Lefebvre RC, Hursey KG, Carleton RA.** Labeling of participants in high blood pressure screening programs: implications for blood cholesterol screenings. Arch Intern Med. 1988;148:1993-7.

42. **Reiss MD, Bookstein JJ, Bleifer KH.** Radiologic aspects of renovascular hypertension. JAMA. 1972;221:374-8.

43. **Weinstein MC, Stason WB.** Hypertension: A Policy Perspective. Cambridge, MA: Harvard University Press; 1976.

44. **Littenberg B, Garber AM, Sox HC.** Screening for hypertension. Ann Intern Med. 1990;112:192-202.

45. **Littenberg B.** A practice guideline revisited: screening for hypertension. Ann Intern Med. 1995;122:937-9.

46. **Hines EA.** Range of normal blood pressure and subsequent development of hypertension. JAMA. 1940;115:271-4.

47. **Bakx JC, van den Hoogen HJ, van den Bosch WJ, et al.** Development of blood pressure and the incidence of hypertension in men and women over an 18-year period: results of the Nijmegen Cohort Study. J Clin Epidemiol. 1999; 52:531-8.

48. **Rosner B, Hennekens CH, Kass EH, Miall WE.** Age-specific correlation analysis of longitudinal blood pressure data. Am J Epidemiol. 1977;106:306-13.

49. **Rabkin SW, Mathewson FAL, Tate RB.** Relationship of blood pressure in 20- to 39-year-old men to subsequent blood pressure and incidence of hypertension over a 30-year observation period. Circulation. 1982;65:291-300.

50. **Svardsudd K, Tibblin G.** A longitudinal blood pressure study. J Chron Dis. 1980;33:627-36.

51. **Borghi C, Costa FV, Boschi S, et al.** Factors associated with the development of stable hypertension in young borderline hypertensives. J Hypertens. 1996;14: 509-17.

52. **Leitschuh M, Cupples LA, Kannel W, et al.** High-normal blood pressure progression to hypertension in the Framingham Heart Study. Hypertension. 1991;17:22-7.

Key Points

Depression

- [ ] There is no direct evidence that screening for depression alone leads to improved treatment or outcomes.

- [ ] There is evidence of benefit of screening for depression when there is a system in place for screening results to be coordinated with effective follow-up and treatment, as well as assessment for other psychiatric co-morbidities.

- [ ] There is no evidence of any significant differences in efficacy of the various screening instruments; thus shorter forms may be more practicable in the primary care setting.

- [ ] The optimal interval for screening for depression is not clear.

Screening for Depression in the Primary Care Setting

David S. Brody, MD, and Abhay J. Dhond, MD, MPH

Publisher's Note: This article has been specially written for *Screening for Diseases*. It has not been previously published.

The rationale for screening for depression in primary care is that it is common, highly impairing, and responsive to treatment. Yet depression is frequently not detected in the primary care setting, and, even when detected, it is not always adequately treated. Brief, easily administered screening questionnaires with adequate sensitivity and specificity are available. If, when, and how these questionnaires should be used has been actively debated in recent years.

To answer these questions, Gilbody and colleagues performed a systematic review of the literature published through 2000 (1). They concluded that there was little evidence showing that screening for depression in primary care was of benefit in improving psychosocial outcomes. Coyne and colleagues have reached a similar conclusion, adding that routine screening should be undertaken only when the resources are available for interpreting the significance of positive screen scores, appropriate and acceptable interventions are available, and potential negative effects of screening can be avoided (2). More recently, the U.S. Preventive Task Force recommended screening adults for depression in clinical practices that have systems in place to ensure accurate diagnoses, effective treatment, and follow-up (3, 4).

This paper will examine the scientific basis for these recommendations, discuss important implementation issues, and identify the issues that must be resolved before a more definitive conclusion on screening can be reached. The specific issues that will be addressed include the following:

1. Is depression important?
2. Is treatment for depression effective?
3. Is screening for depression needed in primary care?
4. How accurate are depression-screening instruments?
5. Does screening with supportive management and follow-up systems result in improved outcomes?
6. What are the risks and costs associated with depression screening?
7. Who should be screened? How often? Who should pay for it?

A Medline search was done to obtain relevant articles published between 1989 and February 2002. Articles were also identified from the bibliographies of recent review articles and retrieved articles.

IS DEPRESSION IMPORTANT?
Prevalence

Next to hypertension, depression is the most common chronic condition encountered in general medical practice (5). It is estimated that approximately 5% of the population experiences a depressive episode in any given year (6). The prevalence of major depression in western industrialized communities is 2.3% to 3.2% for men and 4.5% to 9.3% for women (7). The lifetime risk of developing major depression is 5% to 12% for men and 10% to 25% for women (7, 8). In the primary care setting, structured psychiatric interviews diagnose major depression in 5% to 12% of outpatients (5, 9–11).

Additional patients suffer from milder but still clinically significant sub-threshold levels of depression. Dysthymia is a chronic but less intense form of depression that lasts 2 years or more. The prevalence rates of dysthymia in primary care range from 2% to 8% (11, 12). Minor depression includes patients with two to four depressive symptoms nearly every day for at least 2 weeks, provided that at least one of these symptoms is depressed mood or anhedonia. This category can include patients with a history of major depression who have had only a partial remission or a relapse. The reported prevalence rates for minor depression in primary care range from 3% to 16% (11–14). In some reports, the prevalence of minor depression was nearly twice that of major depression (12–15).

In serious acute and chronic illness, the prevalence of depression is higher than in the general primary care population. After acute myocardial infarction (MI), up to 25% of patients have severe, often recurrent depression, while up to 65% of patients after MI manifest symptoms diagnostic of either major or minor depression (16). The lifetime risk of major depression in diabetics is 33% (17). The prevalence rates for current major depression are similar for type 1 and type 2 diabetes mellitus and range from 10% to 15% (17, 18). Clinically significant depression is found in approximately 23% to 47% of patients after stroke (19, 20). Studies on cancer patients show a wide variability in the prevalence of depression, ranging from 1.5% to 50% (mean 24%) (21). High rates of depression are also seen in patients with other chronic diseases, such as end-stage renal disease, Parkinson's disease, Alzheimer's disease, and AIDS/HIV infection (20). The rate of depression among elderly patients living in nursing homes is estimated at 15% to 25% (22, 23). Approximately 13% of elderly nursing home residents develop a new episode of major depression during a 1-year period of confinement, and an additional 18% develop new depressive symptoms (22, 23).

Natural History

Major depression may have its onset at any age, although it usually begins in the 20s or 30s (6). The natural history of major depression is variable. Depression is often chronic, with alternating relapses and remissions (5, 24). Some patients have only a single episode of major depression, then return to normal pre-morbid status. However, more than half of patients who develop a major depressive episode will have a recurrence (6).

When undetected and untreated, depression frequently becomes chronic. In a study by Rost et al, it was reported that 32% of patients with major depression remained undetected for up to 1 year in the primary care setting (25). During follow-up, more than half of the patients with undetected depression continued to meet criteria for major depression (59.7% of patients at 6 months and 52.8% of patients at 1 year). Moreover, almost half of the undetected patients developed suicidal ideation. Less than one third of undetected patients made a physician visit during the month they reported their worst symptoms. Compared with baseline nondepressed subjects, undetected depressed patients reported nine times more role limitations resulting from emotional problems, three times more role limitations resulting from physical problems, and eight times more disability days at their worst assessment. Coryell et al found that untreated individuals report greater interpersonal problems, more difficulty in enjoying activities, and a decrease in occupational status compared with treated patients over a 6-year follow-up period (26).

While undetected depression appears to be associated with considerable morbidity, the detection of these individuals has not necessarily proven to improve outcomes. Studies have failed to show that the detection of depression in the primary care setting leads to decreased morbidity (25, 27–31). The reason for this finding is not fully understood. It could be that detected patients may not be receiving adequate treatment. It is also possible that there may be unobserved differences in severity of depression between the two groups: the undetected patients may have milder disease compared with the detected group (32). It is also possible that some "undetected" patients have simply been reluctant to inform their primary care physicians (PCPs) that they are being treated by mental health specialists (2).

Impact on Health Care Utilization, Functioning, Quality of Life, and Mortality

Depression has a major impact on functioning and quality of life, morbidity and mortality, and utilization of health care resources. The economic costs are enormous, over $40 billion annually in the United States (33). Patients with depression have higher rates of health care utilization, make more visits to health care providers, and undergo more tests (34–36). The World Health Organization has estimated that depression may be responsible for as much as 25% of all visits to health care centers worldwide (37). Medical illness in patients with psychiatric comorbidity, especially depression, has been associated with longer and more expensive hospital stays and more extensive follow-up after discharge (38–43).

Patients with major depressive disorder or subthreshold levels of depressive symptoms also experience deficits in quality of life, daily function, and perceived health status

that are at least comparable to and usually worse than patients with chronic diseases such as coronary artery disease, arthritis, diabetes, and lung disorders (38, 44). According to World Health Organization estimates, major depression is the fourth most important cause worldwide of loss in disability-adjusted life-years and will become the second most important cause by the year 2020 (45, 46).

Depression associated with a chronic medical disease is particularly burdensome. Depression and heart disease seem to have independent additive adverse effects on functioning, well being, and mortality. The combination of advanced coronary artery disease and depression causes almost twice the social impairment caused by either disease alone (38, 47). Similarly, increased impairment of health-related quality of life has been noted in depression or dysthymia associated with other chronic diseases including diabetes, pulmonary disease, cancer, liver disease, arthritis, and renal disease (44). Moreover, these deficits persist over time and result in substantial and long-lasting decrements in multiple domains of functioning and well-being (48).

Depression increases the risk of death due to suicides and to co-morbid medical problems. Suicide is the ninth leading cause of death in the United States (49); more than 32,000 Americans commit suicide each year (50). Psychiatric illness is the strongest predictor of suicide (51). Among general medical patients, those with depression are more than ten times more likely to contemplate suicide than those who are not depressed (52). Depressed men are more likely to commit suicide than depressed women, with the highest rate among elderly white men (49, 53, 54). The lifetime risk of completed suicide in patients with major depression is 15% (7).

At least 20 methodologically sound studies have found a positive correlation between depression and mortality (55). High levels of depressive symptoms are an independent risk factor for mortality in the elderly community population (RR, 1.24; 95% CI, 1.06-1.46) (56). Major depressive disorder was also found to be an independent risk factor for mortality (RR, 1.59; 95% CI, 1.02-2.06) within 1 year of diagnosis in the nursing home patients (22). The increased risk of death in this population may be linked specifically to cardiovascular mortality (57–59). Depression after MI is an independent predictor of mortality. Depressed patients have 6- to 8-fold higher mortality 6 to 18 months after MI compared with patients who are not depressed (60, 61). In patients with unstable angina, depression is also associated with an increased risk of major cardiac events (62). In patients with diabetes a significant and consistent association has been reported between diabetic complications (retinopathy, neuropathy, macrovascular disease, and sexual dysfunction) and depression (63). In addition, depression can increase the morbidity and mortality associated with a variety of other medical disorders (64–67).

The reason for poor outcomes in patients with depression is not fully understood; however, poor patient adherence to treatment recommendations may explain part of the problem. A meta-analysis of 12 studies revealed that depressed patients are three times more likely to be non-adherent to medical treatment recommendations than nondepressed patients (68). Patients with depression after MI have lower adherence to prescribed pharmacotherapy and are less likely to adhere to recommended behavior and lifestyle changes intended to reduce the risk of subsequent cardiac events (69). Depressed patients have also been shown to have poorer adherence to prescribed aspirin therapy, smoking cessation, and cardiac rehabilitation (70–73). Depression has also been associated with poor compliance in other non-cardiac diseases including asthma, chronic obstructive pulmonary disease (COPD), diabetes mellitus, end-stage renal disease, rheumatoid arthritis, AIDS, and cancer (68, 74–86).

What is less clear is the impact of treating depression on the outcomes associated with the foregoing medical conditions. Lustman et al found that cognitive behavior therapy and supportive diabetes education was an effective nonpharmacologic treatment for major depression in patients with type 2 diabetes and may be associated with improved glycemic control (87). Blumenthal et al demonstrated a 74% reduction in combined endpoints (death, MI, and revascularization) in a small group of cardiac ischemia patients with stress and hostility who participated in a stress management group (88). Frasure-Smith showed that high-stress post-MI patients who took part in a 1-year program of stress monitoring and home visits by a nurse to help them deal with their life problems did not experience the increased cardiac mortality seen in similar patients who did not participate in such a program (89). A subsequent study by this group did not show improved outcomes for patients who received a home-based nurse administered stress reduction program after MI. Post-hoc analysis of this study, however, suggests that the patients who responded to the intervention (i.e., those who decreased their level of emotional distress) experienced decreased morbidity and mortality (90). The recently completed SAD HART study showed that Zoloft was a well-tolerated and effective treatment for depression in post-MI patients and that patients treated with Zoloft had a trend toward reduced cardiac events; the latter outcome, however, did not reach statistical significance (91).

IS TREATMENT FOR DEPRESSION EFFECTIVE?

Effective treatment is available for primary care patients with depression (92–95). Available treatments can be divided into two broad categories: pharmacotherapy and psychotherapy. Psychotherapy is probably as effective as treatment with antidepressants in patients with mild-to-moderate depression (27). However, psychotherapeutic interventions are more difficult to provide in primary care because they are more time consuming and require specific expertise or may depend on easy access to mental health specialists. Thus pharmacotherapy is preferred by physicians and patients who want to be treated in the primary care setting. Antidepressants are effective and are commonly prescribed by PCPs.

In a recent review of the literature, Williams et al found that 51% of patients randomly assigned to active treatment with antidepressants (vs. 32% of patients receiving placebo) reported at least 50% improvement in depressive symptoms (92). No significant difference in clinical effectiveness has been found either between different classes of antidepressants or between individual drugs within a class. The ARTIST study was specifically designed to compare the effectiveness of three SSRIs (paroxetine, fluoxetine, and sertraline) in primary care patients with depression (94). Responses to the three drugs were comparable on all measures and at all time points. The three SSRIs had similar effectiveness for depressive symptoms as well as multiple domains of health-related quality of life over the duration of the trial.

Furthermore, it has been observed that individual patient characteristics do not reliably predict better or worse response to a particular drug or antidepressant class (95). However, dropout rates as a result of adverse effects are lower with newer agents compared with tricyclic antidepressants (8% vs. 13%, respectively; $P < 0.05$) (93). Moreover, compared with tricyclic agents, SSRIs have fewer drug interactions, simpler dosing, and less toxic effects in event of an overdose. As a result, SSRIs have become the most commonly prescribed class of antidepressants (94).

Although effective treatment is available, it is unclear how often primary care patients are appropriately treated for depression. A number of common problems that compromise the effectiveness of depression treatment in primary care have been identified: inadequate dosage and duration of treatment with antidepressant medications, infrequent follow-up, lack of adjustment therapy according to patient response, and poor patient adherence to antidepressant medications (28, 96–101). It is not surprising therefore that a number of studies have found either no benefit or only modest short-term benefit from the treatment of depression in primary care (25, 102–105).

The SSRIs have made it easier for PCPs to provide effective treatment. As a result, prescribing of these medications has increased dramatically during the past 10 years (106, 107). The ARTIST study suggests that PCPs can achieve acceptable outcomes with these medications (94). In this study, the percentage of patients who met criteria for major depression dropped from 74% at baseline to 26% at 9 months; however, a placebo group was not included for comparison.

One concern that has surfaced about the increased number of prescriptions for antidepressant prescriptions written by PCPs is the possibility of over-prescribing. Coyne has pointed out that the rates of treatment exceed the presumed prevalence of depression in some populations and raise the issue of whether patients are being treated with medications they either do not need or are not likely to benefit from (108). No data are available, however, on how often this takes place.

IS SCREENING FOR DEPRESSION NEEDED?

Depression does not have an asymptomatic stage, but patients usually present to PCPs with somatic rather than emotional complaints. The literature suggests that 35% to 50% of the time depression is not recognized in the primary care setting (28, 109–112). The extent to which physicians fail to recognize depression may have been exaggerated, however (113). Most of the studies that have examined this question were conducted more than 10 years ago. The studies that found that half of the cases of depression in primary care go undetected based their findings on depression screening instruments that produce many false positives. In addition, missed cases are more likely to be patients with less severe depression or patients who are reluctant to accept diagnosis or treatment of depression (114). Some missed cases may actually already be receiving care from a mental health specialist (2). Finally, depression is sometimes recognized but not coded or noted in the medical record because of reimbursement issues and fear of stigmatization (115).

Recent data indicate that PCPs are now recognizing depression more frequently. Data from the National Ambulatory Medical Care Survey, a national probability survey of outpatient practices, reveal that depression diagnoses increased from 5 million visits (2.2% of primary care visits) in 1980 to 9 million visits (3.2% of visits in 1999) (116). It is also quite likely that there is considerable variability among physicians in terms of their ability to recognize depression. Interested physicians with good communication skills may be able to detect most cases of depression without the aid of a screening instrument. Others may need either more training in identifying depression or a screening questionnaire if they want to increase their depression detection rate.

WHAT IS THE ACCURACY OF DEPRESSION SCREENING INSTRUMENTS?

Several questionnaires have been developed to identify patients who need further evaluation or to provide confirmatory data on patients who are suspected of being depressed. These questionnaires can be administered either to all patients as a screening tool or to selected patients with a higher probability of depression as a tool for case finding. Mulrow et al reviewed the literature on case-finding instruments for depression in primary care and assessed nine different instruments, which were used in 18 studies involving more than 15,000 patients (117). Length of the instruments ranged from 2 to 28 questions, and average administration time ranged from 2.1 to 5.6 minutes. The overall sensitivity was 84% (95% CI, 79%-89%) and overall specificity was 72% (95% CI, 67%-77%). No significant difference, at these levels of sensitivity and specificity, was found between various instruments that were used.

Analysis revealed that for an estimated 5% prevalence of major depression in the primary care patient population, 31 out of every 100 patient would screen positive. Four out of these 31 would have major depression (true-positives), whereas 27 would be false- positive. Some of the false-positives may, however, have dysthymia or other psychiatric disorders that may warrant treatment or close monitoring. It is estimated that one patient with major depression would be missed (false-negative) for every 100 patients screened. Further diagnostic evaluation would be required to separate the false- from the true-positives.

Commonly used screening instruments include the Short Beck Depression Inventory (7, 13, or 21 questions) (118, 119); the Zung Self-Rating Depression Scale (20 questions) (120); the Center for Epidemiologic Studies Depression screen (CES-D) (10 or 20 questions) (121); the General Health Questionnaire (GHQ) (12, 28, or 30 questions) (122–124); the Hopkins Symptom Checklist (HSCL) (125, 126); the PHQ-9 (127); the Whooley 2-item screen (128); the Williams-1 item screen (129); the PRIME-MD (130, 131); and the Symptom-Driven Diagnostic System (SDDS-PC) (132).

The Beck Depression Inventory, the Zung Self-Rating Depression Scale, and the Center for Epidemiologic Studies Depression Screen are instruments that screen for depression that can also be used to rate the severity of depression and monitor response to therapy. The General Health Questionnaire and the Hopkins Symptom Checklist are nonspecific instruments that screen for psychiatric illness. Both have several versions with different numbers of questions.

More recently, 1- or 2-question screening instruments for depression have been found to be comparable to the aforementioned longer tests. Williams et al compared a single-question case-finding instrument with a longer, 20-item CESD and found that the two instruments had similar performance characteristics (129). The question used is: "Have you felt depressed or sad much of the time in the past year?" When depression is suspected, this screening question about depressed mood can detect 85%-90% of patients with major depression.

Whooley et al found that adding a second question about anhedonia to the screening test increased the detection rate (128). A positive response on the 2-item instrument had a sensitivity of 96% (95% CI, 90%-99%) and a specificity of 57% (95% CI, 53%-62%). The Whooley 2-item test questions are: "During the past month, have you often been bothered by feeling down, depressed, or hopeless?" and "During the past month, have you often been bothered by having little interest or pleasure in doing things?" These shorter 1- or 2-item tests are more likely to be used by PCPs in daily practice and can be incorporated into a routine history protocol.

Table 1. Screening and Feedback Studies

Author/Year	Setting	Design	Interventions	Outcomes
Johnstone/1976	One practice in England	Consecutive patients were screened and assigned to feedback or no-feedback groups	Feedback of results of General Health Questionnaire	At 3 months, feedback patients were more likely to report "feeling well"; no difference in GHQ score at 1 year
Linn/1980	Academic primary care clinic	New patients randomly assigned to feedback or no-feedback groups; outcomes assessed by chart audits	Feedback of results of Zung Depression Scale	Depression more likely to be diagnosed in patients assigned to feedback group (29% vs. 89%); no difference in treatment
Magruder/1990	VA clinic: 8 PCPs	Patients randomized to intervention and control groups	Feedback of screening results	Increased rate of treatment among intervention patients; no effect on depression scores
Dowrick/1995	Group practice in England	Patients with undetected depression randomized to intervention and control groups	Feedback of screening results	No effect on outcomes
Reifler/1996	Resident clinic in urban academic hospital	Patients randomized to intervention and control groups	Feedback of screening results and diagnostic module	Lower utilization in screened patients; no difference in functional outcomes or patient satisfaction
Williams/1999	4 primary care clinics: 80 residents and PCPs	Patients randomly assigned to receive one of two screening questionnaires or usual care	Feedback of screening results	Recovery more likely with feedback but no difference in improvement in depressive symptoms
Spitzer/1999	4 primary care practices and 31 physicians	Patients completed a self-administered PRIME-MD	Feedback of results of PRIME-MD	Among the 3000 patients assessed, there were 74 with a newly established diagnoses of major depression; of these, 10% were treated with antidepressants, and 5% were referred to a mental health specialist

PRIME-MD and SDDS-PC differ from other instruments in two important ways. First, these instruments include both screening and diagnostic modules, and second, they assess depression as well as other common mental health diseases (e.g., anxiety, eating disorders, alcohol abuse, somatization). There are two versions of PRIME-MD. In the original version, the diagnostic assessment is conducted by the clinician as a structured interview (131). The more recent version is completely self-administered and has similar reliability and validity as the clinician-administered instrument (130). PHQ-9 is the self-administered mood module from PRIME-MD.

DOES SCREENING IMPROVE TREATMENT AND OUTCOMES?
Screening and Feedback Alone

Studies that have evaluated the effect of screening and feedback on the diagnosis of depression have generally found that it increases recognition of depression by PCPs by a factor of 2 to 3.4. The impact of this intervention on treatment and outcomes has been more questionable, however (**Table 1**).

Linn and Yager provided feedback on the results of the Zung Self-Rating Depression Scale taken by 74 new patients and found that although depression was more likely to be diagnosed in the feedback group (29% vs. 8%), the treatment rates were quite low in each group (13% vs. 8%) (27). Magruder-Habib et al screened Veterans Administration patients for depression and used the Diagnostic Interview Schedule (DIS) to establish a diagnosis of major depression (133). Providing diagnostic feedback on depressed patients led to an absolute difference in the rate of treatment between feedback and control groups of 24% at 6 weeks and 14% at 1 year.

Spitzer et al administered the self-administered version of PRIME-MD to 3000 patients (130). They identified 74 patients with a diagnosis of major depression that had not been previously recognized by their PCP. After diagnosis, however, only seven of these patients were treated with antidepressants by their PCP, and four were referred to a mental health specialist.

Table 2. **Screening and Feedback Plus Treatment Advice Studies**

Author/Year	Setting	Design	Interventions	Outcomes
Callahan/1994	Academic group practice: 103 residents and PCPs	Elderly patients randomized to intervention and control groups	Feedback of screening results and explicit treatment recommendations	Increased recognition and treatment in intervention patients, but no difference in outcomes
Rollman/2001	10 academic PCPs	Patients who screened positive for depression randomized to usual care with passive or active feedback	*Passive feedback*: PCP reminded of diagnosis at each visit; *active feedback*: PCP given treatment recommendations via electronic medical record	Neither active nor passive feedback led to treatment differences

Johnstone and Goldberg randomly assigned 119 patients with depression, diagnosed by the General Health Questionnaire, to immediate feedback of the GHQ results to the physician or to usual care (134). There was no difference between the groups in the mean GHQ scores at 12 months except for a subgroup of patients with severe depression, for whom feedback improved their scores. Dowrick studied 116 patients (who were initially not felt to be depressed) with Short Beck Depression Inventory scores administered by PCPs working in two English practices (135). Patients were randomly assigned to no feedback or to feedback that was given to providers 1 week after the visit. Rates of intention to treat were low but were marginally higher for the feedback group. Disclosure of cases of unrecognized depression had no effect on outcomes at 6- and 12-month follow-ups (136).

Reifler et al evaluated the SDDS and found that, compared with the control group, screened patients had a lower mean number of visits, but there were no other meaningful differences in outcomes (137). Lewis et al also evaluated the impact of providing feedback from both a screening and a diagnostic assessment (138). Patients randomized to the group, in which physicians received screening plus diagnostic feedback, were slightly less likely than controls to be depressed at 6 weeks (69% vs. 74%), but there was no difference in GHQ scores at 6 months. Providing only the screening scores did not improve any outcomes.

Williams found that screening with either a simple question or the 20-item CES-D did not affect treatment and had inconsistent impact on outcomes (129). Recovery from depression was more likely in the screened groups than in the usual care group (48% vs. 27%); however, there was no difference in patients mean improvement in depression symptoms.

Screening and Feedback Plus Treatment Advice

Two studies have added treatment recommendations to the feedback that physicians receive from feedback questionnaires (**Table 2**). Callahan et al studied elderly patients seen in an academic primary care setting (139). All physicians received an educational talk at baseline. Patients who scored higher than 14 on the Hamilton Depression scale were randomized to either a usual-care group or an intervention group in which providers received feedback from screening plus specific treatment recommendations regarding medications and follow-up. These investigators found that the intervention resulted in a modest increase in treatment but no difference in outcomes.

Rollman et al provided diagnostic feedback on all patients with depression seen in an academic group practice and treatment recommendations via electronic medical record on a randomized sample of these patients (140). The addition of the treatment recommendations did not increase the use of antidepressant medications.

Screening and Feedback with Integrated Interventions

Clearly, screening by itself has not been shown to consistently improve either treatment or outcomes. Only two studies have evaluated the impact of adding treatment recommendations to the feedback on the results of a screening questionnaire. Over the past 10 years, several other strategies have been evaluated (**Table 3**). The most basic approach is to screen for depression and refer patients who screen positive to an onsite mental health expert who assumes full responsibility for treating the patients' mental health disorder.

Several studies have specifically evaluated the use of structured protocols and trained clinicians to treat depression in the primary care setting. Schulberg et al showed that primary care patients with major depression who were randomized to receive either pharmacotherapy or psychotherapy from experts using a structured protocol experienced better outcomes than similar patients who received usual care for their depression from their PCPs (141). Mynors-Wallis et al also randomized primary care patients with major depression to a pharmacotherapy, psychotherapy (problem-solving therapy), or a medication placebo group (142). All treatments were administered in the patients' primary care office or home by trained clinicians using structured protocols. Again, the medication and psychotherapy treatments were shown to be more effective than placebo. Williams et al conducted a similar study involving elderly primary care patients with minor depression or dysthymia (143). Patients were randomized to receive an SSRI, problem-solving therapy, or placebo from trained clinicians using structured protocols. In this study, the SSRI group demonstrated moderate benefit versus placebo, but there was no difference between the problem-

Table 3. **Screening and Feedback Plus Integrated Intervention Studies**

Author/Year	Setting	Design	Intervention	Outcomes
Mynors-Wallis/1995	26 PCPs in England	Patients randomized to one of two intervention groups or drug placebo group	Structured treatments by trained providers involving problem-solving therapy, amitriptyline, or placebo	Problem-solving therapy resulted in greater symptom reduction than placebo; no difference between amitriptyline and problem-solving therapy outcomes
Katon/1995	HMO group practice: 22 PCPs	Patients randomized to intervention or control groups	Physician education; patient education booklets and videotapes; increased number and duration of visits; alternating visits with a psychiatrist; refill monitoring and feedback	Intervention resulted in more adequate antidepressant dosing and greater improvement in depression scores in patients with major (but not minor) depression
Katon/1996	HMO group practice: 22 PCPs	Patients randomized to intervention or control groups	Physician education, patient education booklets and videotape, patient seen 4 to 6 times by psychologist in primary care clinic to provide psychotherapy and assess medication adherence and outcomes, psychiatrists review each patient	Intervention resulted in greater adherence to pharmacotherapy and greater decrease in depression severity
Schulberg/1996	4 academically affiliated primary care clinics	Patients randomized to interpersonal therapy, nortriptyline, or usual-care groups	Structured treatments involving therapy or medication given in medical clinics by trained providers	Patients in interpersonal therapy and nortriptyline groups experienced greater symptom reduction than usual-care patients
Williams/2000	4 primary care practices	Patients randomized to problem-solving therapy, paroxetine, or placebo groups	Structured treatments in medical clinics by trained providers for elderly patients with dysthymia or minor depression	Paroxetine patients showed greater symptom resolution than placebo group; problem-solving therapy did not lead to consistent benefits compared with placebo
Whooley/2000	13 HMO primary care clinics	Clinics randomly assigned to intervention or control groups	Feedback of screening results; patients offered opportunity to participate in educational group sessions	No difference in process or outcome measures
Katzelnick/2000	163 PCP practices	Practices randomized to control or intervention group; high utilizers identified from HMO database and telephone screening for depression	Physician education; patient education materials; pharmacotherapy algorithm; telephone and database monitoring of adherence and response; case review by psychiatrist	Interventions resulted in increased use of antidepressants and greater improvement in depression and functional status scores
Simon/2000	5 PCP HMO practices	Patients who received new antidepressant prescriptions randomized to usual-care feedback only or to feedback and care management	Feedback recommendations based on pharmacy database, telephone monitoring of adherence and outcomes, and practice support	Feedback-only did not result in any improvements in treatment outcomes; feedback plus care management resulted in significant improvement in outcomes compared with usual care
Hunkeler/2000	2 HMO PCP practices	Depressed patients randomized to usual care, nurse telephone monitoring, or telephone monitoring plus peer support groups	Series of nurse telephone contacts to provide emotional support and focused behavioral interventions; series of phone contacts by trained patients who had recovered from depression	Nurse phone contacts with or without peer support improved outcomes up to 6 months
Wells/2000–2001	46 PCP practices	Practices randomized to usual care or one of two quality improvement programs	Local experts and nurses trained to provide clinician education, patient education, standardized assessment and treatment planning, medication adherence monitoring, and improved access to psychotherapy	Quality improvement patients were more likely to receive antidepressants or see a mental health specialist, and were more likely to recover at 6 and 12 months; these improvements were not sustained at the 2-year follow-up
Rost/2001	12 PCP practices	Practices randomized to intervention control groups	Physician and nurse education; screening and feedback; nurses used to assess, educate, and monitor adherence and outcomes	In untreated patients, intervention improved depression symptoms; no benefit seen for patients already receiving treatment

solving therapy and placebo groups. Taken together, these studies show that patients with depression can be effectively treated in the primary care setting by trained clinicians using evidence-based structured protocols. Dissemination of this type of intervention is hampered by a variety of factors, including complex health insurance arrangements that limit the PCP's ability to refer to a specific mental health provider, the availability of space in the primary care office, and the interest and availability of mental health specialists.

Other studies have focused on strategies to support the management of depression by PCPs. The types of interventions that have been evaluated either alone or in a variety of combinations include patient education, physician education, treatment recommendations by the use of algorithms or feedback from mental health specialists, and routine telephone support and monitoring of outcomes and adherence by care managers, usually nurses. In general, the more intervention strategies that are used, the greater is the effect on treatment and outcomes.

Whooley et al conducted a study in which elderly patients were randomized to a usual care group or to an intervention group, which consisted of feedback from the Geriatric Depression Scale and the opportunity to attend six weekly group patient education sessions, led by a nurse (144). There were no significant outcome differences in the two groups at follow-up 2 years later. Simon et al evaluated the impact of providing treatment recommendations and telephone support and monitoring of outcomes and adherence (care management) (145). Patients who received a new prescription for an antidepressant were randomized into a usual-care group, treatment recommendations, or treatment recommendation plus care management group. The investigators found that treatment recommendations alone were not effective, but combining treatment recommendations and care management improved outcomes at 3- and 6-month follow-ups.

Hunkeler et al conducted a similar study, which involved more frequent contacts by care managers, as well as telephone and in-person supportive contacts by trained health plan members who had recovered from depression (146). Patients who received a prescription for an antidepressant medication were randomized into usual care, care management, and care management plus peer-support groups. The study revealed that care management with or without peer support improved some outcomes at 6-week and 6-month follow-ups.

Rost (147), Katzelnick (148), Wells (149), and Katon (150, 151) have conducted studies that involved a more complex series of interventions. All studies resulted in improved outcomes for at least some patients. In most studies, this improvement was maintained for up to 12 months. Studies that featured a greater number of intervention strategies or greater intervention intensity resulted in the best outcomes. Even in these studies, however, long-term benefit was not clear. In one study, most of the improvements seen at 12 months were not sustained at the 2-year follow-up (152). In another study, improvements in the treatment of depression by PCPs were not maintained after the project had ended (153).

WHAT ARE THE COSTS AND RISKS OF SCREENING FOR DEPRESSION?

The direct cost of screening is estimated to be approximately $5 per patient, which includes the cost of producing the screening instrument, patient time required to complete the instrument, and nurse and physician time required to score it and assess the patient (154). This cost estimate assumes that a nurse will be largely responsible for assessing patients who screen positive. A major determinant of the overall cost of screening is the number of patients who screen positive and require further assessment. As noted above, in a practice with a 5% prevalence of major depression, for every 100 patients screened 31 will require further assessment, and of those only 4 will turn out to have major depression (117). The additional time needed to perform these assessments may interrupt patient flow and prevent physicians from providing other, possibly more beneficial, services.

Screening only makes sense if there are resources available to provide a thorough mental health evaluation, treatment recommendations, patient education, and monitoring of outcomes and patient adherence to medications. The cost of these resources may add as much as $300 to $600 per patient to the cost of care (155, 156). More modest but possibly less effective interventions, such as Rost's and Simon's, were found to add $73 and $80, respectively, per patient to the cost of care (145, 147).

One concern about screening is its potential to increase the number of patients who receive SSRIs who either do not need them or would benefit more from another form of treatment. To the extent that PCPs base treatment decisions primarily on the results of a depression screening instrument, many patients who would not meet criteria for clinical depression are likely to be treated with an SSRI. In addition, given the high rate of co-morbidity of depression with other psychiatric disorders (130, 131), such as mania, substance abuse, post-traumatic stress disorder, and eating disorders, some patients with depression who receive an SSRI should receive another form of therapy. The extent to which patients are being inappropriately treated with SSRIs is unknown, but it is likely to be substantial. From 1991 to 1997 the number of SSRIs prescribed by PCPs doubled (106). The cost of SSRI prescriptions continue to increase at a rate of 14% per year, and PCPs prescribe more than 70% of SSRIs in this country (107). It has been documented that in some populations the number of PCP prescriptions for SSRIs equals or exceeds the estimated prevalence of depression in those populations (2).

The inappropriate prescribing of SSRIs not only increases health care costs but exposes patients to an unnecessary risk of side effects from these medications. Wide-scale screening for depression is likely to increase this growing problem, unless adequate provisions are made to perform a thorough and accurate mental health evaluation and to promote evidence-based clinical decisions.

In addition to increasing the costs of treatment and the risk of side effects, screening for depression without performing a detailed mental health evaluation on those who screen positive can also lead to unnecessary labeling of patients who do not meet criteria for a mood disorder. The diagnoses of depression may be associated with stigma in the eyes of the patient and the general public. This may affect patients' thoughts about themselves, their functioning and quality of life, and their ability to get a job. The process of screening may also make physicians less vigilant for depression at visits where screening does not take place. They may believe that a patient who screened negative for depression 3 months or a year ago is not likely to be depressed now, even if there are symptoms suggestive of depression. Over-reliance on episodic screening evaluations may therefore decrease the rate of case findings at visits where screening does not take place.

Primary care physicians have expressed a reluctance to screen for depression, in part because of concerns about negative reaction from patients (157). How much of a problem this really is remains unclear.

Cost-Effectiveness Analyses

Several recent cost-effectiveness analyses have evaluated whether screening with or without additional integrated interventions warrants consideration. Valenstein et al looked at the cost-utility of screening for depression in primary care versus no screening using a Markov model (154). The target population was a hypothetical cohort of 40-year-old adults with an assumed prevalence of major depression of 8%. They estimated that the screening test would have a sensitivity and specificity for the detection of major depression of 84% and 85%, respectively, and that the cost of screening all patients and assessing those who screen positive would be $5 per patient. This estimate was based on a "team model" of primary care, with the physician spending 1 minute and a nurse devoting 6 minutes per patient. Computer-assisted screening instruments could reduce the cost to $3 per patient. They found that annual screening was cost-effective compared with no screening only when there was a high prevalence of major depression, very low screening costs, and implausibly high remission rates.

Screening every 3 to 5 years may be cost-effective but only in settings with integrated interventions, where screening can be done efficiently and high remission rates can be achieved. One-time-only screening may be cost effective in settings without integrated interventions, but this conclusion was tentative and highly dependent on model assumptions. One-time-only screening was more convincingly cost-effective if it was implemented in settings with integrated interventions, resulting in low screening costs and high but achievable remission rates. Only one-time-only screening consistently had a quality-adjusted life-years ratio of less than $50,000. This analysis did not take into consideration the increased risk of unnecessary or inappropriate treatment resulting from screening.

Using data on costs and effectiveness from the Wells trial, Schoenbaum et al calculated the cost-utility of a program that included one-time screening and a series of integrated interventions (158). Relative to usual care, the experimental intervention yielded additional benefits at a cost of $10,000 to $35000 per quality-adjusted life year gained. This analysis, however, did not take into consideration start-up costs associated with training clinicians and nurses, the development of materials used in the study, and the time involved in providing monthly audit and feedback to the clinic or clinicians. The cost of implementing this study was estimated to be $60,000 to $144,000 per practice, depending on the size of the practice.

In a similar analysis that used data obtained from Katzelnick's multi-component intervention, which included one-time screening, Simon et al found a cost per depression-free day gain of $51.84 (CI, $17.37 to $108.47) (159). This study focused on a high-risk population of high utilizers, however.

Although one-time-only screening may be cost effective, it may not be an optimal approach to a disorder like depression. One-time-only screening or long intervals between screening makes more sense for asymptomatic conditions where it may be possible to identify important precursors or risk factors at an early stage when treatment is more effective. Implementing such an approach for depression may miss many episodes after or in-between screenings and would over-select for chronic depressive disorders such as dysthymia. It may also discourage physicians from actively evaluating patients for depression during non-screening visits.

IMPLEMENTATION ISSUES

If screening for depression is to be undertaken, a variety of implementation issues must be addressed. First, should all patients be screened or just those with risk factors or presentations suggestive of an increased risk of depression? Screening only higher-risk patients would increase its positive predictive value but would also increase the number of cases of depression that go undetected. Second, how often should patients be screened? The Valenstein study suggests that it may be cost effective to screen for depression once but not annually or more often (154). Screening only once, however, will not have much impact on the overall recognition and outcomes of depression. Third, who should administer the screening test, score it, and present it to the physician? The studies that have effectively implemented depression screening have used research assistants or support staff in the doctor's office to perform these functions (160). Fourth, if depression screening is to be implemented, what other screening measures should be included? Psychiatric co-morbidities are common and can affect management decisions (130, 131). Screening tests are available, and arguments have been made for screening for other mental health problems, such as domestic violence, panic disorder, and substance abuse, but the cost and benefits of screening for other psychiatric disorders in addition to depression has not been well documented.

Finally, who should pay for the increased costs associated with the screening and management of depression? The U.S. Preventive Task force has recommended screening for depression only when there are systems in place to ensure accurate diagnoses, effective treatment, and follow-up (3). These types of systems are expensive because they typically involve the use of care managers, input from mental health specialists, and physician, staff, and patient education. They have usually been supported by grant funding but, when the grants end, the disease management systems usually end as well. Because of the cost and resources required, these systems have not been widely disseminated outside of the research settings in which they were developed (161). Tools have been developed to facilitate the implementation of these systems in a physician's office (162). Automated depression management systems have also been developed, which can increase their availability and reduce their costs (163). It is not reasonable to expect PCPs to shoulder the burden of the expense associated with the implementation of these systems. Health insurance companies or health care systems may be willing to pay for them if they can be consistently shown to reduce costs or improve outcomes.

CONCLUSIONS

There is no right or wrong answer to the issue of screening for depression in primary care. The value of screening will depend on a number of factors, including 1) the prevalence of depression in the population that is being screened, 2) the physician's ability to identify depression without the systematic use of a screening instrument, and 3) the capability of the physician to effectively use depression screening tools, manage depression, monitor outcomes, and motivate and educate patients to accept the diagnoses of depression and to adhere to its treatment.

Various thresholds can be used to determine which patients to screen. These might include all patients, all new patients, patients with known risk factors for depression (e.g., past history or family history of depression, serious chronic diseases), or patients with a common presentation of depression (e.g., multiple somatic symptoms, vague complaints such as fatigue). As the threshold increases, there will be fewer false-positives, and screening will become more cost-effective, but an increasing number of patients with depression will be missed. How many is un-

clear. Further research is needed to evaluate the impact of different sets of criteria for selective screening.

Serious consideration should be given to using screening instruments that can evaluate a variety of common psychiatric disorders. Psychiatric co-morbidity is extremely common and can affect the management of depression. Multi-disorder instruments such as PRIME-MD have found that at least one third of patients with mental disorders will have an anxiety disorder, eating disorder, or probable drug or alcohol abuse, in the absence of a mood disorder, and 65% of patients with a mood disorder will also have one or more of these additional mental health problems (131). Screening only for depression can therefore miss serious mental health disorders or lead to inappropriate types of treatment.

Physicians who decide to screen must be prepared to evaluate, diagnose, manage, closely follow, and educate patients who screen positive. Some interested and well-trained physicians may be able to do all of this on their own, but most will not. If we are to truly improve the recognition, management, and outcomes of depression in primary care, health care systems, and health insurance companies will need to work with PCPs to implement well-organized systems of care to accomplish these tasks.

References

1. **Gilbody SM, House AO, Sheldon TA.** Routinely administered questionnaires for depression and anxiety: systematic review. Br Med J. 2001;322:406-9.

2. **Coyne JC, Thompson R, Palmer SC, et al.** Appl Prev Psychol. 2000;9:101-21.

3. **U.S. Preventive Services Task Force.** Screening for depression: recommendations and rationale. Ann Intern Med. 2002;136:760-4.

4. **Pignone MP, Gaynes BN, Rushton JL et al.** Screening for depression in adults: a summary of the evidence for the U.S. Preventive Services Task Force. Ann Intern Med. 2002;136:765-76

5. **Miranda J, Hohmann AA, Attkisson CC.** Epidemiology of mental disorders in primary care. San Francisco: Jossey-Bass; 1994:3-15.

6. **Depression Guideline Panel.** Guideline: Overview of Mood Disorders. Rockville, MD: AHCPR; 1993:17-40

7. **American Psychiatric Association.** Diagnostic and Statistical Manual of Mental Disorders, 4th ed. Washington, DC: 1994.

8. **Kessler RC, McGonagle KA, Zhao S, et al.** Lifetime and 12-month prevalence of psychiatric disorders in the United States: results from the National Comorbidity Survey. Arch Gen Psychiatry. 1994;51:8-19

9. **Wells K, Sturn R, Sherbourne C, Meredith L.** Caring for Depression. Cambridge, MA: Harvard University Press; 1996.

10. **Brody DS, Larson DB.** The role of PCPs in managing depression. J Gen Intern Med. 1992;7:243-7.

11. **Spitzer RL, Williams JB, Kroenke K, et al.** Utility of a new procedure for diagnosing mental disorders in primary care: the PRIME-MD 1000 study. JAMA. 1994;272:1749-56.

12. **Moore JD, Bona JR.** Depression and dysthymia. Med Clin North Am. 2001;85:631-44.

13. **Beck DA, Koenig HG.** Minor depression: a review of the literature. Int J Psychiatry Med. 1996;26:177-209.

14. **Crum RM, Cooper-Patrick L, Ford DE.** Depressive symptoms among general medicine patients: prevalence and one-year outcome. Psychosom Med. 1994; 56:109-17

15. **Pincus HA, Davis WW, McQueen LE.** "Subthreshold" mental disorders: a review and synthesis of studies on minor depression and other "brand names."

Br J Psychiatry. 1999;174:288-96.

16. Januzzi J, Stern T, Pasternak R, DeSanctis R. The influence of anxiety and depression on outcomes of patients with coronary artery disease. Arch Intern Med. 2000;160:1913-21.

17. Gavard JA, Lustman PJ, Clouse PE. Prevalence of depression in adults with diabetes: an epidemiologic evaluation. Diabetes Care. 1992;16:1167-78.

18. Lustman P, Clouse R, Freedland K. Management of depression in adults with diabetes: implications of recent trials. Semin Clin Neuropsychol. 1998;3: 102-14.

19. Schubert D, Taylor C, Lee S, et al. Physical consequences of depression in the stroke patient. Gen Hosp Psychiatry. 1992;14:69-76.

20. Sutor B, Rummans T, Jowsey S, et al. Major depression in medically ill patients. Mayo Clin Proc. 1998;73:329-37.

21. McDaniel J, Musselman D, Porter M, et al. Depression in patients with cancer: diagnosis, biology, and treatment. Arch Gen Psychiatry. 1995;52:89-99.

22. Rovner B. Depression and increased risk of mortality in the nursing home patient. Am J Med. 1993;94:19S-23S.

23. NIH Consensus Conference. Diagnosis and treatment of depression in late life. JAMA 1992;268:1018-24.

24. Judd L, Akishal H, Maser J, et.al. A prospective 12-year study of subsyndromal and syndromal depressive symptoms in unipolar major depressive disorders. Arch Gen Psychiatry. 1998;55:694-700.

25. Rost K, Zhang M, Fortney J, et al. Persistently poor outcomes of undetected major depression in primary care. Gen Hosp Psychiatry. 1998;20:12-20.

26. Coryell W, Endicott J, Winokur, et al. Characteristics and significance of untreated major depressive disorder. Am J Psychiatry. 1995;152:1124-9.

27. Linn LS, Yager J. The effect of screening, sensitization, and feedback on notation of depression. J Med Edu. 1980;55:942-9.

28. Ormel J, Koeter MWJ, van den Brink W, et al. Recognition, management, and course of anxiety and depression in general practice. Arch Gen Psychiatry. 1991;48:700-6.

29. Simon GE, Von Korff M. Recognition, management, and outcomes of depression in primary care. Arch Fam Med. 1995;4:99-105.

30. Coryell W, Akiskal H, S, Leon AC, et al. The time course of non-chronic major depressive disorder: uniformity across episodes and samples. National Institute of Mental Health Collaborative Program on the Psychobiology of Depression: Clinical Studies. Arch Gen Psychiatry. 1994;51:405-10.

31. Tiemens BG, Ormel, J, Simon GE. Occurrence, recognition, and outcome of psychological disorders in primary care. Am J Psychiatry. 1996;133:636-4.

32. Coyne JC, Schwenk TL, Fechner-Bates S. Non-detection of depression by PCPs reconsidered. Gen Hosp Psychiatry. 1995;17:3-12.

33. Greenberg PE, Stiglin LE, Finkelstein SN, Berndt ER. The economic burden of depression in 1990. J Clin Psychiatry. 1993;54:405-18.

34. Regier D, Hirschfeld M, Goodwin F, et al. The NIMH depression awareness, recognition, and treatment program: structure, aims and scientific basis. Am J Psychiatry. 1988;145:1351-7.

35. Manning W, Wells K. The effect of psychological distress and psychological well being on use of medical services. Med Care. 1992;30:541-53.

36. Simon G, Ormel J, Von Korff M, et al. Health care costs associated with depression and anxiety disorders in primary care. Am J Psychiatry. 1995;152: 352-7.

37. Kleinman A, Cohen A. Psychiatry's global challenge. Sci Am. 1997;3:86-9.

38. Wells K, Steward A, Hays R, et al. The functioning and well-being of depressed patients: results from the medical outcomes study. JAMA. 1989;262: 914-9.

39. Broadhead W, Balazer D, George L, Tse C. Depression, diability days, and days lost from work in a prospective epidemiologic survey. JAMA. 1990;264: 2524-8.

40. Kathol R, Wenzel R. Natural history of symptoms of depression and anxtiety during inpatient treatment on general medicine wards. J Gen Intern Med. 1992; 7:287-93.

41. Fulop G, Strain J, Fahs M, et al. Medical disorders associated with psychiatric comorbidity and prolonged hospital stay. Hosp Comm Psychiatry. 1989;40: 80-2.

42. Keitner G, Ryan C, Miller I, et al. Twelve-month outcome of patients with major depression and comorbid psychiatric or medical illness (compound depres-

sion). Am J Psychiatry. 1991;148:345-50.

43. Saravay S, Steinberg M, Weinschel B, et al. Psychological comorbidity and length of stay in the general hospital. Am J Psychiatry. 1991;148:324-9.

44. Spitzer RL, Kroenke K, Linzer M, et al. Health-related quality of life in primary care patients with mental disorders. JAMA. 1995;274:1511-7.

45. Murray CJ, Lopez AD, Jamison DT. The global burden of disease in 1990: summary results, sensitivity analysis, and future directions. Bull WHO. 1994;72: 495-509.

46. Murray CJ, Lopez AD. Evidence-based health policy: lessons from the Global Burden of Disease Study. Science. 1996;274:740-3.

47. Wells KB, Burnam MA, Rogers W, et al. The course of depression in adult outpatients: results from the Medical Outcomes Study. Arch Gen Psychiatry. 1992;49:788-94.

48. Hays RD, Wells KB, Sherbourne CD, et al. Functioning and well-being outcomes of patients with depression compared with chronic general medical illnesses. Arch Gen Psychiatry. 1995;52:11-9.

49. MoScicki EK. Identification of suicide risk factors using epidemiologic studies. Psychiatr Clin North Am. 1997;20:499-517.

50. Hirschfield RM, Russell JM. Assessment and treatment of suicidal patients. New Engl J Med. 1997;337:910-6.

51. Rich CI, Runeson BS. Similarities in diagnostic comorbidity between suicide among young people in Sweden and the United States. Acta Psychiatr Scand. 1992;86:335-9.

52. Olfson M, Weissman MM, Leon AC, et al. Suicidal ideation in primary care. J Gen Intern Med. 1996;11:447-53.

53. Fawcett J, Scheftner WA, Fogg L, et al. Time-related predictors of suicide in major affective disorder. Am J Psychiatry. 1990;147:1189-94.

54. Mortensen PB, Agerbo E, Erickson T, et al. Psychiatric illness and risk factors for suicide in Denmark. Lancet. 2000;355:9-12.

55. Wulsin L. Does depression kill? Arch Intern Med. 2000;160:1731-2.

56. Schulz R, Beach S, Ives D, et al. Association between depression and mortality in older adults. Arch Intern Med. 2000;160:1761-8.

57. Barefoot J, Scroll M. Symptoms of depression, acute myocardial infarction, and total mortality in a community sample. Circulation. 1996;93:1976-80.

58. Bruce M, Leaf P. Psychiatric disorders and 15-month mortality in a community sample of older adults. Am J Public Health. 1989;79:727-30.

59. Anda R, Williamson D, Jones D, et al. Depressed affect, hopelessness, and the risk of ischemic heart disease in a cohort of US adults. Epidemiology. 1993; 4:285-94.

60. Frasure-Smith N, Lesperance F, Talajic M. Depression following myocardial infarction: impact on 6-month survival. JAMA. 1993;270:1819-25.

61. Frasure-Smith N, Lesperance F, Talajic M. Depression and 18-month prognosis after myocardial infarction. Circulation. 1995;91:999-1005.

62. Lesperance F, Frasure-Smith N, Juneau M, Theroux P. Depression and 1-year prognosis in unstable angina. Arch Intern Med. 2000;160:1354-60.

63. de Groot M, Anderson R, Freedland KE, et al. Association of depression and diabetes complications: a meta-analysis. Psychosom Med. 2001;63:619-30.

64. Wai L, Burton H, Richmond J, et al. Influence of psychological factors on survival of home dialysis patients. Lancet. 1981;2:1155-6.

65. Drossman D, McKee D, Sandler R, et al. Psychosocial factors in the irritable bowel syndrome: a multivariate study of patients and nonpatients with irritable bowel syndrome. Gastroenterology. 1988;95:701-8.

66. Rovner B, German P, Brant L, et al. Depression and mortality in nursing homes. JAMA. 1991;265:993-6.

67. Rodin G, Voshart K. Depressive symptoms and functional impairment in the medically ill. Gen Hosp Psychiatry. 1987;9:251-8.

68. DiMatteo M, Lepper H, Croghan T. Depression is a risk factor for non-compliance with medical treatment: meta-analysis of the effects of anxiety and depression on patient compliance. Arch Intern Med. 2000;160:2101-7.

69. Ziegelstein R, Fauerbach J, Stevens S, et al. Patients with depression are less likely to follow recommendations to reduce cardiac risk during recovery from myocardial infarction. Arch Intern Med. 2000;160:1818-23.

70. Carney R, Freeland K, Rich M, Jaffe A. Depression as a risk factor for cardiac events in established coronary heart disease: review of possible mechanisms. Ann Behav Med. 1995;17:142-9.

71. Carney R, Freeland K, Eisen S, et al. Major depression and medication

adherence in elderly patients with coronary artery disease. Health Psychol. 1995; 14:88-90.

72. **Guiry E, Conroy R, Hickey N, Mulkahy R.** Psychological responses to an acute coronary event and its effect on subsequent rehabilitation and lifestyle change. Clin Cardiol. 1987;10:256-60.

73. **Blumenthal J, Williams RS, Wallace AG, et al.** Physiological and psychological variables predict compliance to prescribed exercise therapy in patients recovering from myocardial infarction. Psychosom Med. 1982;44:519-27.

74. **Bosley C, Fosbury J, Cochrane G.** The psychological factors associated with poor compliance with treatment in asthma. Eur Respir J. 1995;8:899-904.

75. **Bosley C, Corden Z, Rees P, Chochrane G.** Psychological factors associated with use of home nebulized therapy for COPD. Eur Respir J. 1996;9:2346-50.

76. **Singh N, Squier C, Sivek C, et al.** Determinants of compliance with antiretroviral therapy in patients with human immunodeficiency virus: prospective assessment with implications for enhancing compliance. AIDS Care. 1996;8: 261-9.

77. **Mohr D, Goodkin D, Likosky W, et al.** Treatment of depression improves adherence to interferon beta-1b therapy for multiple sclerosis. Arch Neurol. 1997; 54:531-3.

78. **Brownbridge B, Fielding D.** An investigation of psychological factors influencing adherence to medical regime in children and adolescents undergoing hemodialysis and CAPD. Int J Adolesc Med Health. 1989;4:7-18.

79. **De-Nour A, Czaczkes J.** The influence of patient's personality on adjustment to chronic dialysis. J Nerv Ment Dis. 1976;162:323-33.

80. **Gilbar O, De-Nour A.** Adjustment to illness and dropout of chemotherapy. J Psychosom Res. 1989;33:1-5.

81. **Katz R, Ashmore J, Barboa E, et al.** Knowledge of disease and dietary compliance in patients with end-stage renal disease. Psychol Rep. 1998;82:331-336.

82. **Kiley D, Lam C, Pollak R.** A study of treatment compliance following kidney transplantation. Transplantation. 1993;55:51-6.

83. **Lebovits A, Strain J, Schleifer S, et al.** Patient noncompliance with self-administered chemotherapy. Cancer. 1990;65:17-22.

84. **Rodriguez A, Diaz M, Colon A, Santiago-Delpin E.** Psychosocial profile of noncompliant transplant patients. Transplant Proc. 1991;23:1807-9.

85. **Schneider M, Friend R, Whitaker P, Wadhwa N.** Fluid noncompliance and symptomatology in end-stage renal disease: cognitive and emotional variables. Health Psychol. 1991;10:209-15.

86. **Taal E, Rasker J, Seydel E, Weigman O.** Health status, adherence with health recomendations, self-efficacy, and social support in patients with rhematoid arthritis. Patient Educ Counsel. 1993;20:63-76.

87. **Lustman PJ, Griffith LS, Freedland KE, et al.** Cognitive behavior therapy for depression in type 2 diabetes mellitus: a randomized controlled trial. Ann Intern Med. 1998;129:613-21.

88. **Blumenthal JA, Jiang W, Babyak MA, et al.** Stress management and exercise training in cardiac patients with myocardial ischemia: effects on prognosis and evaluation of mechanisms. Arch Intern Med. 1997;157:2213-23.

89. **Frasure-Smith N.** In-hospital symptoms of psychological stress as predictors of long-term outcome after acute myocardial infarction in men. Am J Cardiol. 1991;67:121-7.

90. **Frasure-Smith N, Lesperance F, Prince RH, et al.** Randomized trial of home-based psychosocial nursing intervention for patients recovering from myocardial infarction. Lancet. 1997;350:473-9.

91. **Glassman AH, O'Connor CM, Califf RM, et al.** Sertraline treatment of major depression in patients with acute MI or unstable angina. JAMA. 2002;288: 701-9

92. **Williams JW, Mulrow CD, Chiquette E, et al.** A systematic review of newer pharmacotherapies for depression in adults: evidence report summary. Ann Intern Med. 2000;132:743-56.

93. **Mulrow CD, Williams JWJ, Chiquette E.** et al. Efficacy of newer pharmacotherapies for treating depression in primary care patients. Am J Med. 2000; 108:54-64.

94. **Kroenke K, West SL, Swindle R, et al.** Similar effectiveness of paroxetine, fluoxetine, and sertraline in primary care. JAMA. 2001;286:2947-55.

95. **Simon G.** Choosing a first-line antidepressant: equal on average does not mean equal for everyone. JAMA. 2001;286:3003-4.

96. **Dunn RL, Donoghue JM, Ozminkowski RJ, et al.** Longitudinal patterns of antidepressant prescribing in primary care in the UK: comparison with treatment guidelines. J Psychopharmacol. 1999;13:136-43.

97. **Lin E, VonKorff M, Katon W, et al.** The role of PCPs in patient adherence to antidepressant therapy. Med Care. 1995;33:67.

98. **Keller KB, Klerman GL, Lavor PW, et al.** Treatment received by depressed patients. JAMA. 1983;246:1848.

99. **Katon W, VonKorff M, Lin E, et al.** Adequacy and duration of antidepressant treatment in primary care. Med Care. 1992;30:67.

100. **Simon G, VonKorff M, Wagner EH, et al.** Patterns of antidepressant use in community practice. Gen Hosp Psychiatry. 1993;15:399.

101. **Katon W, Lin E, VonKorff M, et al.** The predictors of persistence of depression in primary care. J Affective Disord. 1994;31:81.

102. **Ormel J, Van Den Brink W, Koeter MWJ, et al.** Recognition management and outcome of psychological disorders in primary care: a naturalistic study. Psychological Med. 1990;20:909-23.

103. **Brugha R, Bebbington PE, MacCarthy B, et al.** Antidepressants may not assist recovery in practice: a naturalistic prospective survey. Acta Psychiatr Scand. 1992;86:5-11.

104. **Coyne JC, Palmer SC, Thompson R.** Routine screening entails additional pitfalls. Br Med J. 2001;323:167.

105. **Pini S, Perkonnig A, Tansella M, et al.** Prevalence and 12 month outcome of threshold and sub-threshold mental disorders in primary care. J Affect Dis.1999;56:37-48

106. **Hirshfield RM.** American health care systems and depression: the past, present, and the future. J Clin Psychiatry. 1998;59(Suppl 20):5-10.

107. **Hoechst MR.** HMO Pharmacy Summary. Managed Care Digest. 1999; 3:7.

108. **Coyne JC, Thompson R, Klinkman MS, et al.** Emotional disorders in primary care. J Consulting Clin Psychol. 2002;70:798-809.

109. **Perez-Stable EJ, Miranda J, Munoz RF, et al.** Depression in medical outpatients: under-recognition and misdiagnosis. Arch Intern Med. 1990;150: 1083-8.

110. **Von Korff M, Shapiro S, Burke JD, et al.** Anxiety and depression in primary care clinic: comparison of diagnostic interview schedule, general health questionnaire, and practitioner assessments. Arch Gen Psychiatry. 1987;44: 152-6.

111. **Neilsen AC, Williams TA.** Depression in ambulatory medical patients: prevalence by self-report questionnaire and recognition by non-psychiatric physicians. Arch Gen Psychiatry. 1980;37:999-1004.

112. **Thompson TL, Stoudemire A, Mitchell WD, et al.** Under-recognition of patients' psychosocial distress in a university hospital medical clinic. Am J Psychiatr. 1983;140:158-61.

113. **Kroenke K.** Depression screening is not enough. Ann Intern Med. 2001; 134:418-20.

114. **Simon GE, Goldberg D, Tiemens BG, et al.** Outcomes of recognized and unrecognized depression in an international primary care study. Gen Hosp Psychiatry. 1999;21:97-105.

115. **Rost K, Smith R, Matthews DB, et al.** The deliberate misdiagnosis of major depression in primary care. Arch Fam Med. 1994;3:333-7.

116. **Pirraglia PA, Stafford RS, Singer DE.** National trends in depression diagnosis and antidepressant use in primary care. J Gen Intern Med. 2002;17:208.

117. **Mulrow CD, Williams JWJ, Gerety MB, et al.** Case-finding instruments for depression in primary care settings. Ann Intern Med. 1995;122:913-21.

118. **Beck AT, Beck RW.** Screening depressed patients in family practice: a rapid technique. Postgrad Med. 1972;52:81-5.

119. **Beck AT, Rial WY, Rickels K.** Short form of depression inventory: cross-validation. Psychol Rep. 1974;34:1184-6.

120. **Zung WWK.** A self-rating depression scale. Arch Gen Psychiatry. 1965;12: 63-70.

121. **Kirmayer LJ, Robbins JM, Dworkind M, et al.** Somatization and the recognition of depression and anxiety in primary care. Am J Psychiatry. 1993; 150:734-41.

122. **Worsley A, Gribbin CC.** A factor analytic study of the twelve-item general health questionnaire. Aust N Z J Psychiatry. 1977;11:269-72.

123. **Goldberg DP, Hillier VF.** A scaled version of the General Health Ques-

tionnaire. Psychol Med. 1979;9:139-45.

124. **Tarnopolksy A, Hand DJ, McLean EK, et al.** Validity and uses of a screening questionnaire (GHQ) in the community. Br J Psych. 1979;134:508-15.

125. **Hough R, Landsverk J, Stone J, et al.** Comparison of Psychiatric Screening Questionnaires for Primary Care Patients. National Institute of Mental Health. 1983. Final report for NIMH Contract 278-81.

126. **Schmitz N, Kruse J, Heckrath C, et al.** Diagnosing mental disorders in primary care: the General Health Questionnaire (GHQ) and the symptom check list (SCL- 90-R) as screening instruments. Soc Psychiatry Psychiatr Epidemiol. 1999;43:360-6.

127. **Kroenke K, Spitzer RL, Williams JB.** The PHQ-9: validity of a brief depression severity measure. J Gen Intern Med. 2001;16:606-13.

128. **Whooley M, Avins A, Miranda J, Browner W.** Case-finding instruments for depression: two questions are as good as many. J Gen Intern Med. 1997;12:439-45.

129. **Williams JWJ, Mulrow CD, Kroenke K, et al.** Case-finding for depression in primary care: a randomized trial. Am J Med. 1999;106:46-3.

130. **Spitzer RL, Kroenke K, Williams JBW, et al.** Validation and utility of a self-report version of PRIME-MD, the PHQ primary care study. JAMA. 1999; 282:1737-44.

131. **Spitzer RL, Williams JB, Kroenke K, et al.** Utility of a new procedure for diagnosing mental disorders in primary care: the PRIME-MD 1000 study. JAMA. 1994;272:1749-56.

132. **Broadhead WE, Leon AC, Weissman MM, et al.** Development and validation of the SDDS-PC screen for multiple mental disorders in primary care. Arch Fam Med. 1995;4:211-9.

133. **Magruder-Habib K, Zung WWK, et al.** Improving physicians' recognition and treatment of depression in general medical care. Results from a randomized clinical trial. Med Care. 1990;28:239-50.

134. **Johnstone A, Goldberg D.** Psychiatric screening in general practice: a controlled trial. Lancet. 1976;1:605-8.

135. **Dowrick C.** Does testing for depression influence diagnosis or management by general practitioners? Fam Pract. 1995;12:461-5.

136. **Dowrick C, Buchan I.** Twelve-month outcome of depression in general practice: does detection or disclosure make a difference? Br Med J. 1995;311:1274-6.

137. **Reifler DR, Kessler HS, Bernhard EJ, et al.** Impact of screening for mental health concerns on health service utilization and functional status in primary care patients. Arch Intern Med. 1996;156:2593-9.

138. **Lewis G, Sharp D, Bartholomew J, et al.** Computerized assessment of common mental disorders in primary care: effect on clinical outcomes. Fam Pract. 1996;13:120-6.

139. **Callahan CM, Hendrei HC, Dittus RS, et al.** Improving treatment of late life depression in primary care: a randomized clinical trial. J Am Geriatr Soc. 1994;42:839-46.

140. **Rollman B, Hanusa B, Gilbert T, et al.** The electronic medical record. Arch Intern Med. 2001;161:189-97.

141. **Schulberg HC, Bock MR, Madonia MJ.** Treating major depression in primary care practice: eight month clinical outcomes. Arch Gen Psychiatry. 1997; 53:913-9.

142. **Mynors-Wallis LM, Gath DH, Lloyd-Thomas AR, et al.** Randomized controlled trial comparing problem solving treatment with amitriptyline and placebo for major depression in primary care. Br Med J. 1995;310:441-5.

143. **Williams JW, Barrett J, Oxman T, et al.** Treatment of dysthymia and minor depression in primary care: a randomized controlled trial in older adults. JAMA. 2000;284:1519-26.

144. **Whooley MA, Stone B, Soghikian K.** Randomized trial of case-finding for depression in elderly primary care patients. J Gen Intern Med. 2000;15:293-300.

145. **Simon GE, VonKorff M, Rutter C, et al.** Randomized trial of monitoring, feedback, and management of care by telephone to improve treatment of depression in primary care. Br Med J. 2000;320:550-4.

146. **Hunkeler EM, Meresman JF, Hargreaves WA, Fireman B, et al.** Efficacy of nurse telehealth care and peer support in augmenting treatment of depression in primary care. Arch Fam Med. 2000;9:700-8.

147. **Rost K, Nutting P, Smith J, et al.** Improving depression outcomes in community primary care practice: a randomized trial of the Quest intervention. J Gen Intern Med. 2001;16:143-9.

148. **Katzelnick DJ, Simon GE, Pearson SD, et al.** Randomized trial of a depression management program in high utilizers of medical care. Arch Fam Med. 2000;9:345-51.

149. **Wells K, Sherbourne C, Schoenbaum M.** Impact of disseminating quality improvement programs in managed primary care: a randomized controlled trial. JAMA. 2000;283:212-20.

150. **Katon W, Von Korff M, Lin E, et al.** Collaborative management to achieve treatment guidelines. Impact on depression in primary care. JAMA. 1995;273:1026-31.

151. **Katon W, Robinson P, Von Korff M, et al.** A multifaceted intervention to improve treatment of depression primary care. Arch Gen Psychiatry. 1996;53:924-32.

152. **Sherbourne CD, Wells KB, Duan N, et al.** Long-term effectiveness of disseminating quality improvement for depression in primary care. Arch Gen Psychiatry. 2001;58:696-703.

153. **Lin EH, Katon WJ, Simon GE, et al.** Achieving guidelines for the treatment of depression in primary care. Med Care. 1997;35:831-42.

154. **Valenstein M, Vijan S, Zeber JE, et al.** The cost-utility of screening for depression in primary care. Ann Intern Med. 2001;134:345-60.

155. **Lave J, Frank R, Schulberg H, et al.** Cost-effectiveness of treatments for major depression in primary care practice. Arch Gen Psychiatry. 1998; 55:645-51

156. **VonKorff M, Katon W, Bush T, et al.** Treatment costs, cost offset, and cost- effectiveness of collaborative management of depression. Psychosom Med. 1998;60:143-9

157. **Solberg LI, Korsen N, Oxman TE, et al.** The need for a system in the care of depression. J Fam Pract. 1999;48:973-9.

158. **Schoenbaum M, Jurgen U, Sherbourne C, et al.** Cost-effectiveness of practice-initiated quality improvement for depression. JAMA. 2001;286:1325-30.

159. **Simon GE, Manning WG, Katzelnick DJ, et al.** Cost-effectiveness of systematic depression treatment for high utilizers of general medical care. Arch Gen Psychiatry. 2001;58:181-7.

160. **Valenstein M, Dalack G, Blow F, et al.** Screening for psychiatric illness with combined screening and diagnostic instrument. J Gen Intern Med. 1997; 12:679-85.

161. **Rubenstein IB, Jackson-Triche M, et al.** Evidence-based care for depression in managed primary care practices. Health Aff. 1999;18:89-105.

162. **Brody, DS, Dietrich AJ, DeGruy F, Kroenke K.** Depression in primary care tool kit. Int J Psychiatry Med. 2000;30:99-110.

163. **Gray GV, Brody DS.** Automating psychiatric tasks: taking quality to the next level. Disease Management Managed Care Interface. Oct. 2001;65-9.

Selected Preventive Services for Adults*

Service	Age	USPSTF Endorsed	Recommended Frequency	Comments
Blood Pressure	All	Yes (1996)	2 years	More frequent testing recommended if initial BP ≥130/87.
Height and Weight	All	Yes (1996)	Periodically	Recommend calculating BMI: Wt (kg)/Ht (m) 2 (squared) or [Wt (lbs) x 703]/Ht (inches) 2.
Cholesterol (Total and HDL)	≥ 35-65 (men) ≥ 45 (women)	Yes (2001)	Variable	Screening can begin at age 20 in men and women who have risk factors for CAD (DM, fam. hy, smokers, HTN). Screening can stop at age 65 in previously screened individuals, repeated screening in those over 65 is less important.
Colorectal cancer Screening	≥50	Yes (2002)	Yearly	Average risk individuals (endorsed by USPSTF and American College Gastroenterology (ACG) **screening strategies** **Colonoscopy** every 10 yrs (preferred as primary strategy by ACG and offered as alternative by USPSTF). **Flexible sigmoidoscopy** every 5 years along with annual fecal occult blood testing (endorsed by USPSTF and offered as secondary strategy by ACG). **Double contrast barium enema** every 5-10 years (offered as an alternative along with fecal occult blood testing by ACG and as alternative by USPSTF). High risk individuals (Family history of colorectal cancer) a. If first degree relative >60 years of age , begin screening at age 40 and evaluate with colonscopy every 10 years (ACG endorsed). b. If first degree relative <60 years of age, begin screening at age 40 OR10 yrs younger than age of youngest affected relative whichever is first (ACG endorsed). Patients with family history of inflammatory bowel disease and personal hx of polyps are **surveillance** patients and not included in the screening recommendations.
Papanicolaou Test/Pelvic Exam (women)	≥ 18 or first sexual intercourse (women)	Yes (2002)	Variable	Pap smear beginning within 3 years of onset of sexual activity or age 21 (whichever comes first) and continuing every 3 years, and more frequently in high-risk patients (prior cervical or vaginal cancer, history of STDs, intercourse < age 16, 5+ sexual partners, and if mother took DES during pregnancy). Pelvic exams independent of Pap smears are of uncertain efficacy in reducing mortality in gynecological cancers. The USPSTF recommends: **against** routinely screening women older than age 65 for cervical cancer if they have had adequate recent screening with normal Pap smears and are not otherwise at high risk for cervical cancer. **against** routine Pap smear screening in women who have had a total hysterectomy for benign disease. The USPSTF concludes that: **the evidence** is insufficient to recommend for or against the routine use of new technologies to screen for cervical cancer. **the evidence** is insufficient to recommend for or against the routine use of human papilloma virus (HPV) testing as a primary screening test for cervical cancer.
Breast Exam/ Mammography	>40 (women)	Yes (2002)	1-2 years	The USPSTF recommends screening mammography, with or without clinical breast examination (CBE), every 1-2 years for women aged 40 and older. The USPSTF concludes that: **the evidence** is insufficient to recommend for or against routine CBE alone to screen for breast cancer. **the evidence** is insufficient to recommend for or against teaching or performing routine breast self-examination (BSE).

*Adapted from the 2004 Pocket Guide to Selected Preventive Services for Adults produced by the ACP Young Physicians Subcommittee.

Digital Rectal Exam/PSA	≥ 50 (men) (ACS)	No (2002)	Yearly	Recommended yearly by ACS. Long-term mortality benefits of PSA and DRE uncertain; testing and frequency at discretion of physician and patient. Consider screening age ≥ 40 in African Americans due to higher prevalence. ACP does not endorse PSA or DRE for routine prostate cancer screening.
Bone Densitometry	Variable (AACE)	Yes (2002)	Variable (AACE)	Recommended by American Association of Clinical Endocrinologists for women in estrogen deficient states and patients with radiographic osteopenia, hyperparathyroidism, vertebral fractures, or on high-dose glucocorticoids and/or osteoporosis medication. USPSTF recommends routine screening in women aged 65 or older.
Vision and hearing assessment	≥ 65	Yes (1996)	Periodically	
Rubella	Childbearing age (women)	Yes (1996)	Once	Screening for rubella can be done by history of vaccination or by serology.
PPD	All	Yes (1996)	Variable	Recommended for asymptomatic patients with HIV, contacts of patients with known TB, and populations with high TB prevalence.
RPR/VRDL	Variable	Yes (1996)	Variable	Recommended for all pregnant women, prostitutes, STD patients, and contacts with infected persons.
HIV	Variable	Yes (1996)	Variable	Recommended for STD patients, homosexual men, IV drug users, prostitutes, sexual contacts of HIV-infected persons, persons with transfusion history (1978-1985), pregnant women from areas with high prevalence of seropositive newborns.
Gonorrhea	Variable (women)	Yes (1996)	Variable	Recommended for prostitutes, women with history of recurrent gonorrhea, women < 25 years old with 2 or more sex partners in the last year, or high-prevalence areas.
Chlamydia	≤ 25 (women)	Yes (2001)	Variable	Recommended for sexually active women < 25, women with a history of STDs, erratic use of barrier contraceptives, cervical ectopy, new/multiple sexual partners or in high prevalence areas.
CHEMOPROPHYLAXIS				
Folic acid	Childbearing (Female)	Yes (1996)	Daily	0.4 mg folic acid/day recommended for women capable of pregnancy continuing through 1st trimester to prevent neural tube defects. 4mg/day for women with previous pregnancy with neural tube defect
Hormone replacement Therapy	All Postmenopausal females	No (2002)	Periodically	The USPSTF recommends against the routine use of estrogen and progestin for the prevention of chronic conditions (such as heart disease or osteoporois in postmenopausal women. The USPSTF concludes that the evidence is insufficient to recommend for or against the use of unopposed estrogen for the prevention of chronic conditions in postmenopausal women who have had a hysterectomy.
COUNSELING				
Tobacco cessation	All tobacco users	Yes (2003)	Periodically	The USPSTF strongly recommends that: **clinicians** screen all adults for tobacco use and provide tobacco cessation interventions for those who use tobacco products. **clinicians** screen all pregnant women for tobacco use and provide augmented pregnancy-tailored counseling to those who smoke. The USPSTF concludes that:the evidence is insufficient to recommend for or against routine screening for tobacco use or interventions to prevent and treat tobacco use and dependence among children or adolescents.
Alcohol use screening	All	Yes (1996)	Periodically	Persons who use alcohol should be counseled about the dangers of drinking and driving.
Fat, cholesterol intake, and caloric balance	All	Yes (1996)	Periodically	Limitation of dietary fat, especially saturated fats.
Calcium intake	All (Female)	Yes (1996)	Periodically	
Regular physical activity	All	Yes (2002)	Periodically	The USPSTF concludes that the evidence is insufficient to recommend for or against behavioral counseling in primary care settings to promote physical activity.
Injury prevention (motor vehicle, household)	All	Yes (1996)	Periodically	Use of seatbelts, child safety seats, helmets when riding motorcycles and bicycles.
STD prevention	All	Yes (1996)	Periodically	
Contraception	All	Yes (1996)	Periodically	